Community Mental Health Care

To the memory of our fathers, Arthur Salter and Maurice Turner,
who made us what we are.

For Elsevier:
Publisher: Steven Black
Development Editor: Catherine Jackson
Project Manager: Jess Thompson
Designer: Stewart Larking
Illustration Buyer: Merlyn Harvey
Illustrator: Hardlines and David Banks

Community Mental Health Care

A practical guide to outdoor psychiatry

Mark Salter MB BS BSc MRCPsych

Consultant Psychiatrist, Homerton University and
St Bartholomew's Hospitals, East London and
the City Mental Health NHS Trust, London

Trevor Turner MD FRCPsych

Consultant Psychiatrist and Clinical Director,
Homerton University and St Bartholomew's Hospitals,
East London and the City Mental Health NHS Trust, London

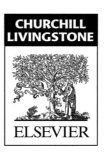

EDINBURGH LONDON NEW YORK OXFORD PHILADELPHIA ST LOUIS SYDNEY TORONTO 2008

CHURCHILL
LIVINGSTONE
ELSEVIER

ISBN: 978 0 443 10254 7

British Library Cataloguing in Publication Data
A catalogue record for this book is available from the British Library.

Library of Congress Cataloging in Publication Data
A catalog record for this book is available from the Library of Congress.

Note
Neither the Publisher nor the authors assume any responsibility for any loss or
injury and/or damage to persons or property arising out of or related to any use of
the material contained in this book. It is the responsibility of the treating practitioner, relying on independent expertise and knowledge of the patient, to determine
the best treatment and method of application for the patient.   **The Publisher**

your source for books,
journals and multimedia
in the health sciences

www.elsevierhealth.com

Working together to grow
libraries in developing countries

www.elsevier.com | www.bookaid.org | www.sabre.org

ELSEVIER   BOOK AID
            International   Sabre Foundation

The
Publisher's
policy is to use
**paper manufactured
from sustainable forests**

Printed in China

Contents

Preface

This book is written for someone who does not at present exist. That strange absence is because the professional community mental health worker, a generic individual appropriately skilled to look after the mentally ill in community settings, has yet to emerge despite more than 40 years of apparent – official even – 'community care'. Our aim is to nurture, educate and, hopefully, inspire a proper name and role for the kind of person who will want to read this book. Nothing less than a new breed of nurse/social worker/therapist can really make community care work.

This new breed of community mental health worker, so far variously known as the keyworker, the care coordinator, the social worker, the CPN (community psychiatric nurse), the professional carer, the care worker or, more prosaically, 'the bloke who comes round once a week to see I'm alright', may have come from any one of a variety of backgrounds. Mental health nursing, local authority 'approved' social work, occupational therapy, clinical psychology, physiotherapy, social therapy or psychotherapy, and voluntary work all provide some of the core experience and skills required for such a post. As a result, today's care coordinators (to use the official term) have very different potential training and agreed skills, and different professional and personal perspectives. This handbook is designed, therefore, to give everyone a common currency of expectation and experience, and it is aimed at being equally helpful to the individual carer (of someone who is mentally ill), the general practitioner and even the trainee psychiatrist.

The driving force behind this book, however, is more than simply telling people the same old story. Skills are essential. Knowledge of mental health at a practical level is vital. Commitment to working with the extraordinary people who live with, and cope with, mental illness is a must. Yet the fragmented nature of community care is like that because it *is* too often a hotch-potch of bickering professionals arguing about who does what while the poor, suffering, user/client/punter/patient (we can't even agree what to call the 'customer'!) sits in a lonely, cold, unfurnished room waiting for someone to turn up. Without a professionalised community worker we will head back to the asylum, back to the dark ages when prejudice and indifference were the rule.

Some may not agree with our views about training, about what needs to be done, about the importance of medication *as well as* personal support, or about the Department of Health (DoH), the Mental Health Act (MHA), the Care Programme Approach (CPA), or other acronymous arrangements. The jargon of community mental health can be seen as precious, simplistic or even downright confusing. There has also been a long-standing battle – in our view outdated and unhelpful – between the so-called 'medical model' and a more 'holistic', socially oriented model. The facts point to a new language of partnership in care between a number of different professionals, demanding a new species of mental health worker. We can't predict a name for this 21st century professional – something around companion, guide or even almoner might emerge – but the essence of her or his skills and tasks are in this book.

This diversity is reflected in the sources of skill, wit and wisdom that we have tapped in the writing of this book. Our undying gratitude is especially due to Nisha Shah and Sue Collinson for their personal support and patience during the extended genesis of this oeuvre, and to Jon Flint for his masterly assistance with the typescript. Our thanks go also to the many patients, carers and colleagues who have contributed, often unwittingly, to helping us clarify our ideas and hopes.

Mark Salter and Trevor Turner
London

Why have care in the community?
(Or how did we get into this in the first place?)

1

Introduction

There has been more written in the last decade about mental health and community care than almost any other subject, whether it be in medical journals, health service publications or the newspapers. Much of it has been critical. The phrase 'care in the community' has even become a kind of joke in the media (Fig. 1.1).

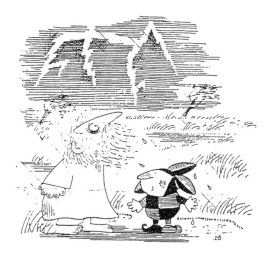

"I told you they'd put us out to care in the community, Lear"

Figure 1.1 ● King Lear and the Fool (from *Private Eye*).

Cartoons abound; stigma accumulates; cynicism about process and motive runs through all the public comment. Yet the true story of modern community care remains largely hidden, just as it should do. What self-respecting journalist would file a story, rooted in day-to-day reality, about a patient with schizophrenia who woke up in the morning in a room of his own, cooked his own breakfast, went off to the day centre, talked to friends and workmates and then had supper with his mum? How unexciting, routine and lacking in colour or deeper meaning.

Obviously a doss of a job for anybody! Instead, such patients reach public aware-ness only when an 'untoward incident' occurs, so that a 'mad axeman' headline can be splashed across the tabloids (Fig. 1.2).

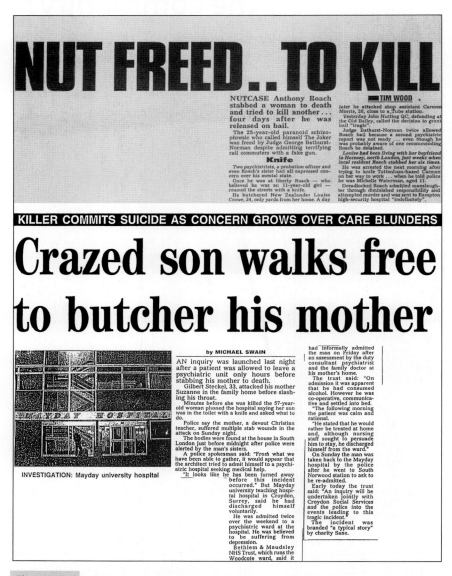

Figure 1.2 ● *Daily Star* (top) and *Daily Express* (bottom) headlines, 16 February 1996.

Then it's quite clear that things are going wrong, that 'something must be done'. The self-righteous can be consulted and comment that the policy is mad. It is the solid, quiet, untrumpeted success of most of community care that in itself is half the problem.

Once upon a time, as the public perception goes, all those who were mentally ill were carefully stowed away in asylums, out of sight and out of mind (Fig. 1.3). By contrast, today the focus is on placing people in the community, to 'normalise' their

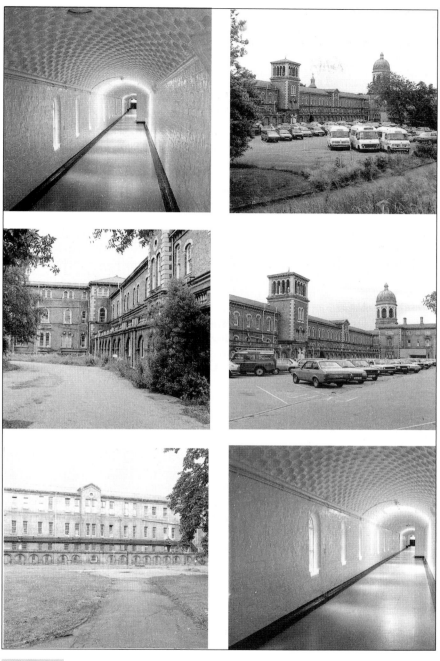

Figure 1.3 ● A typical Victorian asylum, Friem Barnet, with very long corridors, a grandiose exterior and extensive grounds, for air and prayer?

existence. Paradoxically, many people still complain about this, just as they complained about the awful things being done behind the walls of asylums. The difficulty is that, unlike the charitable concern shown for ageing donkeys or neglected children, no one much cares about 'mad folk'. Reasons for this include: 'It's their own fault' and 'What's the point?' As often as not, the discomfort, sheer terror and incomprehensibility of mental disorders just turns people off. They prefer to forget about it, to shut it out from lives already complicated enough by the hurly-burly of the 21st century. Thus, one has to consider a crucial paradox of community care; namely, that the only way you can get the public to care about the mentally ill is to have some awful or colourful event occur, tragicomic or clearly tragical. Such incidents, now euphemistically described as untoward, lead to formal inquiries. Inquiries create cash, resources, concern and even a degree of considered media interest. Even worse, psychosis treated creates psychosis neglected, because no one can see inside the sufferer's head. You have to be untreated, and behave badly, to get the help you need, and to get the help the services need.

But all those working in mental health, whether as nurses, doctors, social workers or care workers, are ever more strictly enjoined to prevent these very untoward events taking place. Suicides, assaults on the public, homicides and other spectacles are embroiled in what is now termed 'clinical risk management'. In particular, the government has insisted on a sensible, although perhaps overbureaucratic, policy that they have called the Care Programme Approach (CPA). This obliges all those providing professional care for the mentally ill to organise care plans based on needs assessment, to appoint key workers (now renamed care coordinators) and to meet regularly to ensure that individuals are properly 'supervised' in the community. Unfortunately, if we in the mental health field succeed in this task, it is likely that, given any historical understanding, there will be a perception of 'all quiet on the mental health front'. Funding and resources will be diverted to other areas deemed to be more in need. Failure may lead to individuals being pilloried, publicly scapegoated and possibly sacked. But, and this is the important point, thanks to these 'failures', the service will continue to be resourced because it will be seen as requiring such resources. You are damned by neglect if you do, damned by publicity if you don't.

The trick therefore, to the cynically minded, is to have untoward incidents occur in spite of doing everything right, and that takes careful planning, considerable experience and (of course) good practice. This book is designed not only to ensure good practice but also to help community care workers find the right balance in dealing with the mentally ill, their colleagues and themselves. Untoward incidents have always happened (see below) and will continue to happen in the foreseeable future, no matter what one does. In fact, they define the nature of mental illness in terms of society and how it responds. If this is understood, then the tasks, interest and excitement of mental health care can be placed in perspective.

Community care in history

The rise of the asylums

Community care probably began because of an untoward incident. You can take your pick in this regard. The Quakers in late 18th century York were shocked at the mistreatment and death of a certain Hannah Mills in the confines of the appalling and secretive (friends' visits were refused) York asylum. As a result, in 1792, they founded The Retreat, a 'quiet haven ... for reparation or safety', based on moral management and the gentle transformation of someone 'out of their wits' into an acceptable, God-fearing citizen. Treatment was a mixture of diet, occupation, prayer and trust, and a rejection of the crude medical methods of the time such as bleeding and purging. Likewise, in 1815, there was a formal inquiry into practices at Bethlem Hospital (also known as 'Bedlam'), the long-established (since the 13th century) and almost only psychiatric unit in London. Again, the findings of what was this time a parliamentary inquiry revealed awful practices and scapegoated the apothecary John Haslam (who was *not* the physician in charge and who had limited responsibility for the management regime), but, most important of all, led to a gradual process of psychiatric reform. Given that back in the 1790s, the ground-breaking French psychiatrist Philippe Pinel had actually unchained the 'insane' (amidst the chaos of the French revolution and the 'reign of terror') and, given that by the time of the 1815 inquiry, George III, because of his 'madness', had been deposed from the throne and replaced by his son as Regent, it is not surprising that sympathy towards mental disorders was growing.

It should also be understood that the 'asylum' that emerged from these particular events, subsequently known as the mental hospital, was designed as a friendly sanctuary, a model of appropriate society, a thoughtful living arrangement to help restore the 'shattered bark' of mental disorder. Meant to be no more than a small community, where ideas, manners, activities and feelings could be carefully modified, it was created from a strange amalgam of 19th century Christian evangelism, Quaker brotherhood, the street visibility of mad folk in an increasingly urbanised industrial world, and a developing understanding that mental illness was not caused by demons, witchcraft or other supernatural effects, but was rather a disease of the mind and even the brain, something that could be treated by appropriate management. The philosophy of care very much reflected today's community approach, seeing the pressures of life as causative and the use of 'normal' surroundings and day-to-day occupations as curative. Therapeutic community living was the design motif, using the catchphrase 'moral therapy'.

At this time the medical profession, in the form of 'alienists' (i.e. doctors with a special interest in medical psychology), took over the management of these asylums for the simple reason that many people had associated physical illnesses and because there was no one else who really wanted the job. It was not a rewarding task, led to considerable stigma and was not especially renumerative, unless you were one of the very few private entrepreneurs who ran their own 'houses' (short for madhouses) and cornered the small but lucrative higher bourgeois market. In a famous novel entitled *Hard Cash* (published in 1867), the popular Victorian author Charles Reade mocked the pretensions and greed of the emerging psychiatric profession. He has a bluff, sensible doctor call them the 'Mad Ox' (i.e. 'mad docs'), making it quite clear that, even amongst fellow medics, they were regarded as unreliable and as crazy as those they were purporting to manage. Furthermore, as soon as building of the new asylums started, arguments began about their costs and their usefulness, and there was considerable suspicion of the motives behind their construction. In other words, the whole psychiatric enterprise met with opposition from most quarters throughout its development. Present problems are nothing new.

Nevertheless, build them they did, and there was nothing that Victorian philanthropists liked more than building institutions, whether asylums, hospitals, schools, waterworks, factories or town halls. Parliament was put under pressure by an increasingly powerful lobby, led by the long-lived Lord Shaftesbury, to pass significant Acts in 1808 (allowing each county to build an asylum) and 1844 (ordering each county to do so), the costs being put on the rates. In essence, specific funds were set aside – 'top-sliced' or 'ring-fenced' to use modern NHS management-speak – just for the care of the mentally ill. This was almost unique, a dedicated provision for the 'pauper insane', all paid for by the government and ratepayers' taxes – a form of National Mental Health Service, free at the point of care, over a century before the beginning of the modern NHS. Unfortunately, with some handsome buildings and grounds – and their own farms and walks, designed to occupy, enlighten and cure their troubled inmates – the asylums proved horribly popular. From having 200–300 inmates, they grew into enormous 3000+ 'museums of madness', isolated communities, largely keeping patients herded in dull security rather than offering any therapeutic advance. Patients did go in and out as their illnesses (e.g. manic depression) waxed and waned, but more and more of them simply accumulated as a chronic lunatic population, with all the problems of institutionalisation, neglect, diseases of overcrowding (e.g. dysentery) and the petty and not so petty tyrannies that fester behind closed doors. Asylums became disposal units for many of society's unwanted souls, relatives visiting less and less as the years went by.

Essentially, the 19th century public had two views of asylums and psychiatrists. On the one hand, there was concern about false imprisonment. Were unscrupulous doctors putting rich heiresses, for example, behind asylum walls so that wicked relatives could steal their money? On the other hand, there were regular complaints about outrages in public committed by 'lunatics', so why didn't the doctors get on and do something about it? A number of contemporary books, for example *The Woman in White* by Wilkie Collins, popularised this concern. A series of laws throughout the 19th century tried to protect the public in the right way, culminating in the highly legalistic 1890 Lunacy Act. There was constant pressure to 'build, build', fuelled by public anxieties; in 1896, the *British Medical Journal* published a leader entitled 'Lunatics at Large', expressing concern at various assaults by mentally ill people on innocent citizens. The asylum population rose remorselessly, rich and poor being all too happy to dispose (humanely as they saw it) of their unwanted, insane relatives. In fact, the Victorians found to their horror that, during the 19th century, the 'normal' population had increased threefold but the population of the officially 'insane' had increased tenfold. In other words, the country was breeding degeneration – and theories of an inherited, degenerate streak were all the rage, with the middle classes terrified of being drowned in a tide of unchecked, lower-class, idiocy-cum-lunacy.

It should also be understood that, at this time, doctors had no control over who came in to these asylums. Patients were simply sent in by magistrates under certificates, and overcrowding led to new wings being added, often in a haphazard fashion. Untoward incidents (poor food, fires, assaults) were regularly reported in the popular press. Nurses were called attendants, and doctors, i.e. junior doctors, assistant medical officers, whereas a physician superintendent, aided by the chief attendant, matron and bursar/housekeeper ran the whole institution as a mini-fiefdom. There were no such things as social workers although there was a person called an almoner, who distributed some charity money to poorer families. Just as the caseloads of community workers silt up today, so the asylums (despite discharging up to 50% of their inmates per annum) silted up with chronic cases, with individuals living and dying in hospital over many years. This inability to prevent more people coming in to the system than it could cope with is, by definition, the permanent problem of caring for those who are socially disabled. Demand always outstrips supply as thresholds change. Contemporary providers and their methods are always blamed.

Despite this increased provision of asylum beds, based on raising a rate (i.e. a local household tax) from each county to pay for building its asylum – or a new extension – and with each parish having to pay a subsidy to keep their 'pauper

6

lunatics' in the asylum (like the catchment area and case management commitments of today), attempts were made to try to provide alternative care outside the institution. This included what were originally called 'cottage asylums', in which patients who seemed quiet and amenable were put in cottages in the grounds and encouraged to live their lives semi-independently. In fact, one leading asylum superintendent, John Bucknill, actually placed his patients in a couple of houses at the seaside, where at first they became objects of curiosity but were soon accepted as part of the town's landscape. Likewise in Scotland, almost uniquely, there arose a system called boarding out, in which patients were placed with families, who were given money for their care. This was rather like the modern use of foster care, whether for children or disabled adults, and by and large it succeeded in its aims. Why it should have worked in Scotland, particularly in the Highlands, rather than in England is difficult to understand. However, the first organisation aimed at helping people who had left the asylum – the Mental After Care Association (MACA) – was founded in England in the late 1880s and still operates today. Notwithstanding all these initiatives, asylum numbers grew and grew into the mid-20th century, with a few dips during World Wars I and II (when staff were in short supply), peaking at around 155 000 in 1956 (Fig. 1.4). Institutions were simply accepted as the normal disposal route, as part of the landscape. What else could one do with incurable disease?

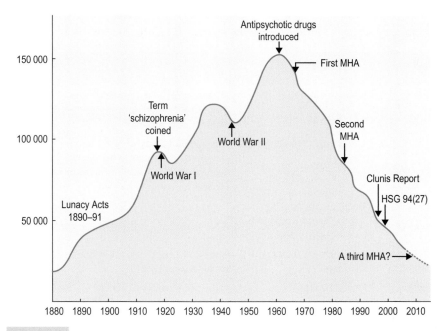

Figure 1.4 ● In-patients resident in psychiatric hospitals in England and Wales, 1880–2010. HSG, Health Service Guideline; MHA, Mental Health Act.

Back to the community

By the early 1960s, the years in which John F Kennedy was President of the United States and Elvis Presley was topping the charts, it had become clear to policy makers at the Department of Health (DoH) that it would be possible to run down asylum bed numbers. In a famous speech in 1961 to the National Association of Mental Health, the Minister of Health, Enoch Powell, signalled the end of the asylum era. 'There they stand', he declaimed, 'isolated, majestic, imperious, brooded over by the gigantic water tower and chimney combined, rising unmistakeable and daunting out of the countryside – the asylums which our forefathers built with such solidity.' The combination of new medications, for example chlorpromazine, introduced in the early 1950s, new ideas about open doors and 'normalising' people who were deemed mentally ill, and the obvious economics (from the government's point of view) of closing down expensive establishments all led to a radically different solution. No longer would the mentally ill have to be put behind walls in large Victorian and, therefore, out-of-date hospitals. Spurred on by the writings of sociologists such as Erving Goffman (*Asylums*, 1962) and the anti-psychiatrists such as RD Laing (who attributed schizophrenia to the capitalist organisation of society), and attracted by the simple humanity of individuals living their own lives in quiet normality, the policy of community care was gradually, albeit somewhat incoherently, established. The Mental Health Acts (MHAs) of 1959 and 1983 promoted this system. Scandals in some of the large hospitals, related to neglect or maltreatment of patients, speeded up the whole process. As ever, inquiries – hospital inquiries rather than untoward incidents – by pricking the public conscience, led the way in generating new approaches to mental health care (Table 1.1).

Table 1.1 ● Key dates and documents in the history of community care, 1959–2002

Date	Document	Comments
1959	Mental Health Act	Abolished previous legislation and magistrates' orders; introduced mental health review tribunals
1962	*A Hospital Plan for England and Wales*	This outlined plans for restricting hospital services to acute care in the district general hospital while developing local authority services for community care
1963	*Health and Welfare: The Development of Community Care* (Ministry of Health)	
1975	*Better Services for the Mentally Ill*	Promoted a continuing shift from hospital to social services care
1983	Mental Health Act	Introduced 'consent' procedures, the Mental Health Act Commission (MHAC), 'approved' social workers and aftercare responsibilities
1988	*Community Care: Agenda for Action* – Griffiths Report	Community care was 'everyone's distant relative but nobody's baby' – funding needed
1989	*Caring for People: Community Care in the Next Decade and Beyond: Caring for the 1990s* (DoH)	No mental hospital closures unless funded alternatives in place but little central finance or commitment. Social services encouraged to buy voluntary and private sector services

Table 1.1 ● *(Continued)*

Date	Document	Comments
1990	The NHS and Community Care Act	The legislation implementing *Caring for People*; thus, local authorities now responsible for assessing need and delivering care packages. This included the Care Programme Approach (CPA)
1990	*Care Programme Approach (CPA) for People with a Mental Illness Referred to the Specialist Psychiatric Services* [HC(90)23/LASSL(90)11] (DoH)	DoH outline of CPA and its central role in aftercare
1994	*Guidance on the Discharge of Mentally Disordered People and their Continuing Care in the Community* [HSG(94)27/LASSL(94)4] (DoH)	Mandatory formal inquiries to be set up for any 'untoward' incidents
1995	Mental Health (Patients in the Community) Bill	New powers for aftercare via supervised discharge (a new Section 25 of the MHA), including patients being required to live at a specific address and attend for treatment, etc.; however, no powers for compulsory treatment against a patient's will
1999	*A National Service Framework (NSF) for Mental Health*	Outlined standards of care, how they would be developed and how performance would be measured
1999	Green Paper on Reform of the MHA	Included compulsory treatment in the community but closer attention to patients' rights
2000	The NHS Plan	Promised funding for new mental health teams (e.g. assertive outreach, home treatment) in the community
2002	Draft mental health bill published	Opposed by a broad Mental Health Alliance because of, among other concerns, very loose criteria for detention, community treatment powers and a new DSPD category (dangerous severe personality disorder)

9

Although some commentators, especially the more traditional psychiatrists, expressed concern, in general this move into the community was welcomed. It was welcomed by patients, families, social workers, many nurses and doctors, and politicians, the last happy at the apparent reduction in the financial burden on the NHS, as costly beds were closed and hospital sites sold off to house builders. As bed numbers declined, so did formal sections under the MHA, at least until the late 1970s. Research into the impact of community care, famously in Wisconsin (Stein and Test, 1980) and Sydney (Hoult, 1986), showed it to be cost-effective, clinically effective and family-effective. That is to say, in reasonably stable communities, provided there was some sort of hospital backup and a nicely committed community care team, there was no need to resort to hospital for many relapses in mental illness. The most extreme example of putting this belief into practice took place in Italy in 1978 – influenced by the guru-like psychiatrist Franco Basaglia – when all admissions to mental hospitals were banned amidst an outpouring of liberationist and left-wing philosophy, despite many inmates having nowhere else to go.

The key features of this turnaround can be summarised as a series of core principles for those wishing to help the mentally ill, whatever the era, whatever the politics and whatever the limitations of money available (see Box 1.1).

Box 1.1 Key lessons from history for helping the mentally ill

1. Find and wisely use a new treatment, of whatever sort. The effectiveness of drug therapy can be demonstrated, in part historically, by the fact that it is clearly associated with a reduction in the asylum population

2. Keep humanity to the fore. Allowing people to choose their own curtains and what time they have breakfast will usually win out over solutions that opt for control and institutionalisation

3. Get someone to give you the money. This is particularly difficult, but a subtle combination of appealing to people's consciences and arousing their fears about wandering madmen and fears that 'it could happen to you' is the best approach

4. Get a member of the royal family to go mad. The best example is George III, but several members of the royal family have been helpful advocates

5. Make sure that 'madness' is seen as an illness rather than something for which people can be blamed. Witches get burned at the stake, patients suffer but get treated. The anti-stigma campaign has to be repeated every decade, and for every generation

Modern times and the rising tide of 'untowardness'

Taking people with chronic mental illnesses out of hospitals was at first extremely successful. A number of thoughtful studies (e.g. the TAPS reports from Friem Hospital) have indicated that many individuals can live in friendly surroundings of a personalised and domestic nature and do not need total institutions. Putting these individuals into the community (and surveys showed that many of them wanted to leave) improved their social networks to a remarkable degree. It gave them access to other services that were not health oriented, to normal meeting places such as cafes or cinemas, and could be seen as helping to reduce the stigma surrounding people who are mentally ill. Unfortunately, during the 1980s, the rising unemployment and vagrancy rates, the gaps in provision for the less well off and the obviously poor, and the excessive reduction of hospital beds, whether for rehabilitation or respite, started to change the picture. Cuts in the NHS naturally led to cuts in the 'Cinderella services', those specialties that are easily outgunned in the battle for resources. Mental health is one of these, and always will be.

Amongst the homeless, now part of the street scene in the inner cities, about 30–40% will usually be suffering from some form of severe mental illness. Many of these make up that group of patients called, quaintly, the 'new long-stay' in psychiatric surveys. That is to say, they have never stayed in hospital for a long time but have simply gone in and out with each relapse, through the so-called 'revolving door'. Burdened by chronic illnesses such as schizophrenia or manic depression, often lacking insight and vulnerable to drug or alcohol abuse as well, they appear on the streets in various forms, pathetic, threatening, muttering to themselves or shouting at the voices that constantly plague them. Several have climbed into the lion's den at London Zoo, in spectacular fashion, but more often they end up in prison. Cynical descriptions of community care thus became commonplace, for example 'another person, somewhere else', or 'an intellectual pastime of sociologists' or 'outdoor relief'. The apparent failures of the policy became all too visible for the public to have much faith in it.

In particular, just as hospital scandals had fuelled the drive for care in the community back in the 1960s and 1970s (and of course in 1792 and 1815), so various untoward incidents started to erode faith in community care. This rising climate of untowardness, even in the 21st century, shows how the asylum still has a hold over our thinking. We can see this in our legislation, the mental health laws currently in use in England, Scotland and many other Western countries being effectively asylum acts, their blueprints drafted in a bygone era when incarceration was at its peak. We may see it too in the structure of our treatment services. Fifty years into the age of community care, many professionals still prefer to hold clinics in hospitals rather than in community centres or general practices. In spite of plenty of evidence for the efficacy of family, social and other psychological interventions for major mental illnesses, it is drug therapy, monitored by hospital-based professionals, that remains the mainstay of treatment.

Successive governments have done little better. In the UK, between 1960 and 1990, no less than four White Papers recommended devolution of mental health care into community-based units. Yet the actual funding for these plans fell far short of what most regard as necessary for the widespread provision of effective community care, despite the money that should have been available from selling off over 120 asylum sites, almost all in prime suburban housing areas. No one now knows where all this money went; successive NHS reorganisations make it very difficult to trace particular sales/assets. Some certainly did go into new buildings, e.g. smaller, modern facilities or aftercare homes. Some undoubtedly was used by desperate health authorities to shore up underfunding elsewhere.

Over this same period, however, society has greatly changed. Technology, particularly the contraceptive pill, the motor car, the jumbo jet, the television and the computer, has given new lifestyles to millions. With this has come a tremendous growth in consumerism, and a major shift in emphasis from social responsibility to individual rights. As the public has come to see health in consumerist terms, deference to health professionals has given way to demands for information about treatments and outcomes. Alongside this shift towards individualism has grown an increasing disquiet. So successful have we become at sustaining the comfort of the individual that it has become accepted that comfort is a right, rather than a welcome by-product of our civilisation. Lapses in its provision are taken as evidence of failure, which is now met with increasing dissatisfaction, protest and, above all, a need for action to be taken to address the problem. This accounts for the increased popularity of inquiries, and even 'charters', in many problematic areas of public life, as well as the fashionable concepts of risk, risk evaluation and risk management, as we shall see in later chapters.

Oblivious to all these changes, psychiatric hospitals with their 'hospital beds' have continued to close. In addition, a very small number of the recipients of the new 'care in the community' (in the 1970s, this phrase carried a more optimistic connotation than it carries today) have continued to act as they have always done, causing unease and, very rarely, harm to others. This harm has certainly occurred no more often than it did before 'decarceration', but in a society changed out of all recognition from that era, such events now draw an increasingly individualised response. Major incidents involving mentally ill people are increasingly known by the name of the protagonist rather than by the institution in which the event occurred. We have moved from the age of hospital scandals to an age of personalised care failure, of 'scare in the community'.

By the early 1980s, therefore, many mentally ill people were being managed with minimal resources, in the uncontrolled setting of the community, using ideas of care derived from a custodial era. Staff consisted of largely separate social service departments employing local borough social workers, voluntary agencies of varying reliability, GPs and district nurses in primary care, and a few newly labelled community psychiatric nurses (CPNs), tempted from the inpatient wards by extra pay and the hope of a quieter life. None of these had much specific training in the home care of mentally ill people, and/or their families, outside the formal structure of asylums. Coordination of services was minimal (in fact, many health workers and social workers despised each other) and theories of normalisation and avoiding dependency often meant that patients were left to look after themselves. Care was now carried out in full view of an increasingly curious public whose age-old fear of mental illness was readily inflated by sensationalist media coverage. The stage was thus set for a major event.

The onset of the 'serious incident culture'

That event came in July 1984. Sharon Campbell, who suffered with a psychotic disorder, murdered her social worker, Isobel Schwarz. After a long campaign by the victim's father, an inquiry was held. Its report was not published until 4 years after her death (Spokes Report, 1988). It described how numerous failures of inter-agency communication, combined with poor coordination and delivery of services, had been instrumental in the social worker's death. Its findings were subsequently enshrined in a new government policy document, which outlined the CPA [in official terminology, this formal guidance was called HC(90)23/LASSL(90)11]. Essentially, it recommended that care for the seriously mentally ill (SMI) could be improved by identifying those named individuals responsible for the care of a patient in a written, mutually agreed care plan that would be subject to regular review. Thus the terms 'key worker' (and later 'care coordinator') and 'responsible' (borrowed from the language of the MHA) entered the professional's day-to-day vocabulary.

Although the CPA was explicit in its definitions of just who was responsible for the care of the patient, it was far less clear whether its use was mandatory, and whether the government was willing to provide the funding to pay for all the extra work that the new system entailed. The government remained vague on these points. It was assumed that government suggestions on the CPA were for guidance only, given the language used in the official document. Across the country, implementation of the CPA remained piecemeal. Then, in late 1992, several incidents occurred in quick succession. Michael Buchanan killed a retired police officer and Christopher Clunis killed a newly married bystander, Jonathan Zito, on a railway platform. Both assailants suffered with schizophrenia. Weeks later, another patient, Ben Silcock, was severely mauled after entering the lion's enclosure at London Zoo. The event was caught on amateur video and broadcast widely. For a time, it seemed as though a mental health catastrophe was always in the news.

Spurred on by the public reaction to these events, the government response was prompt. Reports were obtained from the clinicians attempting to care for Silcock, Clunis and Buchanan. Senior staff were summoned to Whitehall. The results of their deliberations were published in August 1993 and became known as Mrs Bottomley's ten-point plan, after the then Health Minister, Virginia Bottomley, herself a former mental health social worker. This document defined the shape and substance of virtually all government policy on the issue of community mental health for the rest of the century. Because of vociferous protests from patient groups, who painted lurid pictures of medication forcibly administered 'on the kitchen table', as well as more realistic concerns over contravention of the European Convention on Human Rights, it dodged the central issues of increased funding or greater powers of treatment for patients in the community. Instead, the government suggested, sufficient improvements could be made by better training and communication, by more effective targeting of vulnerable individuals and the implementation of improved information systems, including the use of a supervision register to focus resources on those most in need. All those familiar with the chronic underfunding of community psychiatry at once recognised the resource implications of these measures, yet any commitment to spend more on mental health care was absent from the document, which spoke only of encouraging the development of such facilities.

Over the next three years, policy statements, guidance documents and even new legislation churned out of the DoH. When finally introduced, the supervision register was met with disinterest and even defiance by many clinicians, who viewed it as a kind of public blacklist, enhancing stigma and subverting confidentiality, but not helping one jot with providing care. This opposition did little to soften the government stance on the issue but did at least clarify the official position on resources; the new tools for shoring up community care were *not* to be allocated any extra funding. The tinkering with the MHA, which became law in 1995 (the Patients in the Community Act 1995), was similarly received and even labelled 'anti-therapeutic' by some, as it conferred no extra resources or therapeutic powers whilst at the same time legally binding carers to give care that they would have provided in any case. It did enable responsible medical officers (RMOs) to order patients to live at a particular house or home, to enter that home as and when they wished, and to take and convey patients for treatment, e.g. to a hospital or day centre. It did *not* empower any form of therapy or medication.

While these debates went on, fresh incidents continued to make headline news. In April 1993, Johnathan Newby, a young volunteer, was killed (by a patient who was drunk) whilst alone on duty at a community care home in Oxford. In the summer of that year, *The Independent* newspaper published its own inquiry into the killing of Jonathan Zito by Christopher Clunis under the headline 'The Scandal of the Schizophrenic Killer that Nobody Stopped'. September of that year saw the murder of a young occupational therapist by a patient who was still detained under a section of the MHA. This in fact took place in a modern purpose-built psychiatric unit but in an isolated area, out of sight of other staff. Media coverage of such events grew steadily to become the principal source of public knowledge – and opinion – about the care of the mentally ill. The phrase 'care in the community' had taken on an adjectival connotation of failure and neglect. The public, faced with the emotive issue of the apparently common, random slaughter of normal, decent citizens, began to assume that homicide was somehow prima facie evidence of failure of care.

Life after Clunis

This assumption was enhanced by the publication of the seminal Ritchie Report of the inquiry into the care and treatment of Christopher Clunis in 1994, which received widespread media coverage (Fig. 1.5). The report set out, in obsessional detail, the 'catalogue of failure and missed opportunity' in the care given to Clunis over the years that led up to the homicide. Numerous carers were named and criticised, although no single person or service was singled out for blame, not least because Clunis moved from borough to borough, was constantly non-cooperative, and tended to frighten those trying to help or assess him. Rather, the problem was seen as 'cumulative'. The report echoed the Spokes Report in its identification of a tendency to downplay or underestimate the significance of violent behaviour in the patient's history. It also identified many shortcomings in the system of care: scant resources; poor training in the skills of risk assessment, record keeping and communication; and inconsistency in diagnostic and treatment approaches. It also criticised the government, saying that its guidance on CPA was 'difficult to understand and couched in unhelpful jargon'. Its recommendations were no less explicit: the urgent need to increase the number of acute inner-city beds and aftercare hostels; the need to provide adequate staffing levels in hard-pressed, hard-to-fill social services posts; improved training in risk assessment, with urgent cases receiving full assessment in 3 hours; and training in communication and record keeping. It even went so far as to suggest that patients carry crisis cards in the event of a further crisis.

Throughout its 146 pages, the Clunis Report (by now, reports were popularly known by their protagonist rather than their author) carried the assumption that the way to avoid future disasters lay in improving the current system. It gave little or no consideration to the historical, political or social reasons why the services had been allowed to get into such an ill-organised, poorly resourced and demoralised mess in the first place. It did not address the impossibility of keeping track of – let alone supervising – reluctant disorganised individuals, free to roam at large and often encouraged to do so by hostel staff keen to offload 'difficult customers'. Nor did it question whether any of the fundamental assumptions about the provision of care to vulnerable, unpredictable people in the community might be in any way flawed. A radical rethink about community mental health law, or a return to some sort of custodial care on a useful scale, remained out of the question.

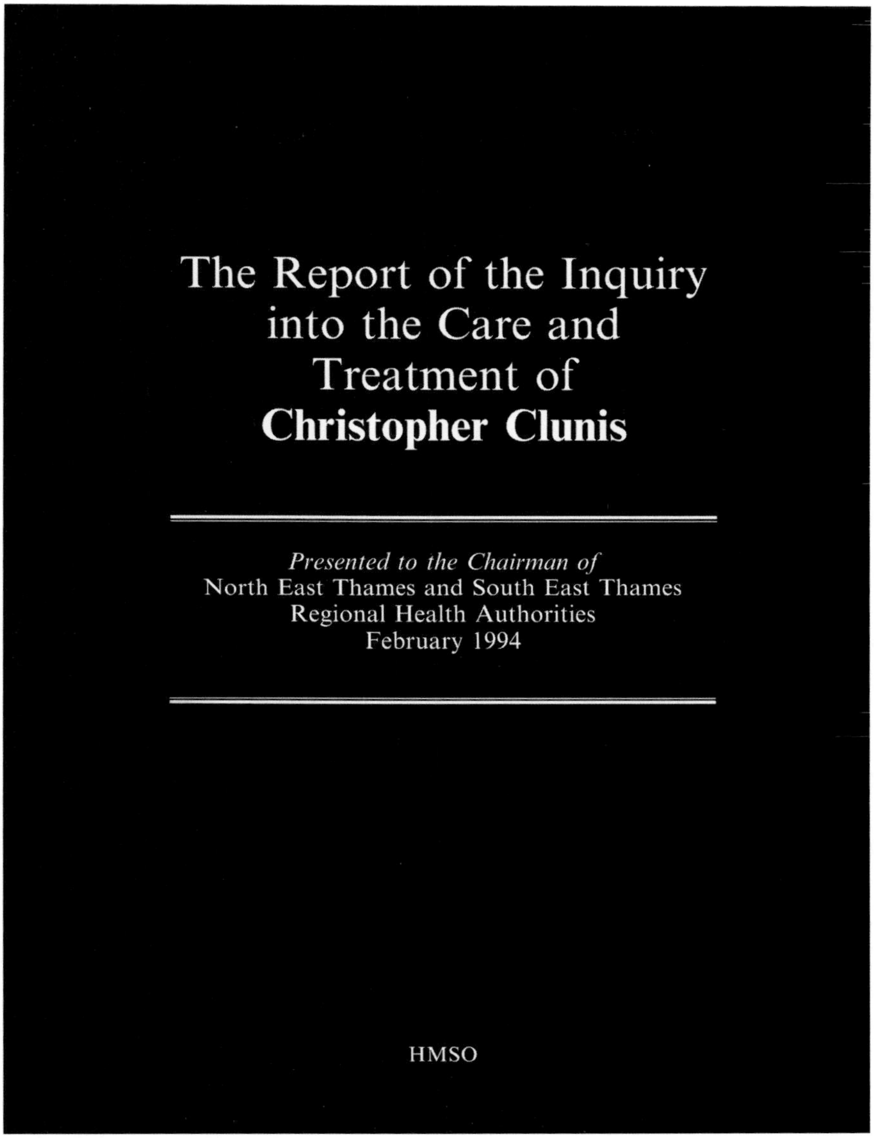

The Report of the Inquiry
into the Care and
Treatment of
Christopher Clunis

Presented to the Chairman of
North East Thames and South East Thames
Regional Health Authorities
February 1994

HMSO

Figure 1.5 ● The Ritchie Report, also known as the Clunis Report (Crown copyright), a turning point in the history of care in the community and its risks.

These attitudes defined the government response to the Clunis Report, which came in the form of yet another *ex cathedra* protocol, HSG(94)27, a discharge guidance. This document paid heed only to the Clunis recommendations that had no direct funding implications. In essence, it consisted of civil servants telling doctors, nurses and social workers how to do their job; fewer incidents should be achieved within the pre-existing framework by professionals learning to use planned discharge from hospital and by applying the CPA more consistently; supervision registers, already assumed to be in place, should be modified to give special significance to factors indicating a risk of suicide, self-neglect or dangerousness to others. The core issue of resources, in particular the need for joint management and funding of key health and social service agencies, was, as ever, not addressed, other than in the vaguest of terms.

Paragraph 34 of the government guidance document was particularly germane to the lot of the care worker. In all cases where a homicide – but not a suicide – occurred, a full, formal, external inquiry was now mandatory. By being seen to conduct rigorous inquiries into the clinical care – or lack of it – that led up to a serious incident, the government could appear to be doing something to address the rising public concern that something must be done. Through the process of inquiry, failures of care could now be traced to specific individuals, made identifiable by an improved CPA process, which required a named care worker and a responsible medical officer. The possibility that these inquiries might be an ineffective way to address the basic flaws in a chronically under-resourced system or might have harmful effects on the already precarious morale of overstretched, undertrained carers didn't seem to occur to many people.

In the years that followed the Clunis Report, trusts and health authorities took up the guidance with gusto. Between 1994 and 1996, no fewer than 20 reports were issued into community homicides involving people with mental illness. By 2002, over 120 had been published according to the Zito Trust (founded by Jayne Zito, the wife of Clunis's victim), a charitable organisation dedicated to enhancing family/victim's rights and encouraging a return to more asylum-style care. At first, this stream of reports seemed helpful. Shortcomings in service provision were found everywhere, not just in run-down inner cities. The reports highlighted the need for more consistent use of reliable, standardised risk evaluation and better coordination and communication. In some cases, they led to direct improvements in service provision. But as the reports accumulated, other less helpful findings began to emerge. The aims and terms of reference of the inquiries became increasingly broad and legalistic. Some went so far as to rewrite the MHA. All of the reports seemed to reach very much the same conclusions and recommendations. Few people bothered to read them, let alone act on all of their recommendations. None of those charged with the job of inquiry have bothered to return (or have been asked to return) to the scene to check that their recommendations have been acted upon. Perhaps worst of all, the inquisitorial climate that they engendered began to exert an increasingly corrosive effect on the morale, motivation and practice of the care workers in the front line.

By the final years of the 20th century, care workers unlucky enough to be involved in an untoward incident found themselves facing something rather like the witch-hunts of the 17th century; thrown into a pool, you were proven innocent if you drowned and burnt at the stake if you survived. The modern version meant public criticism, retraining or worse, otherwise the inquiry would be seen as a cover-up. People began to suspect that the fervour for inquiry was doing more harm than good. Suspicion turned to certainty with the publication in November 1998 of the report into 'Lukewarm Luke' – so-called because of the patient's nickname. This two-volume, 700-odd-page monster of a report, which cost in the region of £750K to produce, can be regarded as the tasteless cherry on the unpalatable cake of serious incident culture. Its published conclusions were no different from the reports that preceded it, but the most important conclusion went unpublished: inquiries do not change anything very much. Rather, they reveal what happens when apparently rational methods are applied to an irrational matter. Different parties hold such widely different interests in the matter that it is impossible to reach a coherent truth about the event. Hindsight is blindsight.

The very act of looking back on events once you know their outcome, or even try to imagine their outcome, makes it, by definition, impossible to view such events objectively.

To the hapless professionals, an inquiry is effectively a form of local audit the potential of which to drive change is far in excess of what should normally be expected from a single case study. For the bereaved, the inquiry serves a more propitiatory role. To the media, it is a great chance to sell newspapers. For the government, inquiries have been a good way of drawing attention away from the decades of neglect by creating the idea that something is finally being done. It is hardly surprising, therefore, that by the late 1990s, inquiries had come to be seen by many as an irrelevant distraction from the long-ignored issues of underfunding, stigma, irrationality and neglect that have underlain the problems of community care all along. And so it goes, up to the present ...

Future hopes and fears – a new Mental Health Act?

Nevertheless, since 2001 in particular, in what might be termed a post-inquiry culture, there has been at least a genuine attempt to improve both funding and resource organisation for community-based care. This has derived partly from some especially lurid assaults on celebrities (e.g. George Harrison, Jill Dando), partly from the more specific need to reform the MHA in the light of the Michael Stone case (the convicted murderer of Liz and Megan Russell and attempted murderer of the then 9-year-old Josie Russell) and partly from welcome efforts by the Labour Party, in its second and third terms, to improve public services across the board. Thus, a National Service Framework (NSF) was published in 1999, after a lengthy consultation of stakeholders from voluntary, user and statutory services. The NSF outlined what the government expected of every health authority in terms of mental health service provision (i.e. 24-hour access to care, specific assessments for carers, etc.). From this, a further NHS Plan was developed, promising many millions of pounds investment in new services from April 2002 for the following 3 years. A National Patient Safety Agency (NPSA) was also set up, which was designed to pull together data from all forms of audit and inquiry, hopefully to enhance lower-risk care.

The driving force for change, of course, has been public concern about risk, the case of the personality-disordered Michael Stone being a key event. His apparently motiveless assault on the innocent Russell family in a quiet Kent lane in 1996 – he was only convicted eventually in 2001 having successfully appealed against his first sentence – was not only horrific but made more so by the knowledge that he was already well known to mental health services. He had an established diagnosis of antisocial personality disorder but could not be treated under the 1983 MHA because of what is known as the 'treatability' clause (see Chapter 9). This states that if someone is detained for a psychopathic disorder (the 1959 term for antisocial personality disorder, as the 1983 MHA simply repeated the language of the previous 1959 MHA), treatment can only be carried out if it 'is likely to alleviate or prevent a deterioration of their condition'. This clause does not apply if a patient is being detained under the much more usual category of mental illness, such as schizophrenia or depression, and reflects the considerable legal, medical and philosophical concerns about the whole notion of personality disorder (PD)/psychopathy as a genuine psychiatric condition. Unlike other illnesses, it does not come on with a change in symptoms or how you feel, or any overt psychological impairments (e.g. hearing voices, loss of memory). Rather, it is a persistent, maladaptive pattern of behaviour which means that you start to behave badly as a child or teenager, not complying with the accepted social rules (running away from home, stealing at random, getting into fights), and, as a result (usually), develop a recidivist, criminal career. Poor impulse control, broken relationships and drug/alcohol abuse are also characteristic.

In the case of Michael Stone, who had a background of previous violence and criminal convictions, the pattern was quite typical and he had been assessed by psychiatrists when in custody. Had he had a mental illness, he could have been detained for treatment under the 1983 MHA and transferred from prison to a medium secure unit (MSU) to ensure that treatment. But because his behaviour was ascribed to PD, the only legal resort was to wait for him to break the law again, then convict him, perhaps for a longer period, to enable various standard rehabilitation approaches to be tried. Most regular criminals satisfy all or some of the antisocial PD criteria, so such an approach could be appropriate. However, the nature of his crime (assaulting a mother and her children with a hammer) and the strident public safety agenda – alongside media sneers at woolly-minded, cowardly psychiatrists ducking out of their responsibilities by using a legal loophole – generated Home Office fury. The then Home Secretary, Jack Straw, had a very public row with the then President of the Royal College of Psychiatrists, Robert Kendell, and in a December 2000 White Paper, Reforming the Mental Health Act, a new category of dangerously severe personality disorder (DSPD) was introduced. Such high-risk patients – and this issue took up the whole second half of the paper – were now going to be detained if they were deemed to 'pose a significant risk of serious harm to others'. That is, their personality characteristics would *in themselves* lead to preventative detention, rather than their being detained once they had committed the crime(s) that usually resulted from these personality characteristics. This approach was essentially a psychologised version of 19th century criminal anthropology, whereby the shape of your head or low-set ears were considered as overt marks of criminality. The government was proposing detention *before* the crime.

Despite widespread criticism, the government has ploughed on with its DSPD agenda, including treatment for the protection of others, in its draft MHA bill. This bill also set out a single definition of mental disorder – making it possible to detain people for drug/alcohol dependence or sexual perversion, both carefully excluded before – and gave powers to doctors that depended on treatment being 'required', 'necessary' or 'appropriate' rather than likely to 'alleviate or prevent'. Although acknowledging privately that the difference between mental illness and PD is very difficult to explain to the public, government ministers consider that the 2000–4000 people who make up the DSPD category (most of whom are in custody anyway) must be dealt with. Pilot treatment projects have been started in several units. Unfortunately, other aspects of the new bill that might have been more progressive, although still controversial, such as routine tribunals for all detained patients within 4 weeks, and tribunals being given powers to impose a form of community treatment order (for example, you need not stay in hospital but you must see your doctor/CPN and accept regular medication), have all become confused with the DSPD issue. The government has become untrustworthy in the eyes of most mental health agencies (patients, voluntary groups, professionals). No one believes that resources will be forthcoming and, at the time of writing, matters are in limbo. The MHA bill was not included in the Queen's speeches of 2003 or 2004 – indicating either that the government no longer sees it as a priority or that it harbours doubts as to its validity, or a mixture of both. Amendments, or perhaps a rewrite, are likely.

Despite these legal delays – and there is no doubt that a better legal framework, based around a non-stigmatising notion of incapacity rather than mental health alone, could greatly improve the delivery of community-based psychiatric care – other approaches, related to new specialist teams, have been pushed aggressively. Again, the stimulus for these new resources is not just altruism; apart from Michael Stone, there have sadly been other high-profile cases. For example, assaults with swords always get the headlines. Thus, the 1996 attack on a nursery school in Wolverhampton by the machete-wielding (and severely unwell) Horrett Campbell led to seven children being seriously injured. The 1997 attack on a church congregation in Thornton Heath by a naked samurai sword-wielding computer consultant (with a hitherto blameless home life and no known history of previous psychosis) was likewise much publicised, and the assault on the Cheltenham MP (and murder of his agent) by Robert Ashman – also wielding a samurai sword – also generated headlines galore, not least because Ashman, despite being obviously psychotic while in custody, tried to represent himself in court and had to be deemed 'unfit to plead' before being dispatched to Broadmoor. Again, he had no previous history of mental illness, unlike the less fortunate Andrew Kerman, shot dead by panicky police in Liverpool while waving a samurai sword in the street. He was known to have schizophrenia, was known to be relapsing, and the police had been to his house to take him to hospital (but he somehow escaped with the sword).

Such cases highlight very well the issues of 'How do you prevent patients relapsing, especially when they lack insight and don't engage in treatment?' and 'How do you diagnose patients early so that they do not reach states of intense fear or agitation?' Both issues reflect the pervasive impact of stigma on all aspects of mental illness, especially when it comes to the severe psychoses. As we observe in the next chapter, patients and their families often do not wish to acknowledge their condition, and public attitudes are hardened by repetitive 'mad psycho' stories. For example, the Jill Dando murder hunt (she was shot outside her own front door) not only engaged up to one-third of London's detectives for a year or more but also led to psycho headlines when Barry George was convicted in July 2001 (Fig. 1.6). Staff at a local mental health day centre that he attended regularly were not aware of his apparent intentions. The recommended systematic risk assessment of another high-profile case (that of Michael Abram, who seriously wounded the ex-Beatle George Harrison in December 1999) did not come up with any obvious risk of violence. Abram was quite properly acquitted of attempted murder on the grounds of insanity in November 2000, although detained for treatment in an MSU, and the health authority report of October 2001 agreed on the usual serious failings in terms of his care programme (i.e. no proper follow-up, lack of coordination between agencies). The problem in Abram's case was of dual diagnosis: schizophrenia and hard drug taking. He was known as an eccentric, but not violent, resident of Huyton, Liverpool, and kept on falling between the boundaries of drug dependence and general psychiatric teams.

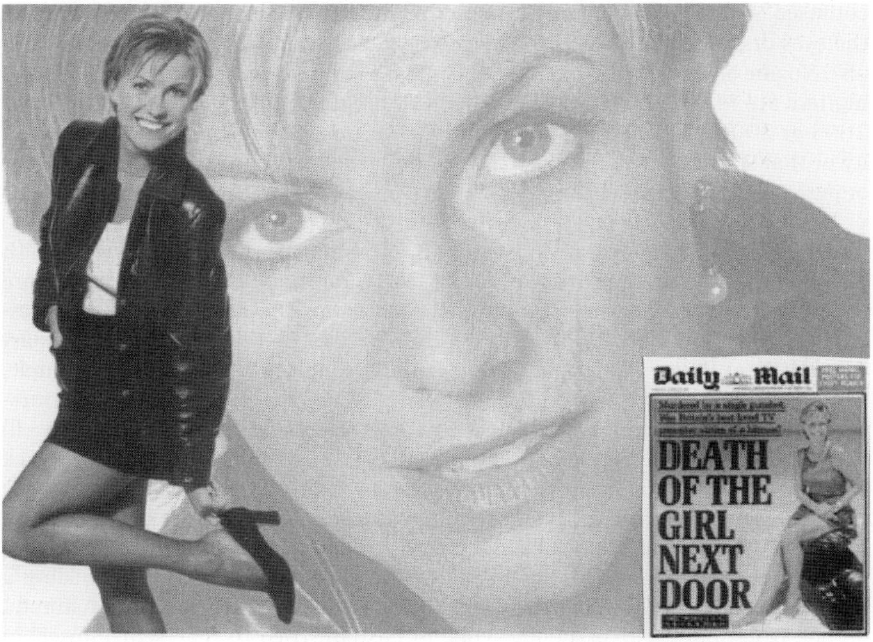

Figure 1.6 ● *Daily Mail* front page, 27 April 1999. In July 2001 Barry George was found guilty of the murder of the popular TV presenter Jill Dando. The fact that he had a psychiatric history played a major role in his conviction, but the extent of the evidence used by the prosecution still provokes controversy.

New types of service?

Given this challenge of providing accessible services that bridge the gaps and engage even the most reluctant patient, the NHS Plan has come up with three types of specialist teams and a commitment to provide 1000 or more psychologists for increased support at the primary care level. The specialist teams that are being funded include: assertive outreach (AO); crisis response (CR); and early intervention (EI) (see Box 1.2).

Box 1.2   The aims and roles of the new specialist teams

Designed to fill the gaps in current services, theoretically they should:

1. Maintain contact with and prevent relapse in those with serious mental illness who are difficult to engage (AO) via 'assertive' support and easy availability

2. Provide 24-hour crisis support for those in need, at home (home treatment) or perhaps in a specific 'crisis house' (CR), thus avoiding hospital admission

3. Engage in treatment of those with first-onset psychosis, especially schizophrenia, providing family psychoeducation and psychological intervention (cognitive behavioural therapy) alongside modern medication (EI)

These teams will have specialist staff, will have clearly defined roles [i.e. no more than 8–10 patients per AO worker, unlike the 20–30 or more per community mental health team (CMHT) worker] and are designed to work alongside current resources. The government is prepared to commit additional funds to community care, but only on its terms. No more ill-defined money disappearing into pet projects, on overspends or staff shortages – it has to be used exclusively on these specialist teams and will, it says, be closely monitored.

How well these new – and welcome – resources will fit alongside the acute wards and CMHTs (which are to continue) is yet to be determined. For example, in London and other inner-city areas, staff shortages in the less glamorous jobs could get worse as the bright new teams (AO, CI and EI) cherry-pick the best staff. Arguments will almost certainly develop over whose responsibility a particular patient is – interfaces between the teams will lead (as they have done in areas where such arrangements were piloted) to boundary disputes, with everyone trying to keep away from the most difficult, chronic, demanding PD-type patient. The 2002 *Dual Diagnosis: Good Practice Guide* from the DoH will also make demands to integrate services for dual diagnosis patients, who could end up bouncing between CR, CMHT, hospital ward, day unit and even AO. Furthermore, the evidence for these new teams being more effective than traditional CMHTs (in the UK and Europe at least) is very limited if not non-existent. They certainly have been positive in the USA and Australia, but these countries have very differently configured 'standard' psychiatric services, with private care and insurance funding arrangements generating very patchy community care resources.

Nevertheless, if these new teams, or at least locally refined versions of them, can be reproduced, and the government does commit the funding, there is now a chance – for the first time in decades, we would contend – for a true community care mental health worker to emerge. To provide such care in the UK in the 21st century will require a greater range of skills. The bumpy road from asylum to community over the last 50 years has had no real philosophical underpinning, apart from the general notion that institution equals bad and community equals good. This may or may not be so, depending on your illness, your family and how people react to you, and there is now a gradual turning of the tide towards various subtle – and unsubtle – forms of reinstitutionalisation. These may be private care homes, 24-hour staffed hostels, low-security rehabilitation units or 'wards in the community', but whatever they are called, they do reflect a need for sanctuary for some people.

Keeping patients well, as history shows us, requires a mix of money and therapeutic skills, a knowledge of social, welfare, cultural and housing arrangements, an awareness of basic medical and medication aspects, and a hard core of common sense. Yet, the very titles of the reports from the National Confidential Inquiry into Suicide and Homicide by People with Mental Illness (DoH) tell their own story. The 1999 report was called *Safer Services*, that of March 2001 was *Safety First*, and that of 2006 was *Avoidable Deaths*. History requires a lot of reading, but checking out just one of these will nicely summarise the world in which community care now exists.

Here and now

As a result of this strange journey through history, politics, sociology and psychopharmacology, current policy, in fact, remains at a crossroads, though

21

overtly, about outreach and crisis intervention. There is still strength in the desire to promote a community-based treatment service. In terms of acceptability, the avoidance of care behind institutional walls, and the over-riding need to reduce costs, seems generally sensible. Many people would question, of course, whether it really is cheaper. Hostels staffed 24 hours a day by trained nurses are just as costly as chronic wards on hospital sites. Assertive outreach teams are manpower intensive. The public's view about *not* locking up people who might be dangerous is becoming darker and more critical.

It has been suggested that we have forgotten the true functions of asylum. These include sanctuary, food and shelter, acceptance of unusual behaviours, professional treatment and the provision of structure for lives in chaos. Given the complications of modern life (Could you fix your DVD player? How easy do you find it to fill in your income tax form?), is it fair to expect people disordered in thought and emotion, and distracted by hallucinations, to cope with modern living? In particular, there is nothing more frustrating, whether you are a homeless patient with schizophrenia or a tourist lost in a foreign country, than to encounter the complexities of modern bureaucracy. You are directed to an office, someone asks you some questions, you are passed on to another office, you wait for quite a while, little clear information is given to you, and you have to fill in lots of forms. The benefits system changes almost annually, and the combination of poverty, poor housing and the disabilities of illness easily wear one down.

What does emerge, however, from looking at how we got to the current situation, is that people who suffer from mental illness require help from people who do not suffer in this way. In particular, they require help from people who have skills, empathy, energy, positive personalities and a willingness to do something different and useful with their lives. Whenever patients are asked what they need, during any era in history, their requests are remarkably simple. They want somewhere nice to live, someone to talk to and help with their problems, and something to do with their day-to-day lives. These may seem simple requests but it takes considerable training and an up-to-date knowledge of medicine, society and the psychology of giving help to deliver a reasonable service.

Some people may think that all history shows us is that nothing changes, that the revolving-door debate goes on and on, and that the mentally ill will always be stigmatised and kept away from the 'normal' people of society. But although it is true that the history of one patient with schizophrenia, particularly someone suffering from a revolving-door lifestyle, represents a microcosm of the whole history of psychiatric care, a number of other truths can be established (see Box 1.3). Above all, get to treatment early. There is powerful evidence that getting help early for serious mental illness prevents the awful deteriorations seen in the back wards of the old asylums. This is why Chapter 2 is all about how to get people into treatment.

Box 1.3   Nine truths from the story of community care

1. The whole business of treating 'mad folk' (or whatever they are termed) has always involved many people, with differing skills, in a range of places.

2. Mental illnesses really do exist. Seeing them as merely social constructions (that is, as a kind of make-believe created by the inequities of society at a particular time) does not account for the extraordinary overlap between mental and physical illnesses, the acknowledged benefits of modern treatments (especially drugs) and the simple question of how one would expect disordered brains to behave.

3. People suffering from mental illnesses (we prefer to call them patients, indicating suffering, rather than clients, suggesting the payment of money for help) require help and ways to help them exist. Whether this form of help is called treatment, therapy, care, cure or containment does not really matter, provided the aim is to benefit the patient rather than to enhance the reputation of the person doing the therapy.

4. Every argument, incident or problem related to resources in mental health has always happened before. The same debates occur again and again, although dressed up in a different language.

5. There is a regular pendulum between custody and community care. Whichever is the current fashion will be criticised, and whichever is out of fashion will be seen as a kind of 'golden age' when all was sunny and good.

6. It has long been accepted, since Hippocrates, nearly five centuries before Christ, that if you want to 'minister to a mind diseased' you generally have to call a doctor. Priests, counsellors, friends and relatives may all be helpful, but the need for professional care has always been deemed essential. Nowadays, fortunately, such professional help need not just come from a doctor. A professionally trained community mental health worker, with the proper social, medical, nursing and occupational skills, is often the one who is really required.

7. Anyone who works with the mentally ill gets tarred with the same brush. It is part of the deal so to speak, the 'germ theory' of psychiatric care. It is as if one is infected by one's work, with the stigma attached to fears of going mad. Phrases such as 'It takes one to know one' or 'You're the only sane psychiatrist I know' are typical of the attitudes prevalent in the business.

8. Although it is accepted that racist and sexist language (and attitudes) are not healthy, it has become commonplace for what might be called 'mentalist' language to be freely used. Journalists write about 'psychotic killers', and people whose habits one dislikes are called 'sad'. Distinguishing the features of mental illness from behaviours seen as bad or immoral is a key task of the modern mental health worker.

9. Community care is not perfect and is easily mocked. But remember, although it may have its untoward incidents and public embarrassments, at least they are taking place in the open where they can be seen and where things can be done about them earlier rather than later.

References

Hoult J (1986) Community care of the acutely mentally ill. *British Journal of Psychiatry* 149: 137–44.

Stein LI, Test MA (1980) Alternatives to hospital treatment. 1. Conceptual model, treatment program, and clinical evaluation. *Archives of General Psychiatry* 37: 392–7.

Getting into treatment

2

Getting treatment for a psychiatric problem is usually a problem in itself. The first section of this chapter, therefore, is concerned with the rocky road that leads to treatment. Next, assuming that contact is made, we consider the many possible agents of help to whom patients may turn, or perhaps find themselves propelled. To patient and new care worker alike, this variety of response can be bewildering. Thus, that crucial first contact can all too easily turn into something of a lottery. Getting into treatment can happen at home or away, so some thought must be given to the fine art of domiciliary (i.e. home) visiting. Last but not least, not everyone with a mental illness in need of help – particularly a serious one – is willing to see it that way. In such situations, a working knowledge of the way in which a patient may be given compulsory help is essential, and this topic is also covered in more detail in Chapter 9, which deals with the Mental Health Act (MHA).

Rocks on the road to care

Mental mythology

Deep down, everyone thinks that they are a psychologist. This can be inferred from conversations overheard in supermarket queues, the psychobabble of management trainees or the expert who is wheeled out to explain the latest inexplicable human horror on the news. Given the essentially egocentric nature of human minds, this is hardly surprising. I am the owner of a mind, I know how my head works, therefore I can make a fair stab at how someone else's head works. Presto, I'm a psychologist. It is remarkable how tenaciously we cling to our numerous pet theories of human nature even when all rational consideration of the evidence should have long ago made us keep quiet and call for help. This is compounded by a related myth, namely that people who study human nature do not *really* know what they are talking about. Were you to develop the tiredness, thirst and frequent urination that turn out to be diabetes, would you waste any time in seeking medical help? But when someone develops symptoms of tiredness, pervasive gloom, weight loss and early waking, all manner of theorising can go on, sometimes for years, before the unfortunate patient finally receives professional help. This is not to say that such theorising is necessarily unhelpful, but rather that it is simply human. All of us, in order to keep our sanity, have to look for meaning in things and, by and large, we tend to choose meanings that fit our hopes and expectations. Very few of us prefer the explanation that we are going out of our mind.

Consider a young man who develops a profound depression and retreats to his bedroom shortly after breaking up with his girlfriend. He can be heard talking to himself loudly at nights. His mother may satisfy herself with the belief that the girl has upset him profoundly. His mates, with a different picture of what he's like, might put it down to all the dope (i.e. cannabis) that he smokes. His employer may well see it in terms of the fact that the job proved too much for him. What they have all done is commit the time-honoured mistake of confusing cause with effect. When B happens, we automatically start to search for A and, having found it, we identify it as the cause. Because A happened before B, we easily assume that B happened because of A, as if, for example, breakfast causes you to set off for work. Life events seem to make sense. But the idea that the young man may be in the early throes of schizophrenia, aggravated by cannabis, which has led to the loss of his girlfriend and job, often lies outside the frame of reference used by his social network.

For the parents in particular, such explanations carry other advantages, for example avoiding the disquieting thought that 'maybe it's all our fault': a dodgy inheritance or a failure of upbringing. The psychological theorising that held sway over the aetiology of schizophrenia throughout the 1960s and 1970s did much to perpetuate this unrealistic fear. But parents do still feel guilty about how their children turn out. And presumptions of childhood abuse are very fashionable these days as explanations for all sorts of abnormal behaviours or personal problems.

Cultural misunderstanding and stigma

This face-saving rationalisation of mental illness may also occur at a cultural, rather than a family, level. Consider the ultra-orthodox Jewish family who allow their youngest daughter's manic depression to go unseen and untreated for a decade until their other seven children have found suitable marriages. Consider the cultural variations that may provide other explanations for odd behaviour. Why seize upon mental illness when the juju, a hex, a djinn or obiah are more plausible and more acceptable? Nor has the increasing psychologisation of our own culture rendered it immune to such aetiological mythologizing: 'Prozac made me a subway bomber'; the popular belief that psychotherapy will somehow miraculously reveal the cause of a mass murderer's shocking behaviour; 'shopping addiction syndrome'. Unsubstantiated theory is alive and well, and always has been.

For others, the fear lies not in an unwillingness to face up to the possibility of mental illness but in what will happen as a result. The idea that treatment is synonymous with 'being taken away and doped up' or 'being turned into a zombie' remains common. For many, mental illness still conjures up an image of irrevocable loss. These ideas derive not only from ignorance about the nature of mental illness itself but also from ignorance about the effectiveness of many modern treatments. Treatments are, of course, far from perfect, in particular the drug treatments for the major psychoses. It is quite common for patients, relatives and friends alike to confuse the side effects of these drugs with ongoing signs of the illness, in spite of hours of patient education. The belief that 'all you've done is to drug him up' very easily extends into the rationalisation that there was nothing wrong in the first place. People often have short memories for unpleasant things, and many patients simply do not recall what they were like when psychotic.

These differing views on the causes and treatments of mental illness, combined with self-deception, ignorance, fear and trivial explanations – schizophrenia is just a split personality – can all serve to delay or prevent the moment when the individual, or those around him, may decide that the time has come to seek help. While such ideas hold sway, it simply doesn't occur to anyone that a professional may be able to provide help. An essential element of the care worker's skill, therefore, lies in developing a foreknowledge of such individual, familial and cultural considerations and evolving a language with which to address them. Workers must not only know these as facts, or as obstacles simply to be negotiated in the first tricky assessment interview, but also need to stay with the much more active process of trying to see it from that other point of view. Such an incorporation of knowledge into practice takes time and effort.

The best way to achieve this is to keep your eyes and ears that little bit more widely open whenever in such a situation. Make notes if necessary. Research the background literature. Check out adverts in the local and professional press for cultural awareness days and demand the time off to attend them (see Chapter 7). Also, try to avoid the trap of thinking that you only need to know more about other cultures' attitudes to mental illness. Your own culture is changing just as quickly. Cultivate a watchful eye for subtle giveaways of mentalist thinking in the press, radio and television. Like fire hydrant signs, they're everywhere once you start looking for them. TV soaps, films and magazines not only constantly portray people with mental illnesses but also reveal attitudes to mental health and mental health workers that are often quite damning.

The other great block to engagement in treatment lies not in the belief and value systems of others but in your own. As a care worker, you will be exposed to all manner of suffering, day in and day out. It is a simple fact of the way in which our minds and brains work that, in time, they adapt to constancy. A young soldier reacts to the chaos of battle very differently from the veteran. As a care worker, it can become all too easy to forget that, for the patients and their families, a serious mental illness is a uniquely frightening experience. As time goes by and experience is accumulated, it becomes harder to empathise with individual distress. Just how such negative detachment can be avoided is hard to explain in mere print, but remaining aware of it must surely be a sound starting point. Striking a balance between staying calm amidst the chaos and not being supercilious about a family's apparently inappropriate or overanxious behaviour is the golden goal of care work. So, forewarned about some of the roadblocks (see Box 2.1), who and what lies down the road?

Box 2.1   Obstacles on the path into care

- Lack of insight by patient/family/peers, worsened by the illness symptoms
- Alternative theories of what is wrong, e.g. diet, stress, physical disorder
- Stigma: shame of disclosure; fear of persecution; fear of being laughed at/avoided/blamed; fear of being seen as weak
- Fear of treatment: drug side effects; mind control; incompetent psychiatrists
- Confusion of cause and effect, e.g. job loss, broken relationships

Mental illness: first ports of call

The general practitioner (GP)

In the UK, the GP is the gatekeeper of the NHS and for good reason. No one else is so well placed to keep an eye on the health of the population. Some 90% of the patients on a GP's list will consult with that GP over a 3-year period. So it seems reasonable that someone seeking help for a mental health problem might start with their GP. Unfortunately, there are one or two problems here. GPs are often so busy being gatekeepers that they are in a hurry. Few have time for the 20-minute chat that is needed to gain a useful picture of a mental health problem. In the UK in 1995, the average GP consultation lasted 4.5 minutes and, even by 2001, it was less than 7 minutes.

Another problem is that GPs vary greatly in their interest in and experience of mental health. The pressured and physically focused nature of their work allows many cases to go unseen; of those who are detected, only 5% are referred on to specialist services anyway and, of these, about one-third fail to show up for their appointment. Furthermore, GP lists are not stable. A rural GP in the leafy shires may get to know his or her patients well over the years but, in the inner city, with its high rates of migration, poverty, vagrancy and mental illness, such stability is rare. About one-quarter of the patients on some GPs, lists move on every year. And as more GPs take responsibility for their budgets, they have to make tough decisions. Who would you refer with your last pound: a rude, smelly, hallucinating vagrant or a cute little kid with a headache?

In spite of these difficulties, a large number of patients who go on to involve mental health workers find their way into the system via GPs. And quite a few are known *only* to their GP, often not wanting to see anybody else. The main message for the care worker, therefore, is that GPs are important, so get to know the ones in your area. There are various ways to do this. For example, find out which are the larger group practices in your area. These usually employ a practice manager, more often than not overworked but with an uncanny knowledge of the whereabouts, interests and foibles of all the doctors in the practice. A one-off meeting with him or her can be invaluable, if only to find out when all the GPs will be in one place at one time, ready to hear a pitch from a friendly mental health worker over a sandwich. A little time spent here will be well repaid: the GPs are the ones who will still be looking after your patient long after the present crisis is over. Likewise, keeping the GP informed about what you are doing – brief factual notes, for example half a dozen lines, every few months – pays dividends over time: 'Ah, so you're the person who sees him every week ...'

The local social services department

The local social services department might not seem like the most obvious choice as the first port of call for someone with a mental health problem. Unless, that is, you work in a social services department. People often present here not so much because of the problem itself but because of its consequences. People with mental illnesses have problems living life: benefits, fuel bills, giros, rent arrears, childcare problems, the list is endless. In the light of what has been said about differing perceptions of mental illness, many see these social dilemmas as the sole cause of the problem: 'Never mind therapy, what about my gas meter?' In contrast with the local psychiatric services, quite a few regard the local social services department as a stigma-free place where you can get something done, for example obtain money or maybe even a new home.

In many parts of the country, social services are working ever more closely with their counterparts in mental health. As discussed in Chapter 1, over the past decade, the pointlessness of the divide between medical and social aspects of mental health care has led to the creation of community mental health teams (CMHTs). Nowadays, in many CMHTs, doctors, nurses, psychologists, social workers, occupational health workers and assorted other health-care professionals share the same managers. CMHTs do seem to be an effective way of coordinating resources, yet further up the administrative ladder, health and social services are each still wary of putting their hard-won resources into what they see as the bottomless pit on the other side of the health/social service divide. Reliable contact with the local social service departments outside of the CMHT is essential, not only because of the work that they will send to you as a care worker but also because a lot of what they have to offer is likely to form an important part of any treatment in its broadest sense, for example providing community grants, bus passes, childcare, reports for housing, and so forth. The bottom line is that it is important to get to know how the local system works: names, faces, phone numbers and who does what, in and out of hours.

The local hospital casualty department

A large number of patients with mental illness present via accident and emergency (A&E) departments (Fig. 2.1). Evidence suggests that this is on the increase for many

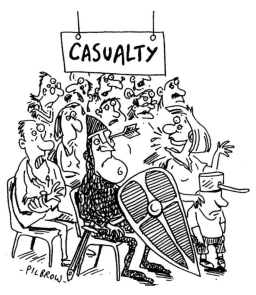

"Been here long?"

Figure 2.1 ● King Harold in A&E (reproduced with permission from *Private Eye*). *Plus ça change*: patient expectations are changing faster than we can deliver services.

of the reasons discussed in Chapter 1. A&E is becoming increasingly seen as the place to go for a prompt crisis intervention. But not that prompt: local A&E departments are probably some of the most hard-pressed NHS units in the country. The shortage of junior doctors is a serious problem. Waiting times of several hours for assessment by a nurse are common. Like GPs, casualty officers also vary widely in their predilection for identifying and handling mental health issues and are often more adept at handling the physical manifestations, such as drug overdosage, acute alcohol withdrawal, self-laceration, acute confusional states, etc. However, there is always a duty psychiatrist on call (or there should be) and this resource is what makes A&E so useful. The local A&E department is really the front line and, at around 11:30 on a Saturday night, its resemblance to a battlefield is not metaphorical.

Go along, introduce yourself and ask to spend an evening or two just observing what goes on. It is impossible not to learn something. The attitude of A&E departments to mental illness is slowly changing, possibly because the shift towards community-based care is causing more cases to turn up there. Lectures and seminars on the management of psychiatric emergencies appear with increasing frequency on the educational programmes of A&E departments everywhere. Try to go to one or, once you have some experience under your belt, why not give one? Other A&E departments are taking a more active approach by recruiting a mental health worker, usually a community psychiatric nurse (CPN), to serve the clinic around the clock. A substantial number of psychiatric admissions come in via A&E, both new and old patients, so it is a key place to work in and learn from.

The police

The police tend to make contact with cases at the more colourful end of the mental illness spectrum, usually as a result of behaviour that may be politely termed anti-social. Given that, to some, mental illness may be defined as a potential for generating social disruption, this is unsurprising. Until recently, the police, particularly in the inner cities, had something of a reputation for prejudice against the mentally ill. Apocryphal tales tell of horrors enacted in the back of a police van or a custody suite. This may be as much a function of the prejudice that many hold about the police as a reflection of reality, but what is unquestionably clear through this fog of suspicion is that they do a tough and thankless job and that it is simply not human to remain unhardened by such a job. The police are well aware of this and, perhaps spurred on by reports of recent investigations into the handling of mentally ill offenders – such as the Ritchie Report into the care of Christopher Clunis – have appointed mental health liaison officers to all police authorities. These officers are there to talk to you and help you with your work. They can also arrange for you to spend an evening out on a response patrol. Once you have spent an evening watching the world from beneath a blue flashing light, your attitude towards the police will never be quite as two-dimensional again.

Because of the sometimes understandable prejudice that many people hold about the police, particularly young men of ethnic minorities, there is a danger that you may come to be seen as an extension of their authority, somehow an agent of repression rather than of help. In our experience, such stigma tends to be short-lived and is far outweighed by the advantages of closer ties with the police. Remember who you will have to rely on when it comes to kicking down the door of a relapsing patient with a Rottweiler at 5:00 PM on a Friday. Also, be clear that when dealing with potential violence, whether in the street, at the office or at a patient's home, it is an absolute rule to ask for police advice and/or help. This is their job and they will always help if given due notice, for example with a problem home visit or in looking for someone who is at risk and out on the streets. Help them to sort out disorganised psychotic people misplaced in police cells and they will help you when you need them. More details on working with the police are given in Chapter 8.

Psychiatric emergency clinics

Not every area has a psychiatric emergency clinic. These clinics are effectively the psychiatric equivalent of hospital A&E departments and, in areas where they still exist, the local A&E doctors will testify to the lower level of mental health cases seen when it is open. They may account for almost half of the admissions to the local psychiatric hospital. Emergency clinics in many ways represent the best of worlds, in that they are easily accessible and they can be more sympathetic to the needs of mentally ill people. Advice, education, drug treatment, short-term follow-up to take the steam out of a crisis, referral on to specialist clinics, admission, all of this can be arranged, often within hours of the presentation.

The police often prefer these facilities to hospital A&E departments for use as a place of safety to which they may send patients detained under Section 136 of the MHA. Waiting times tend to be shorter than in their A&E counterparts. Perhaps their one disadvantage is that, by being so readily available, they may inadvertently encourage a 'crisis only' type of presentation when, in fact, a more measured response over time is required. A request for psychiatric help does not necessarily mean that there is a psychiatric emergency. Fortunately, few patients misuse the service in this way and, paradoxically, such crisis-centred patterns of use can signal the need for more individualised help. It is a simple task to find out whether there is an emergency clinic in your area. If there is, and the message should be becoming clear by now, go and visit it. See for yourself how it works.

Non-statutory (i.e. voluntary) services for the mentally ill

Voluntary services vary tremendously from area to area. This is both their strength and their weakness. Organisations may have a given remit, for example to help members of a specific ethnic minority or to target those with a particular difficulty, such as the Manic Depressive Fellowship. Not all provide a direct care service, some instead concentrating on pointing their customers in the right direction. Some have rules, based on ideology or pragmatism, which may make working with a community team less than easy. The Samaritans, for example, undoubtedly provide a valuable service for those in despair but have a code of confidentiality so strict that they would never dream of making a referral unless their client specifically requested it. Similarly, Alcoholics Anonymous (AA) is indisputably effective in helping some patients with severe drinking problems but regards itself as a self-sufficient organisation, the idea being that, if you're really with AA, you shouldn't need additional help with a drink problem.

In areas where a particular need is intense, for example in localities inhabited by people who hail from a particular ethnic group, organisations have a habit of springing up like mushrooms. But, like mushrooms, they do not last for ever and require careful cultivation if they are to grow properly. Organisations fuelled solely by a particularly energetic individual, or established as the result of a showcase piece of one-off funding, may well not be there when you need them. Never believe anyone (least of all the government) who tells you that a short-term project is here to stay. Some organisations clearly have a much longer life than others, MIND (National Association for Mental Health) in particular, but attitudes to mainstream services vary considerably, from the usefully cooperative to the downright hostile. Fashion and politics tend to run amok in this business: beware, in particular, the guru with 'the solution'. In the long run, it is really only the hard-pressed statutory services that one can truly rely on – these are probably the most worthy beneficiaries of any organisational zeal you may have left after a hard day's work.

Everywhere else

This is not as silly as it sounds. The sheer ubiquity of mental illness means that, at some point, almost everyone meets someone who needs mental help. The lone woman on the tube home, sobbing uncontrollably; the milk piling up outside the old man's door; the landlord worried about a reclusive tenant; the local shopkeeper giving bread to the unkempt lad who talks to himself. Obviously, you cannot have a professional relationship or contact with everyone in your area, but it is important to realise that all those in a patient's social network potentially hold a crucial piece of information that just might help you help your patient. Whether it is the rabbi, the mullah, the vicar, teacher, milkman, neighbour or take-away owner, do not forget to speak to everybody, even if it seems a bit daft at first. You never know what you might find out.

The DV (domiciliary visit), also known as the home visit

So far, we have assumed that the patient has been the one to make the first move into treatment. Frequently, it is the other way round. Physical illness or frailty can immobilise a patient but, more often, it is the patient's mental rather than physical state that proves to be the problem. Anxiety, suspicion, ambivalence or, most commonly, scant insight into the fact of the illness itself will, sooner or later, take you up a garden path or along the balcony of a council block in search of the correct front door. What is behind that door quite often turns out to be one of the reasons why we do this job in the first place. If there is one part of your work most likely to leave you with stories to tell your grandchildren, the odds are that it will involve a DV and, just like any gripping tale about a mission into the unknown, it needs a decent beginning, middle and end (see Box 2.2).

The beginning

The perfect DV begins long before you go through the door. Therefore, rule one is to have a plan. If you don't really have a clear idea why you are there as you walk up the path, you're doing it wrong. Try to decide what you want to achieve before you set out.

Box 2.2 Domiciliary visit checklist

Start
- Enough information
- Good reason for going
- Risk assessed
- Personnel identified
- Police or no police
- Anti-stab jacket
- Correct address
- Timing: surprise or announced
- Locksmith
- Access guaranteed
- 135 warrant (a court order granting entry to someone's home)
- Section papers
- Mobile phone
- Inform base where you are going
- Method of recognising patient

Middle
- Physical and mental state of patient and dwelling
- Adequacy of security/food/water/shelter
- Attitude of neighbours

End
- Plans for next contact
- Reaccessibility
- Closure of property
- Write notes/letters, especially to GP
- Thank key players

It could be anything from a 'hello, how are you' fact-finding mission to a kick the door down and come into hospital mission. Whatever it is, know it before you go.

The raw material for your plan is information. Gather together every scrap that you can. The referral note and who it is from (GP, housing, social services) is the obvious starter, but look for what it omits. Is there any known previous psychiatric history? How long has the problem been going on? Has anyone else been through the door recently? What do the neighbours say? Have you asked the landlord? It is impossible to gather every single scrap of information before the visit, but painstaking attention to detail at this stage can avoid all manner of problems later on. Once you have gleaned all that you can, ask one of the most important questions of all: what are the chances of things turning nasty? The basic rule here is that nothing predicts nastiness like nastiness. Have things ever got nasty before? Of course, the great majority of DVs are friendly, unproblematic affairs but never overlook risk assessment and playing safe.

By now, you should have some idea of your objective and who is going to help you achieve it. Identify your team. No one should ever perform a first-time DV on their own. If it is just a hello, then you and a colleague will suffice. If, on the other hand, you think that the person is going to have to come into hospital and may be unwilling to do so, you're going to need the people who are legally allowed to insist on admission. This is covered at the end of the chapter. Fit the personnel to the task in hand, whether it is to sort out housing problems, to administer medication or just to assess the mental state.

Next, focus on the practical things. How will you gain access? Do you have a key to the outer door? Might a helpful relative, friend or neighbour be at hand? A good relationship with the police or local housing department is useful at this point, both such agencies having their own unique and occasionally dexterous ways of opening closed doors. Think also of equipment: not only appropriate documents such as identification and the case notes, but also the obvious, but easily forgotten, things such as spare appointment cards, calling cards and blank paper. If it is likely to come to admission under the act, make sure that someone is carrying the pink pages (official MHA forms) before the visit. The other item, so indispensable that one wonders how we ever managed without it, is the mobile phone (fully charged, of course).

Once you've established your plan and identified your team, don't forget to tell them. It is astonishing how a firm commitment on a Monday can be a half-forgotten chore by Wednesday. There is no such thing as too much communication. Do not confine your plan sharing just to those on the trip. Always let your base know where you'll be and when you'll be there. Now that your team is briefed and you have everything that you need, you're ready for action.

The middle

Allow yourself a realistic amount of time to get to the job and arrive at a sensible time. Even the sickest people are usually at home first thing in the morning, but a 9:00 AM visit conducted under the nagging feeling that you've got to be in two other places by 9:30 seldom runs smoothly. Whether you announce your arrival or not is a strategic decision. For the avoidant patient, the element of surprise is often vital, but someone well known to him should be part of such a visit. Would you let in two or three complete strangers who arrived unannounced?

Next, think of geography. The front door of a neat terrace giving on to a well-lit street should be straightforward, but some estates are designed by architects with an interest in disorientation and fortification. With time, you'll get to know the architectural foibles of your area, but conscious reconnoitring can save precious time spent wandering lost along windswept walkways.

Pause before you knock on the door. Accumulated mail, signs of forced entry, all sorts of subtle signs, for example a large inverted crucifix sprayed on to the door, can sometimes provide intriguing hints at the diagnosis. Beware of peering nonchalantly, front-on, through the letter box. You never know when a meat skewer or unpleasant liquid might be waiting for you. A careful diagonal approach is always safer. One colleague, gingerly lifting the flap front-on, was horrified to see an evil pair of eyes staring back at him. He didn't see the mirror until he was on the way out.

Assuming that the door opens, do not just talk. Scan. Try to get a glimpse past the patient at the state of the place. Without seeming too conspicuous, try to take in a good whiff. When a door is being opened to the outside world for the first time in ages, the smell can be very strong. A friendly smile, saying who you are (with identification upfront) and why you have come ('Your GP asked me to pop round') are all instant starters.

Verbal contact with your patient is of course the aim. There are right and wrong ways of doing this and your immediate feel for the situation will already be pointing you in the right direction. If there is a group of you waiting outside, try to keep the numbers visible at first glance down to a comforting minimum unless, that is, a show of strength is part of your plan. Open questions such as 'How have things been recently?' are more likely to invite fuller diagnosis-laden replies than closed questions such as 'Are you well?', which can be replied to fully with a single frustrating 'Yes'. Try to think of any way in that you can. 'We hear that you're short of cash' can open the tightest of doors.

Once inside, keep your eyes, ears and nose open. Is the place heated? Is it damp? Is it secure? The central question is: can the patient hack it, living there? Look at the state of the television, a common source of angst for many patients with acute schizophrenia. Look for old bottles of pills on the mantelpiece. Are there light bulbs in the sockets and do they work? Most important of all, check the kitchen. Trying not to look too judgemental, see what is kept – or growing – in the fridge.

Even if everything seems fairly innocuous, always try to keep the possibility of a sudden outburst at the back of your mind. Do not ever let a Yale latch snap shut behind you and keep half an eye on any instrument that might be turned into a weapon. Screwdrivers can turn nasty. Again, these are exceptions, but do not hesitate to leave if the tension seems to be rising. Offers of help elsewhere and graceful withdrawal are perfectly sensible.

The end

By now, you will have formed some idea of the likely outcome of your DV. This may vary from a simple agreement to maintain contact or to start some form of treatment through to compulsory admission. Whatever you decide upon, communicate it clearly. Leave a version of it in writing with names, contact numbers and follow-up appointments with times, dates, places and a map of how to get there. All of these increase the chances of the patient engaging in treatment. The key message here is never to leave the patient without agreeing on the next contact. If the patient is to come into hospital, do not treat acceptance as a foregone conclusion that he or she will actually get there. Good care workers should see their charge safely into the skillfully planned ambulance or minicab before they move on to their next job.

Immediately after the visit, record it. Detail of the sort that proves crucial later on has a habit of fading fast from the memory. It is almost impossible to record the utterances of thought-disordered patients more than 10 minutes after they have spoken. Taking notes at the time is usually acceptable (tell the patient what you are doing, of course), but a letter to the referring agent (GP or whoever) is a must. If you can use a dictaphone, do it there and then on the way home. If you can't use a dictaphone, learn how to: it will change your life.

It should be repeated here that nearly all DVs go smoothly; most turn into friendly chats over a cup of tea. It is when they don't that a care worker's thoughts turn to the subject of compulsory detention. There are two key questions to ask at this point. Will the patient willingly come into hospital? If the answer is no, then ask whether the patient will be a risk to him- or her-self or anyone else if left alone. If the answer to this is yes or even only probably, a MHA section should be considered. To accomplish this, you will need an approved social worker (ASW), a psychiatrist and another doctor, preferably the patient's GP, assuming he or she has one (there are exceptions to this that are beyond the reach of this chapter but are covered in Chapter 9). In addition, the nearest relative (if available) can also sign an application and should be consulted by the ASW.

Deciding whether to section a patient is not always easy. There may be disagreement on the extent to which recent events (as much as the actual mental state at the time of the visit) are relevant to the decision. The different professional perspectives of doctors and social workers sometimes create differences on this issue. At assessment, a patient may be able to give a plausible account that is very much at odds with the testimony of the ashen-faced relatives who have endured weeks of his or her illness at close quarters. Taken at face value, such an account may well be grounds to decline a section. Fortunately, the care worker will hardly ever have to make this difficult, and potentially dangerous, decision alone. The information that a care worker may have accumulated about the case, however, is often crucial in the decision-making process, because the oldest rule in determining risk is to look at what behaviours have preceded the assessment: slaps turn to blows; thoughts of self-harm move to plans; self-neglect accumulates detritus.

When attempting to persuade an unwilling patient to consider the advantages of hospitalisation, it is important to bear their mental state in mind throughout the conversation, especially if there is evidence that the patient is psychotic. The precise meaning of this term is discussed more fully in the next chapter, but several aspects are relevant during a DV. First, if a patient is distressed by a belief that others are out to get him or her, this distress is likely to be amplified by an authoritarian, coercive approach. Many a section has been saved by consciously adopting a delicate manner from the outset of the visit towards a paranoid, persecuted state of mind. Second, a common mistake that is made when talking to a deluded individual is to believe that, with time, the person can be talked into insightful cooperation. This belief fundamentally misunderstands the nature of delusional thought. Generally, the length of time spent talking someone into hospital bears little relationship to the chances of getting them in. If you haven't scored by half-time, the odds are that you are not going to. That is to say, after about half an hour, it should be clear what to do. Prolonged 3-hour debates are nearly always fruitless, create considerable frustration for all and waste valuable time. If you really don't know, you can always come back later or the next day.

What next?

The process of therapeutic change begins long before the first point of contact with a care worker. In fact, it often begins at the instant that the patient, or those close to him or her, decides that there is a problem. By the time that a patient first meets you, his or her assumptions, beliefs and expectations of treatment are already well established. The first moment of contact, be it at home or away, is therefore crucial. As in chess, you can tell an interesting game by the first few moves. Practising your opening gambits increases your chances of engaging the patient. It is then possible to embark on the next stage of the therapeutic chess game: the fact-finding process known as diagnosis.

Numerous people have numerous opinions as to how this is best carried out. Some say it should be abandoned altogether. We reject such a notion, instead subscribing firmly to the belief that if something is wrong with the functioning of someone's brain or mind, sooner or later, the best person to talk to about it is someone who sees a lot of such problems. That person is called a psychiatrist, which is why the next chapter is all about psychiatric diagnosis.

What's the matter?
(Or an alternative way of looking at psychiatric diagnosis)

3

Introduction

There is no doubt that most people are rather suspicious of psychiatrists, and particularly suspicious about the business of trying to put names to mental illnesses. This is not least because of the long and complex words that are used, apparently designed to boost the standing of the psychiatrist rather than help the patient. People see terms such as psychosis or neurosis and extensions of these terms such as manic depressive psychosis or obsessional compulsive neurosis and wonder if they are at all helpful. What is the real point of such diagnoses? What is the difference between them and, for example, labels? Is there even such a thing as a mental illness? We all have problems living, but trying to pigeonhole them or package them as medical disorders that can only be understood by doctors, isn't this just that old dinosaur, 'the medical model'? Are psychiatrists not just spin doctors for the inadequate, the immoral, the incompetent?

Much of this concern goes back to the cherished myth that mind and body are somehow separate. That is, parts of your body can break down and be healed, but can your soul (or mind or spirit or psyche), that unique sense of self that makes up who you are, really be repaired, just like a car? Isn't it quite normal to feel upset when a close friend dies or when you see awful things reported on television? Should we call this form of being upset depression? Is it really helpful to give someone in such a situation a psychiatric label? Such questions can lead to answers that suggest that psychiatrists, like other doctors, need diagnoses to extend their empires, to make themselves more indispensable and, of course, to improve their income. And what about the giant pharmaceutical companies, who seem only too happy to talk up the number of new illnesses, so that more people can swallow their products and maximise their profits?

There is no doubt that medicine does tend to trumpet its advances while overlooking its limitations, the serious gaps in how much we know and how much we can do. The pressure to create funds for research, the difficulties in admitting to one's weaknesses and the old human tendency to focus on things that one has achieved (while ignoring things unfixed) are all part of this. At the heart of the matter, however, there has always been a need in medicine to tell the truth *and* to maintain hope, because the demoralisation of being told as a patient that you have something that is incurable can often be too much to bear. And that is the point of diagnoses, of trying to find out and clarify what is the matter. Because if the picture is clear – the how and the why and the what – patients and their problems can start to be understood, historically, personally and socially. 'Tell me where I stand, doctor?' is the common request, and diagnosis is the process of finding out where people stand.

Why have diagnosis?

$$Hx \pm Ex \pm Ix = \Delta$$

The basic reason for trying to establish a correct diagnosis for a patient suffering from an illness is to ensure that a clear and correct treatment plan is put in place. For the individual patient, this is the only rationale that matters. If we know what the matter is, we should know what to do about it. The standard procedure, taught in the earliest years of medical school, is to take a full history (Hx) of what has happened, to examine (Ex) the patients closely in terms of their physical and mental state or with special tests or investigations (Ix; for example radiography), and to put it all together to make a diagnosis (Δ). Of course, there may not be a diagnosis – there may be nothing physically or mentally wrong with the patient. This can lead to problems if the patient thinks he has an illness but the doctor does not. The pressure to prescribe a pill, organise yet another investigation or ask for a second opinion can make for a very muddled response. This is why many people who think that they are unwell, but for whom no diagnosis can be established, are referred to a psychiatrist as a last resort. Do they then suffer from hypochondria, or is this just a label? Sometimes they are labelled as hysterical, particularly if they are women. Whatever the language, using psychiatry as the dumping ground for such muddled interactions is the common result of poor diagnostic practice.

For example, a young woman with severe weight loss, down to 4.5 stone (63 lb/28.5 kg), comes into hospital because she is vomiting, in pain and has headaches. She is assessed with the whole battery of modern investigative techniques, for example blood tests, fibre-optic tubes inserted into her stomach and colon, whole body scans and ultrasounds of every possible organ. All tests are carried out and repeated if the results are equivocal. It emerges during testing that her marriage is in a mess, she was possibly abused in her childhood and she had treatment for depression and eating difficulties when a teenager. She insists it is a physical problem. She has no appetite and can't keep food down. The nurses cannot equate her behaviour in the ward with her apparent symptoms. She is assessed by the psychiatrists who consider that the key problem may be anorexia nervosa, a set of attitudes and feelings (in particular, an intense morbid fear of fatness) that are well-known to present in this way. The patient is transferred to the psychiatric unit, much to the relatives' disapproval. A few hours later, after arguments between all and sundry, she discharges herself. She isn't mad; her family know that there is something wrong but surely it's a bowel problem and not a mind problem? The patient, family, nurses and doctors are all in despair because they cannot agree what is the matter.

Yet even in such difficult situations it is still worth making a diagnosis. If someone is very depressed, for example, they can often develop strange beliefs about what is happening to their body. Treat the depression and the beliefs go away. The task of the doctor is to peel away all the – usually fascinating – personal idiosyncrasies to reach the core problems. The extraordinary thing about many psychiatric diagnoses is how common they are, regardless of where you come from. Symptoms may be presented in a different way or different aspects of them may be emphasised but, whether a patient is from Iceland, Iraq or India, a depressive illness will respond to proper antidepressant therapy. Defined diagnoses also enable good quality research to be carried out because you can compare like with like (from Reykjavik, Baghdad or Delhi) in different treatment approaches. It can often look like labelling, mystification or doctors preening themselves on their knowledge (and sometimes it is), but the whole power of modern medicine is the highly structured and rational process of diagnosis-based treatment. The modern phrase for it, evidence-based medicine, is much loved by both up-to-date doctors and the more cynical NHS managers, not least because of concerns that some medical activity is more about style than practice.

The most important thing about a diagnosis, however, is that it makes it possible to move into therapeutic action. It can be seen as the springboard to getting people better, and has been so ever since Hippocrates invented clinical assessment in ancient Greece. 'Know the man' and 'First to do no harm' were two of his precepts. Some diagnoses are much less clear cut and established than others, which makes for difficult judgements. But although the challenge of getting the diagnosis right is a particular fascination, with close similarities to what detectives do in crime thrillers, the real benefit comes from enabling someone to get better. Generally, people want a nice clear defined box to put themselves into and be helped out of, particularly when they are in pain, frightened, confused or fearful of dying or going mad.

Do mental illnesses exist?

There is a popular view that categories of mental illness are much less robust than those of physical illness. The diagnoses of measles or cancer of the lung are much more readily understood. Thus, with measles, the infectious virus is known; it results in very specific symptoms, which last for a defined period of time and then go away. The cause, pathology (i.e. how it damages different parts of the body) and course are very clear. With lung cancer, much the same is true, although the cause is not quite so certain; it is known that smoking damages the lining of the lungs and, in some people, this damage seems to progress to cancer cells. In fact, our knowledge of different illnesses varies considerably, right down to those colds and coughs and infections that the doctor tells you must be caused by a 'virus', even though they seem to come and go in their own sweet way and are much more bothersome in some people than others.

But, in a sense, all modern illnesses are mere holding stations in the history of medicine. They are based on known symptom clusters, whereby certain experiences seem to go together more often than not, and on similarities of outcome. As research progresses, diseases tend to vary in definition and classification, different subgroups emerge and new treatments eliminate certain presentations. The problem with medicine is that there is no such thing as always and no such thing as never. Most people who get measles get the typical rash, but a puzzling few don't. That is why some people don't know they have had measles even though blood tests can show they have had it. Philosophers might even argue that such individuals have been infected by the measles virus but have not experienced the disease entity known as measles, with its fever, discomfort, spots and maternal concern, and being bed-bound and having time off the from the usual duties.

With mental illnesses these issues are particularly poignant. How can you trust the doctor who tells you that you have a schizophreniform psychosis of psychogenic origin? What does this mean? The boundaries of mental illness are much less clear and, despite billions of pounds spent in research, the biochemistry of common problems such as depression and anxiety is still not known. There are

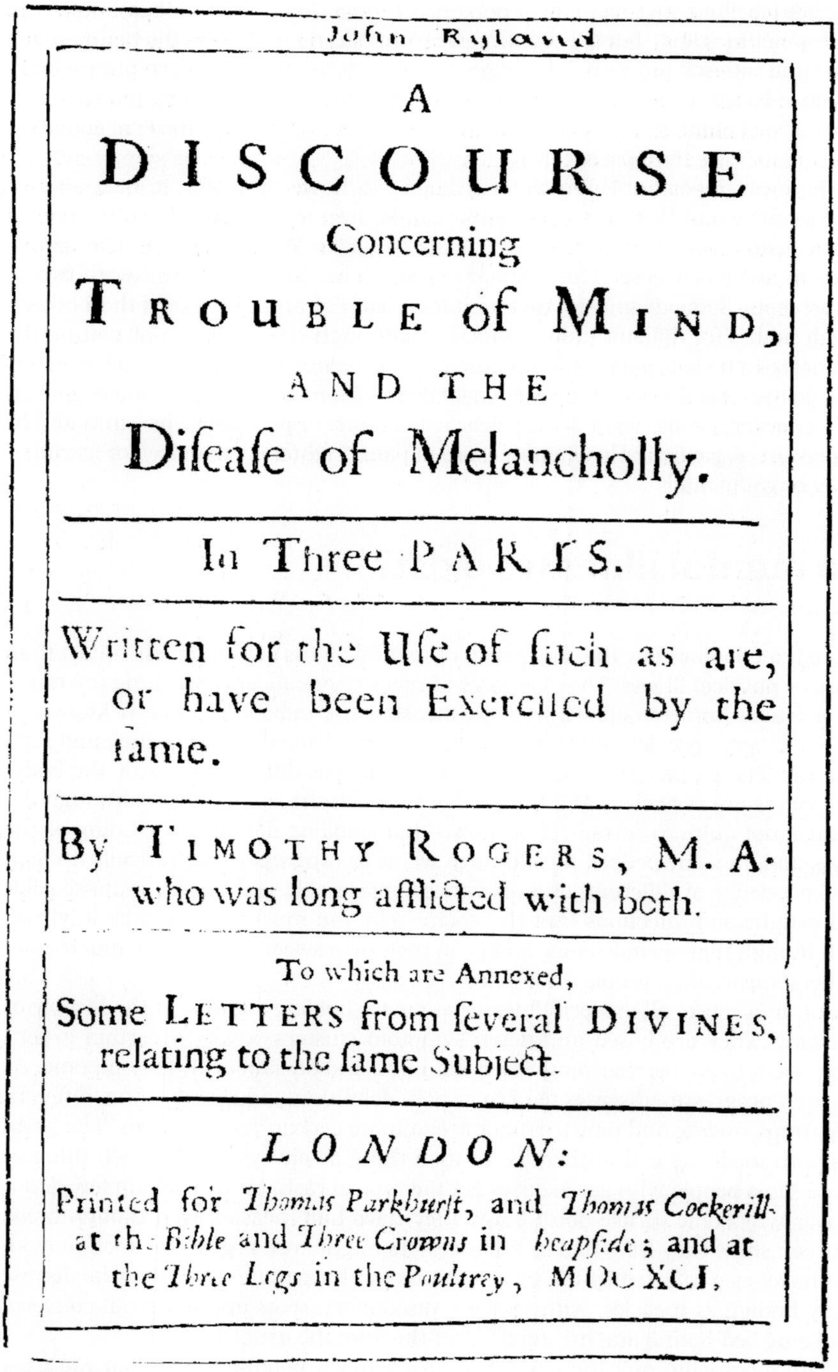

John Ryland

A
DISCOURSE
Concerning
TROUBLE of MIND,
AND THE
Difeafe of Melancholly.

In Three PARTS.

Written for the Ufe of fuch as are, or have been Exercifed by the fame.

By TIMOTHY ROGERS, M. A. who was long afflicted with both.

To which are Annexed,
Some LETTERS from feveral DIVINES, relating to the fame Subject.

LONDON:

Printed for *Thomas Parkhurft*, and *Thomas Cockerill* at the *Bible* and *Three Crowns* in *heapfide*; and at the *Three Legs* in the *Poultrey*, MDCXCI.

Figure 3.1 ● Frontispiece of *A Discourse Concerning Trouble of Mind*, a 17th century attempt at a psychiatric textbook?

no defining blood tests or scans that can tell for sure if a person is psychotic. The names of mental illnesses seem to change over time and seem particularly susceptible to social fashion. Nowadays, we talk of post-traumatic stress disorder (PTSD) or child sexual abuse (CSA), whereas we used to talk of neurasthenia or the nervous child. Oddly enough, if you discard these labels and look at what people suffered from historically, it is clear that the main psychiatric symptoms (and diagnoses) have been the same for hundreds of years. Timothy Rogers wrote *A Discourse Concerning Trouble of Mind and the Disease of Melancholy* in 1691, describing sleeplessness, racking pain, 'apprehension of God's displeasure', gloominess and 'anxieties of the soul' (Fig. 3.1). His symptoms were exactly those of what we now call major depressive disorder.

A particular problem has been the rich language introduced by Sigmund Freud (1856–1939) and the psychoanalysts. In their admirable attempts to understand how people thought and reacted, they created diagnostic categories so loose that almost anyone could be fitted into them. In a notorious research experiment, written up in a paper entitled *On Being Sane in Insane Places*, an American psychologist (Rosenhan, 1973) sent a number of his students to various hospitals. He told them all to give exactly the same story, of a voice saying 'thud' in their head, to see what would happen. Every single student got admitted as a voluntary patient and all were diagnosed as suffering from schizophrenia or something similar. One stayed in for more than 3 months. This was in spite of the fact that none of them indulged in abnormal behaviours or activities, apart from keeping notes about their stay and sticking to the aforesaid story. Even this note keeping was viewed as being potentially deranged – 'indulges in excessive writing behaviour' wrote the nurses – as 'patient' and 'therapist' sat looking at each other writing notes in the ward, day after day after day. This was very much an American cultural phenomenon though, based on private hospitals, using ill-defined terms and (probably) needing all the customers they could get. It was also clear by the 1960s that psychiatrists in Soviet Russia were using equally vague terms, such as 'latent' schizophrenia, to explain the activities of political dissidents. This corruption of psychiatric diagnostic practice, interestingly enough in the megastates of the USA and the USSR and in clear contrast to practices elsewhere, led to a major international effort to ensure tighter diagnostic criteria.

This process, organised by the World Health Organization (WHO), has been largely successful. Psychiatric diagnosis is extraordinarily reliable, which is to say that were you to take a hundred psychiatrists, from anywhere in the world, and ask them to examine a group of patients, they would agree on the diagnosis in 80% or more of cases. This may still seem short of the mark, but is in fact very good compared with many surgical or medical diagnoses. For example, were you to present to the casualty department with severe stomach pain, the diagnostic reliability would be about 50%. This is why up to half of the appendices removed during emergency operations may show no evidence of having anything wrong with them at all.

Versions of psychosis

Within psychiatry, there has always been a healthy tendency for there to be a strong group of dissenters in any generation. This is entirely understandable. The stigma of mental illness creates a considerable rejection of those working in the trade. In the 1960s and 1970s, a radical group of anti-psychiatrists, centred

43

around the charismatic Dr Ronald Laing, suggested that schizophrenia was an understandable reaction to the terrors and madnesses of modern life, Cold War politics, etc. Who was more deranged, the pilot of an aircraft carrying a nuclear bomb (and prepared to use it under orders) or the innocent hallucinating schizophrenic, driven to distress by the game playing of his overcritical family? A film called *Family Life* (made by the radical director Ken Loach in 1971) was especially popular on the student/art house circuit because it portrayed a girl becoming psychotic amidst the subtle psychobullying of her unsympathetic family. However, although the sentiments may have been understandable, the natural distress caused to many families trying to cope with relatives suffering from schizophrenia was immense. Modern research has now largely established that schizophrenia is a disorder of brain function that can be helped by medication, and one most important function of diagnosis is to remove the sense of blame from troubled relatives. As we have stressed elsewhere, seeing mental illness as a health problem can be very protective towards its sufferers, something that 'anti-psychiatry' rather fails to do.

If we consider just what might happen if the brain does go wrong, and of course any organ in the body can go wrong and have pathology, what symptoms would appear? In this sense, diagnosis can be seen not only as a helpful way of understanding problems (and as the only road to proper research) but also as a critical and economic necessity. What we think and what we feel reflects very much how our bodies, brains included, are working. It is by looking at these various brain functions, such as thinking and feeling, that we wish to illustrate what is meant by psychiatric diagnosis. In this sense, the human brain should be seen as an awe-inspiring object, shimmering with reactivity to the various smells, sights and sounds of the space outside it. Given the considerable mysteries of the cerebral hemispheres, think of *Star Trek* as really being about inner space, that personal universe of primitive fears, mother love and inspirational ideas, all somehow connected up by complex patterns of neuroses, neurochemistry and neuroelectricity. Shakespeare's central nervous system wrote *Hamlet*.

How the brain works

Because this is not a textbook, we will not list all the various diagnostic categories with their standard details, though we do outline the major ones later in this chapter. Rather, we will go through some of the normal functions of the brain, such as thinking and feeling, and try to explain how these processes can break down. Such breakdowns can be temporary, can create symptoms of illnesses or can even be normal aspects of human experience. Perhaps the most important thing to understand is that most of the strange things that happen to people when they are mentally ill can happen to anybody. For example, if you put someone into a sensory deprivation apparatus, such that they cannot see, hear, smell or feel what is going on around them, the great majority will start to hallucinate. Likewise, if you inject people with certain drugs you can also usually make them hallucinate. By hallucinate, we mean the experience, for example, of seeing things that do not exist.

It is also commonplace to describe psychiatric illnesses as either *psychoses* (in other words, very severe, such that you're not aware of the reality of what is going on around you) or *neuroses*. These are both old words meaning disorders of the soul (psyche) and disorders of the nerves respectively. For some mysterious reason, their meanings seem to have crossed over historically. Thus, today's serious mental illnesses (psychoses) are now accepted as being disorders of the central nervous system (CNS), including the brain. The less severe illnesses, the neuroses, tend to overlap with those problems of living that have no obvious basis in physical disruption of the nerves. Thus, the later term 'psychoneurosis' (coined by the Freudians), suggesting the psychological aspects of these conditions, is strictly speaking more accurate in its causal attribution.

A standard glossary of diagnostic terms [from the *International Classification of Diseases*, 10th edition (ICD-10)] is included at the end of this chapter for ease of reference. We, though, have broken down our explanation of psychiatric symptoms into the categories of thinking, perception, believing, feeling, memory and the sense of self. After all, this is what brains do, so understanding malfunction in these activities is the key to understanding psychiatric disorders.

Thinking

Thinking is a puzzle. We all do it, and we know exactly what it feels like when we do it, but it is very hard to describe just what it is that we do. Thinking seems to have something to do with meaning, symbols and connections; it's the activity that connects up the different parts of your mind. Think of the line that connects up the numbered dots in children's puzzle books, so that when all the dots are connected a picture emerges. Thinking enables you to make sense of incoming information, to compare it with what you know or remember and to come to conclusions that may even be new ideas. All this happens in your head or, to be more precise, in your brain. It does not, as far as we know, happen in the stomach or the liver. There is a good analogy, however, between the brain and the liver. One takes in information, analyses it and produces thoughts, whereas the other takes in blood and lymph, processes nutrients and impurities, and produces vitamins and bile, etc. If your liver doesn't function, you turn yellow, so-called jaundice; if your brain doesn't function well, you tend to take a rather limited (or even jaundiced) view of the world. The combined process of taking in information, thinking, remembering and producing ideas is called cognition, a term used increasingly in terms of therapeutic strategies.

The act of thinking is usually private and under one's own control. Unless we tell them, no one else knows what is going on in our minds and, by and large, we prefer it that way. Generally speaking, there is a continuous, forward flow of thoughts from A to B to C and so on. Sometimes we think quite quickly, for example when excited or under pressure, whereas at other times, for example when tired, we tend to find it hard to think or concentrate and sometimes our minds seem quite empty. Sometimes we are easily distracted and our thoughts seem to be very slow, as if wading through mud. Sometimes there seem to be too many thoughts in our mind, all jumbled up and leaping all over the place. Sometimes problems are too difficult to sort out, and this difficulty in thinking is accompanied by feeling low or angry. Thoughts almost always have an emotional colouring to them and the separation between thinking and feeling is a touch artificial. In addition, it is a general rule that, when we are feeling depressed, we don't just think about depressed things but the process of thinking itself is depressed, that is, it is slowed down or disconnected.

Not being able to think straight is not that unusual; it happens to us all every now and then. Trying to sort out things that you don't know anything about, trying to cope when feeling very angry or sad or trying to remember things under pressure, for example in an exam, all result in some form of thinking problem. However, when there is no obvious reason for being unable to think straight, and when it seems to go on for much longer than usual, for example day after day, it is usually a sign of illness. Muddled or distracted thinking, such as not being able to keep up with the simplest television programme, is typical of depression. Sometimes the mind goes empty constantly, so-called thought block, and this could be a sign of a more serious illness such as schizophrenia. By contrast, thoughts that are speeded up and that jump all over the place are usually associated with forms of mania or anxiety, or they may be caused by drugs such as amphetamines ('speed', an obvious name for something that speeds up your thoughts) or cocaine. Of course, such muddled patterns of thinking in a patient may emerge just from listening to people talk like them or about them. However, if, as the care worker, you can't actually follow what patients are talking about (and trying to write down exactly what someone is saying can be very illustrative), it is likely that they are suffering from thought disorder (see Box 3.1). Some forms of thought disorder are what we call a 'first rank' (i.e. indicative and important) symptom of schizophrenia, but beware the muddles in speech caused by dementia, brain damage or plain stupidity.

Box 3.1 Illustration of different forms of thought disorder

Acute schizophrenic illness

Now, be seen. I am a snu, in no way. Bottom sucking in here, a recognition of a hemisphere, your hemisphere, that I cannot countenance in any way, a king or a lion. A lion and a pu. In no way, amen, a lion of your countenance, and conceptioning in God preincognito, a snu in no way again, amen.

Acute manic illness

Ah, Doctor Rowlands, with teeth like that you look like a rat, roland rat, water rat, ha ha. Look at that, the water on the floor, water, wind, earth and fire. Fire and iron, elemental iron. We have got a Morphy Richards, I took a shine to it.

The first example illustrates the 'formal thought disorder' of an acute schizophrenic illness. Note how the leaps between the ideas seem inexplicable from the point of view of the listener. The utterance also contains neologisms (new words) and repetitions that may (or may not) have profound significance for the speaker. Although it is tempting to interpret metaphorically, it is often very hard to make clinically useful sense of the content of formal thought disorder.

The commonest form of thought disorder seen in mania (second example), however, displays a clear followable 'flight of ideas'. Although the associations between words and ideas are clearly loosened, the sense is possible to follow through puns, rhymes, assonance and double meanings. Note also the euphoric mood and the overfamiliar manner towards the interviewer.

A particular problem in thinking may be the sense that you are not quite in control of your own thoughts. This can take several forms. Those suffering from obsessional disorders tend to find that certain repetitive thoughts come into their mind, which they know are theirs but which they would rather not think about. They try to put them out of their mind, to distract themselves, without success. The thoughts keep coming back, just like a facial tic. Sometimes they can work out various ways of getting rid of them, for example with rituals like washing their hands many times to remove the thought that there were germs on them, but this is rather exhausting. In fact, they become crippled by these constant thoughts (called obsessions), which tend to dominate their mind. However, at least they know that they are *their* own thoughts, although their obsessional repetitions or mental slowness (the term rumination is used for this constant pattern of thinking) may mimic thought disorders. Oddly enough, some obsessions *do* have accompanying physical twitches or even vocal grunts, showing just how intimately our brains and muscles are connected.

There is an extension of this experience in which patients feel that their thoughts are not their own. It is as if someone else has actually inserted their thoughts into the patient's mind, just as if they had injected some alien substance into their brain. This can be most disconcerting, such that patients even feel that their actions are being controlled, for example by a computer or radio waves, and that what goes in can also come out. Thus, they may actually feel as if their thoughts are being sucked out of their heads, so-called 'thought withdrawal'; when their thoughts are outside of their mind, it seems, quite clearly, that anyone else can pick them up. In other words, the patients feel that people know what they are thinking and can literally read their minds, as if their thoughts are being broadcast to the world. This can make for considerable difficulties, and some patients even try and cover up their heads, ears and eyes to stop it happening. It may also be very difficult for them even to describe what is happening. For example, if a patient is experiencing their thoughts being broadcast to the world and a care worker or psychiatrist asks questions such as 'What's on your mind?', the patient's first reaction is to assume that the care worker or psychiatrist is rather stupid. As far as the patient is concerned, the care worker or psychiatrist obviously knows anyway and is just trying to catch him or her out. Perplexity, distrust and incoherence become the dominant themes in the patient's mental state.

What is vital about all these experiences is that they are typical of the common mental illnesses, such as depression or schizophrenia. They are also easily understood if one accepts that thinking is private, coherent and something that one can usually do, and that any persistent disruption of thinking is likely to be a symptom of illness. If we take the old saying of the French philosopher René Descartes, namely 'I think therefore I am', and paraphrase it as 'I cannot think therefore I am not well', it suggests that people who are 'not well' in this way are highly likely to have a mental illness.

Perception

People often get muddled by the word perception. The simple answer is that it is the registration of a stimulus, which perhaps doesn't get one any further. If we take the analogy of being on the Starship Enterprise, we can consider it as a two-stage process. Thus, an object is displayed on the sensor screens in the spaceship's control room. From being an ill-defined lump, it is gradually transformed by the computers into something of a distinct shape and size, for example another spaceship. The first noticing of the object would be termed a sensation, but the noting of the object *as well as making sense of what it is* would be called a perception.

As we all know, humans have five major senses: sight, sound, touch, taste and smell. The organs for these senses, of various shapes, are stuck onto the brain. The most important ones, the eyes (a direct part of the brain, out on a stalk), ears and nose, consist of strange protuberances, which are much elaborated upon whenever we try to depict what aliens would look like. Using these organs, we can work out what is going on in our world, with various degrees of subtlety. Given the evolution of the human brain's attachments, it seems likely that the most primitive sense is the sense of smell, followed by sight and then probably hearing; we know that babies are listening even before they are born. There are eight wiring relays in the hearing mechanism, which indicates not only its complexity but also its liability to be damaged or disrupted. That is, because much more processing takes place during hearing, it is subject to increased complications. The more parts in the machinery there are, the more there is to go wrong, and Fig. 3.2 illustrates the potential unreliability of our perceptual apparatus).

The reasons for describing this complex neurological setup are important and quite simple. The commonest form of disrupted perception is the experience of 'hearing voices' or, to be more technical, auditory hallucinations. This means that you hear things, or seem to hear things, and they seem absolutely real, but they are not actually there. It is as if someone has broken into your telephone line, making your telephone ring even when no one is actually calling. The problem is that such experiences are probably very common. About 30% of ordinary people experience auditory hallucinations on the edge of sleep, which are often quite vivid. A smaller number of people may experience them as part of their normal consciousness. It is also clear that people can hear not only voices but also all sorts of clicks, grunts and groans. In addition, drugs, tiredness, emotional stress or physical illnesses such as fevers can also bring on auditory hallucinations.

In schizophrenic illnesses, disorders of perception (hallucinosis) are usually in the hearing field, but they can occur in any of the other four senses: visual, tactile (touch) and olfactory (smell) hallucinations occur in 20–30% of such illnesses. Even more problematic, we probably all have a sixth sense, a 'sense of presence', the sense of knowing someone is there even though you have not heard them or smelt them or seen them. If this particular form of perception is heightened, all sorts of things can happen, and ghosts, fairies and other supernatural phenomena all start to make sense. Furthermore, if one considers that the sense of touch is probably broken up into lots of smaller parts, such as balance, vibration, heat, etc.,

Figure 3.2

Visual perception is not as reliable as it appears. Close your left eye and stare straight ahead at the spot with your right eye. Now, without moving your open eye, move the page slowly towards or away from you. Sooner or later the image of the spot will fall upon the blind spot on your retina and will disapear from view. Your brain, not wanting to let you down, will make up the remainder of the image by 'borrowing' from either side of the spot. Because this currently contains a line, your brain takes this as its cue and sketches a continuous line across your field of view. Your brain has told you a fib to keep you happy.

it is possible to see how complex a hallucination can be. Most are simple enough, like feeling a hand stroke your back or smelling something burning, but they can amount to threatening scenarios of intense detail.

Disorders of perception can be put into two main groups. The most understandable are those in which the perception has been physically interfered with. People who are blind or deaf know all about this, although it is interesting that the latter often experience tinnitus, a strange collection of hums, hisses and other sounds that they know to be unreal but which seem to be part and parcel of having a damaged ear mechanism. Likewise, individuals with impaired vision can 'see' all sorts of strange things, which their brains seem to make up when they haven't got real sights to fasten upon. The strange distortions produced by cataracts in the eye are perhaps best understood by going to look at a painting by Turner (no relation). The commonest form of perceptual block occurs after a stroke, when an arm or a leg loses all sensation. Likewise, many people who have head injuries lose their sense of smell and taste. Especially bizarre is the 'phantom limb' experience of people who have lost a leg. Although they know that they no longer have a leg, they can still feel it, feel pain in it and even feel their toes wiggling. The patterns of perception are so deeply laid down in the brain that the brain can't seem to let them go.

In terms of mental illnesses, it is perceptions working overtime that are more important. Thus, if you hear a voice saying 'you smell' while walking down the street, it's quite likely that you will get rather upset by such rudeness. Remember, these voices seem absolutely real. They come from outside. They are not thoughts talking to you inside your head, inside your mind (these experiences can occur, but they are quite different – and patients *know* that they are different from the outside voices). Given that you are experiencing such unpleasant comments, or perhaps strange smells, and they seem to be following you around, it's not unlikely that you may react in a rather unpredictable manner. Some people withdraw, hermit-like, others try to remonstrate, a few may lash out. All are distressed and try to respond in some way, because *it really is happening.*

One of the great things about *Homo sapiens* is that he or she tends to look for explanations of events. We need to make sense of our world. Apply this principle to someone with auditory hallucinations, and it is most likely that they will start with what is around them. The first person to be checked out will be the neighbour, whom the patient may believe is banging on the wall or shouting through the wall. If comments are mocking or unpleasant then they may seek redress. Other patients might decide that their families are talking about them behind their backs; often these complaints can be easily dismissed as being understandable. For example, one patient complained that people were often teasing her in the home in which she lived. This was understandable given that she was a teenager living in a supported but relatively strict children's home. It was only when she explained that people were teasing her when she lay in bed at night that it became clear that she was experiencing auditory hallucinations. Another old man felt harassed by noisy neighbours playing loud music at night. He complained to the police, the council, the Tenants Association and anyone else who would listen. People were sympathetic until he started describing the 1001 bizarre sex acts performed every night in the flat above, and the camera coming through the ceiling to record his every move. Other patients complain of cars hooting at them from outside or of lights being flashed at them deliberately, or keep sending for a gas engineer to fix the leak because of the constant smell that keeps pervading their home. Remember, these are real experiences, reinforced by the persistence of the hallucinations and, thus, the normal coincidences of daily life are often elaborated into a special personal significance.

Sometimes people develop remarkably elaborate explanations for their hallucinations. They may decide that it's the electricity board computer system wiring them up wrongly. They may decide that the police or MI5 are harassing them or that there is a family out there deliberately checking them out and bothering them. This may lead to disputes, in public or in private, or to increased social withdrawal to get away from all the harassment. Often they cannot explain what has happened to them because they are not merely 'hearing voices': from their point of view, they really are experiencing what is going on. Depending on their background, different people will put a different slant on things. In addition, different explanations have been given through history. Explanations from medieval times largely related to demons and angels; for the Victorians, it was steam engines and telegraphs; and those from the modern period are related more to computers, high technology or conspiracies of gangsters or governments.

Whatever the story, at the heart of all these elaborations lies an abnormal perceptual system in somebody's brain. The more bizarre the conclusion, the more easy it is to understand as a mental illness. If it is somewhat banal, such as the girl being teased, it can lead to arguments over whether it really is real. Being harassed by neighbours in certain inner-city housing estates or being racially abused are, unfortunately, common events. It may be impossible to decide that the complainant is hallucinating, given such a background. Part of the detective interest in understanding mental illness is sorting out just these dilemmas. Although auditory hallucinations are the most common, people may also experience strange sensations that they find hard to clarify or a sense of being touched, or even bitten or stroked, by all sorts of people or agencies. This can even amount to the feeling that a snake is crawling around inside your body or being convinced that someone is having sexual intercourse with you as you lie in bed. Such intrusive experiences lead on, quite naturally, to a whole range of strange ideas and the elaboration of variably abnormal beliefs.

50

Believing

As outlined above, ideas or beliefs are natural products of the brain, just as urine is produced by the kidney or breath by the lungs. Beliefs and ideas are produced to make sense of what is going on around us, or of what is going on inside us. Their content is as infinite as the imagination itself. Out of the fuzzy fog of the brain's activity, images or thoughts emerge, just like the fine-tuning of a television set. Sometimes you get the picture right with no volume, sometimes you just get the volume, and different people can reach different conclusions from the same material. New ideas are rather exciting. We even call these brainwaves, the classic example being that of Archimedes leaping out of the bath yelling 'Eureka, Eureka' (the Greek for 'I've found it'). He had just worked out Archimedes' principle, that the volume of an object equals the volume of water displaced by that object. Producing such new but true ideas is part of the remarkable, natural creativity of mankind. It is what makes us different from the rest of the animal kingdom. Producing ideas that are incorrect is very common, but hanging on to them tenaciously, despite contrary evidence and the disagreement of one's peers, usually indicates that there is a fault in the brain's idea-making processes.

These generally false beliefs are called delusions. They can be held with varying degrees of conviction, and we probably all have mini-delusions about ourselves, particularly related to how clever or good-looking we are. But serious delusions will seriously interrupt our ability to make sense of the world, to relate to other people or even to look after ourselves properly. The nature of one's beliefs varies, of course, from country to country, culture to culture and age to age. Falling in love is probably the delusion that we all most commonly share. We start to believe all sorts of extraordinary things about another person, literally blinded to their faults, and, as a result, act in a rather odd fashion. A similar commitment to religion or politics can be variably extreme, but the *contents* of our ideas, as opposed to the *way* in which we reach our conclusions, is less important in terms of the symptoms of a mental illness. Nevertheless, it is a truism to point out that fanatics, holding extreme views at the furthest ends of the religious or political spectrum, do more often than not present with delusional thinking about the world. One of the commonest delusions has of course been the conviction that one is Jesus Christ or the Messiah. No one can disprove that this is so, and even putting half a dozen Messiahs into the same room to argue about it does not lead to clarification. Each one regards the others as liars or mad.

What is most important about delusions, however, is that such abnormal beliefs have become the primary hallmark of madness down the ages, although they are probably secondary to other aspects of brain disorder, as outlined above. For example, if you hear voices that seem like those of angels and your thoughts are being broadcast to the world, it would not take much in the way of Bible reading or being raised in a religious environment to make you start to think that perhaps you do have Christ-like powers. In contrast, if you were brought up in Haiti and started experiencing the feeling of thoughts being taken away from you, and things seemed to be biting at you all the time, you might decide that voodoo was being practised upon you. If one defines culture as the sharing of ideas, it is clear that distorted beliefs, just as much as accepted beliefs, will be modified by the cultural environment in which one lives; a substantial proportion of the US population is willing to accept the possibility of alien abduction. It isn't *what* you believe that makes you mad but rather the way in which you reach that belief and the way in which you hang on to it regardless. It is form, rather than content, that signifies.

It is also clear that the stranger the belief that someone has, the more readily it is seen as being 'mad' by the world around them. So, if you decide that you're a green-blooded Klingon from the planet Zog and you act out this role with conviction, most people will think that you are mad. This belief goes against your social or cultural background, it dominates your mind and you can't be talked out of it. If, on the other hand, the belief is rather more subtle, such as the statement 'a lot of people in the village don't like me, I can feel it somehow', but you do not elaborate on the reasons for it, it may be that it's true (or it may be that you are just as deluded as the Klingon). In fact, if you behave according to this conclusion, however you may have reached it, the chances are that people will start to dislike you because you are likely to be rather surly towards them. Out of this will emerge the strange phenomenon of a delusion that is true, and it will not be seen as a delusion because it isn't particularly rare or bizarre. Thus, the more banal or unelaborated your false belief, the more likely other people are to believe it and accept it at face value. One can see how delusional ideas can fester for years in people's lives, only gradually distinguishing them from other less troubled individuals.

Certain abnormal beliefs are more common than others. Apart from persecution, one of the most dangerous is that of morbid jealousy, whereby a person becomes convinced that their partner is having an affair with someone else. They begin to check on their whereabouts, check sheets for semen stains or even employ a private detective. Once the idea of unfaithfulness has crossed one's mind, everything the other person does serves to reinforce the belief. Shakespeare's play *Othello* is a perfect description of this process and the horror of the consequences.

Similar in nature are the beliefs around erotomania. This involves the conviction that somebody else loves you, usually someone who is in a powerful, socially unattainable position such as a pop star or a prince. Everything that person does reinforces the belief. Most public figures are constantly bedevilled by the letters of such believers, feeding the current fashion for personal guards and anti-stalking campaigns. Other more grandiose delusions can lead to people developing followings and becoming like gurus (Fig. 3.3). Most frightening in this respect was the religious fanatic David Koresh, whose rantings about Armageddon and stockpiling of armaments led to the tragedy at Waco in Texas. Delusional thinking, in the setting of a powerful charismatic personality, can sometimes change the course of history.

Equally strange is the so-called Capgras delusion wherein one believes that a spouse or close friend has been transformed into another person. She may look like your wife, talk like your wife and act like your wife but you *know* that she is different somehow. The problem with such troubled ideas is that an outsider cannot see the disordered thoughts or perceptual derangements. There is (as yet) no external sign, blood test or even a brain scan to show that someone's thinking is out of order. Conversely, sometimes people can be convinced that parts of their own body are changed or deformed, or that there is something living inside them making them do things. They will seek explanations, investigations such as brain scans and, sometimes, operations, persistently undeterred by normal results, normal examinations or constant reassurance that nothing is wrong.

Perhaps the most difficult task for those managing the deluded is working out how to deal with these strange ideas. Should one collude with them, pretending to believe that they are, for example, the Messiah? Should one try to argue them out of such beliefs? The general rule is not to collude, yet not to argue. Putting this into practice is difficult, especially when the patient is angry, and we offer practical hints in Chapter 8. People who hold such delusions are normally, but not always, suffering from schizophrenic illnesses, and one of their many endearing characteristics is that they know when they are being lied to. They really can sort out who is telling them the truth. Far better to honestly disagree, to accept that we all have, amidst the flotsam and jetsam of our brains, various beliefs that other people disagree with, but to try to ensure that sufferers get help. The most difficult beliefs to deal with are those relating to religion, politics and sex, which may explain why it was a general rule amongst the British army in India never to discuss any of these topics when at dinner with colleagues. Consider what most fights are about and this can be seen as a very sensible policy.

Feeling

Alongside all this thinking and perceiving and the creation of ideas is, of course, the complicated business of emotions or feelings. They provide a kind of background tone, a climate or connective tissue, to everything that our brain is otherwise doing. Our mood state, therefore, tends to reflect what we think about, what we remember, how we respond to other people and how efficiently we think and do these things. We can have too much emotion, leading to tears or excessive laughter, or too little emotion, resulting in a kind of negative, flattened-out state. Perhaps the best analogy is to think of mood states as being like the weather. They are changeable, they tend to have set patterns and they tend not to be always under our control. Many cultures have neither specific terms for moods nor do they separate thinking from feeling. Pain, or other physical concomitants, or explanations in terms of gods or the supernatural are used instead to describe how they 'feel'. Like thinking, emotion is so easy to recognise but so hard to define.

The best people to talk about moods are probably poets. Musicians are also pretty good, and the use of music to set the emotional tone of, for example, a film is

Figure 3.3

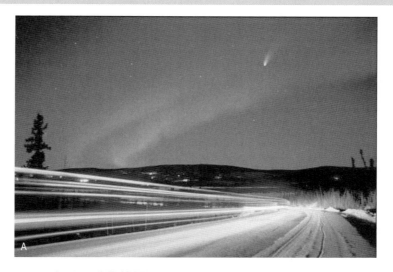

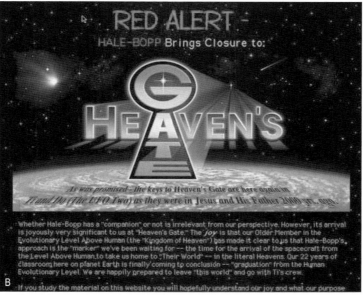

(Continued)

53

Figure 3.3 (*Continued*)

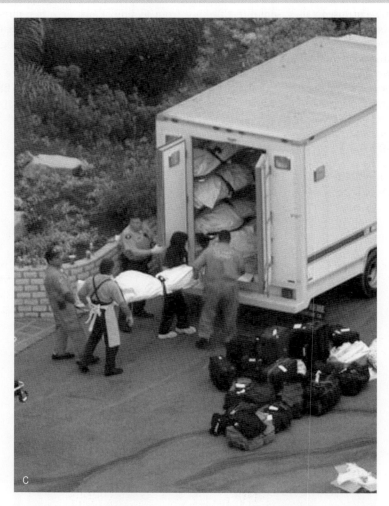

The power of a shared delusional system. In March 1997, 39 men and women were found dead at a ranch in California, having committed suicide in accordance with a shared belief that a spaceship hidden behind the Hale–Bopp comet awaited them. As they put it on their website shortly before their deaths, 'The joy is that our Older Member in the Evolutionary Level has made it clear to us that Hale–Bopp's approach is the "marker" we've been waiting for ... our 22 years of classroom here on planet earth is finally coming to conclusion ... we are happily prepared to leave this world and go with Ti's crew.'

quite deliberate. There are also many English words for moods. We have used three already (feelings, emotions, moods), but is there a difference? The only formal difference, from the psychiatric point of view, is that moods are states described subjectively whereas the term 'affect' is used to describe how someone else's mood comes across to or 'affects' an observer. Roughly speaking, mood and affect should be the same but, if they are not, it may well be that a patient's emotional state is disordered, unwell even.

It is also true that, in the end, we trust our emotions rather than our (more logical?) thinking. It is the old battle between hearts and minds, but most people do prefer the phrases 'I feel' or even 'I believe' to 'I consider' or 'I am of the opinion'. Feeling is seen as being warm and human, thinking as rather cold, android-like and distant. Most of us empathise better with Captain Kirk than with Mr Spock.

Our mood states tend to affect us more obviously in terms of what we do and how we get on with things during the day (Fig. 3.4). If we feel cheerful, then what has happened in the past, what might happen in the future and what is happening now all seem to be reasonably okay. However, if we're feeling depressed, past events take on a regretful sinister tone; everything around is as dull as ditchwater and the future is bleak and hopeless. And we do have many variable mood states, from the sad or happy to the anxious, irritable or bitterly angry. These will vary depending on what we're doing and what time of day it is; they may even vary according to the seasons. But when one mood state tends to be prolonged, intense and out of kilter with the rest of one's life, there is a good chance that it is a sign of mental illness.

We should also note that mood states are strongly linked to our biology. Physical reactions and experiences are so closely tied in to how we feel that we use terms like 'gut-wrenching despair' or 'heart-stopping excitement'. Disordered moods will naturally affect basic functions such as sleeping, eating or sex. People who are high, in a state of so-called mania, don't need to sleep much, talk all the time, laugh and make other people laugh or sometimes get into tempestuous rages for no reason. One can measure such mood changes using standardised questionnaires, but we all have inside us a kind of personal 'affectometer', by which we can measure not only our own state of feeling but also the states of others.

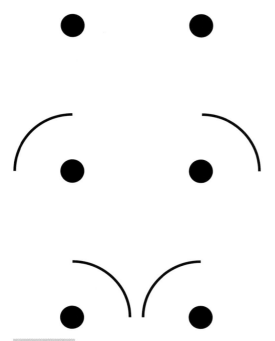

Figure 3.4 ● These simple line drawings illustrate how easily mere squiggles can exert an emotional effect on the brain, leading us to the conclusion that emotion is hardwired into the brain.

The problem with this is perhaps that certain words get overused: the worst case in this respect is the use of the term 'depressed'. In a society that seeks to medicalise so many of the problems of living, and in which happiness is viewed as a right, it is used to cover all sorts of states of mind, from being upset at losing one's cat to the terminal despair of bereavement in an elderly widower. Many physical illnesses can mimic this kind of depression as well, making it easy to misdiagnose, for example, some forms of cancer. The weight loss, loss of appetite, slowness of thinking and apparent despondency are mistaken for an emotional illness. More commonly, however, the opposite happens, with doctors hunting desperately for a serious organic illness when the real problem is a true depression. Likewise, drugs can make us depressed or high, and our favourite drug, alcohol, is notorious in this respect. But perhaps the nicest thing about assessing someone's emotional state is that one has to literally feel it rather than think about it. The trick is to be able to put experiences into context and to separate feelings that are understandable from feelings that seem to be arising out of disordered brain functions. Trying to do this if one has emotional problems oneself is, of course, disastrous. One needs to be clear-headed, or perhaps clear thinking *and* clear feeling, to be able to do this kind of work. The classical Greeks had a philosophy that insisted 'know thyself' – part of psychiatry's problem is that too many therapists are trying to heal themselves while they are meant to be healing others.

Memory

Most people spend most of their time thinking, perceiving, believing and feeling. Memory is something that is largely accepted, only being a bother when it does not seem to be working properly. If emotions are the music or climate that set the tone of our activities, memory is the whole backdrop. Memory makes us who we are, that strange mixture of things that have happened to us, things that are happening to us and what we have inherited from our parents and families. It is the core of our personality, enabling us to react to what is going on and giving us a vast databank by which to judge events. It is also quite wonderful, a marvel of design, the zeitgeist of human genius.

The brain is an infinite-capacity, instant, multisensory, cross-referential storage system, full of maps, plans, books, tapes, videos and holograms of all that we have experienced and learnt. Provided that our attention and concentration span is sufficient, we can cope with all the variable inputs of the day-to-day world and use this memory with stunning effect. However, people who are confused either can't think straight (see above) or perhaps can't make the connections between what is happening and what they know. That is, their brains are starting to fail and their memories, in particular the more recent ones, cannot be recalled. This is nothing less than the worst of human tragedy – without our memory, we are nonviable creatures.

Testing memory is very simple. You can ask someone what happened recently – by and large, there is a short-term 'desktop' working memory (which should tell you what day it is, etc.) and a longer term 'library', with variable access depending on one's mood, thoughts and level of consciousness. The latter is very robust, the former rather flaky. Both are very much part of the hardwiring of the brain, and ease of access tends to fade with age. In general, the greater experience of older people means that it doesn't trouble them too much, but seriously impaired memory function is usually a sign of some form of dementia.

There are standard tests, such as the mini-mental state examination (MMSE; see Box 3.2) that can easily assess how well one is in this respect. One has to be careful because depressed people can seem to lose their memory (this is called a pseudodementia); however, the memory will return when the depression is resolved. Mainstream dementia, the two major causes of which are Alzheimer's disease and impairment of blood supply to the brain (for example because of high blood pressure or a stroke), is unfortunately progressive and very much what is termed an organic disease. In other words, brain scans and other tests show clear structural abnormalities. One of the commonest, but often unrecognised, causes of such brain damage is excessive alcohol consumption, although brain tumours, a number of metabolic diseases and head injuries can all have a similar effect.

Box 3.2   The mini-mental state examination

- The mini-mental state examination (MMSE) or Folstein test is a brief 30-point questionnaire test that is used to assess cognition. It is commonly used in medicine to screen for dementia. In a time span of about 10 minutes, it samples various functions, including arithmetic, memory and orientation. It was introduced by Folstein *et al.* in 1975 and is widely used with small modifications.

- The MMSE test includes simple questions and problems in a number of areas: the time and place of the test, repeating lists of words, arithmetic, language use and comprehension, and copying a drawing.

- Any score over 27 (out of 30) is effectively normal. The normal value is also corrected for degree of schooling and age. Low to very low scores correlate closely with the presence of dementia, although other mental disorders can also lead to abnormal findings on MMSE testing. The presence of purely physical problems can also interfere with interpretation if not properly noted; for example, a patient may be physically unable to hear or read instructions properly or may have a motor deficit that affects writing and drawing skills.

On assessing this part of a person's brain function, psychiatrists usually talk about the cognitive state. The assessment is carried out using a simple series of questions, employing the MMSE, designed to check on the various aspects of memory, orientation and concentration span. Anybody can learn to do these and several simple questions can quickly clarify a person's problems. Remember, impaired memory can lead to all sorts of odd behaviours, such as shoplifting, irritable outbursts, getting lost and wandering. Diagnosis still requires that a history be taken and questions asked, and dementing illnesses are the perfect example of how modern technology has at last caught up with psychiatric evaluation. Tests such as brain scans or post-mortem analyses can provide the proof of a psychiatric diagnosis, just as physicians use blood tests today to diagnose, for example, diabetes.

The sense of self

Lastly, this aspect of what brains do – this self-awareness or self-recognition – is the one that is most obvious to us (Fig. 3.5). When you are awake and aware, you know who you are. Not knowing who you are, a very strange experience, is like waking up in a strange hotel room for the first time. It can also take various forms, temporary or prolonged, and is perhaps the least understood of all the brain's activities. It could even be said to be that function of the brain which makes us think that we have a soul, the part called spiritual.

One aspect of this sense of self is perhaps best described by the term 'initiative'. This is the sense of wanting to get on and do things, of personal drive, of interest in the world around. Losing this sense of 'I want' is not uncommon when you are exhausted, whether by a very busy day or by a series of difficulties. It can be a typical symptom of depression. Psychiatrists have even thought up some fancy words to describe it. One of them is 'anergia', which means lack of go or lack of energy. Another one is the term 'anhedonia', which means a lack of interest in enjoying things, having no sense of hedonism. This dominance of the negative, so to speak, can have many causes, including physical illnesses. However, it is usually quite distinct, presenting as indecisiveness, a sense of nihilism ('What's the point?') or a general sense of not being bothered by things that one should bother about, for example keeping reasonably clean.

Perhaps more relevant to the particular sense of 'I' is the feeling that you are not in control of what you are doing. This has been called the 'loss of ego function', a somewhat pompous term to describe a very troubling, disillusioning experience. The most distressing form occurs in those suffering from schizophrenia, and is termed passivity experience. Sufferers feel that they are not in control of their thinking, their emotions or even their bodily actions. Something or somebody

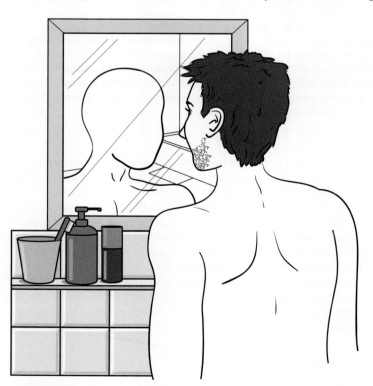

Figure 3.5 ● A distorted sense of self. Not recognising your 'self' is one of the weirder schizophrenic symptoms.

else seems to be making them think certain thoughts or even moving their bodies around like puppets. Such behaviour can be most odd – adopting strange postures or indulging in unusual movements or patterns of speech – and is very alarming to relatives. Some people come across as a kind of empty shell, others (particularly younger sufferers) spend hours looking at themselves in the mirror, pulling at their faces, trying to find out just who they are. It is as if the spark of personality has been taken out of an individual. Such patients often come across as dull and pathetic, but can also be frightened, aggressive or disoriented.

Such behaviour used to be put down to institutionalisation, an effect of people being kept in asylums for too long. We now know that this is not the full story, that it is, unfortunately, part and parcel of prolonged illnesses, usually schizophrenia but sometimes severe depression. A partial variant of this experience, of somehow not knowing who you are, can also take place in people who are very anxious. Such individuals get panic attacks, when they can be rooted to the spot, their hearts thumping and being unable to breathe, convinced that something awful (often they are not quite sure what) is going to happen. This intense panic can last for minutes or hours, and can be accompanied by what is called 'depersonalisation' or 'derealisation'. This is a strange sense of not being real, or a sense of the world around not being real and being cut off from it. Some people talk about a veil coming between them and the world, others find it hard to put into words at all. They feel unreal, detached and terrified that they will never get back to their real selves. Again, there is usually no outward sign of this state, just a rather perplexed and inarticulate person looking scared. It happens to all of us, now and then, when we're especially tired, nervous or hung-over. An extreme form of this anxiety leads to states of hysterical dissociation, in which people feel so cut off from the world that they forget who they are (hysterical amnesia) or develop physical symptoms mimicking strokes (hysterical paraplegia) or voice loss (aphonia).

Perhaps the most extraordinary distortion of this sense of self is the feeling that certain people get of having more than one personality. This has led to some doctors (particularly psychiatrists in California) describing a 'multiple personality syndrome', although most British psychiatrists do not agree with such theories. There are also notions of a 'split personality', as outlined in the novel *The Strange Case of Dr Jekyll and Mr Hyde* (by Robert Louis Stevenson). Such changes in personality, however, are not usually diagnostic of any particular psychiatric disorder. They are more a wish fulfilment and there is clear evidence that people 'learn' their new roles, often helped by 'suggestion' from their psychiatrist/therapist. There is a strong whiff of charlatanry about all this, but such conditions do point to the importance of the sense of self as a function of the brain, they show how changeable it can be and, in particular, how it can be impaired or even eliminated by illness, disordered emotional states, dissatisfaction with ordinary life or influential others (Fig. 3.6).

The main diagnostic categories

The common diagnoses used in standard psychiatric practice today are generally agreed all over the world and reflect the patterns of disordered mental functioning that emerge from the outline given above. They are traditionally divided into the psychoses and the neuroses, the former being defined by symptoms that put the sufferer out of touch with reality. We will not attempt the Socratic – and much

Figure 3.6 ● Your brain at a glance

A rough guess at the complexity of your brain

Never mind the universe, there's something just as complicated sitting between your ears. Your brain has about 10^{14} neurons, each of which sends thousands of messages to thousands of its neighbouring neurons via thousands of different chemical messenger/receptor systems, all of which are bathed in hundreds of salts, hormones, gases and other chemicals which can put each of those billions of neurons into hundreds of thousands of different states. And all this changes every hundredth of a second, every moment of your life.

To put it another way, the brain is so incomprehensibly complex that there is plenty of room in it to account for much more than mere senses, thoughts, feelings, memories and emotions; Shakespeare's central nervous system wrote *Hamlet*. There is easily enough space in here for creativity, consciousness, superstition and, if we are honest about it, even the idea of God himself. Small surprise, then, that when the brain goes wrong, it does so in some pretty spectacular ways

The frontal lobe

It is hard to say exactly what goes on in this part of the brain, but whatever it is, it's important. Individuals who suffer damage to this area undergo drastic change of personality, either becoming disinhibited or zombified, depending on the precise location of the damage. The frontal lobe appears to be where the brain exerts its ability to categorise and switch between tasks, ideas, words and countless other phenomena. As a result, it seems to play a major role in coordinating thinking, emotion and behaviour. Some workers have gone so far as to name this area as the seat of consciousness, but this is probably taking the unitary idea of consciousness too far. The notion of a coherent, single sense of self is likely to be an illusion thrown up by our brains to stop us getting confused and the psychoses probably involve a disturbance of this process

Perceiving: handling incoming data

Seeing and hearing are the most refined senses in our species. The eye is an outgrowth of our brain. The ear has the most complex connections of all our sense organs. In fact, we are more of an acoustic than a visual species. Hearing is the first sense to return after loss of consciousness, and we rely on our ears even more than our eyes in order to live. Put a towel over your television, or turn the volume down, and watch the six o'clock news. See which one you miss the most. Sensory data is processed in many areas of the cortex of the brain, before it is incorporated into the subjective experience of sensation. Different senses have different primary cortical reception areas, but how it ends up as subjective experience is anyone's guess

Memory

The storage space of this soggy lump of electrified fat sitting in your head is staggering. No one has yet been able to define its capacity and, at the moment, this is theoretically infinite. How it achieves this is becoming clearer. There appears to be a narrow, attentive funnel through to a holding station for small chunks of precise, high-quality data, which we can only hold on to for a short time. The upper parts of the midbrain and their connections to the central walls of the hemispheres seem crucial to this process. The long-term store is probably to be found in specialised glutamate-containing cells in the convolutions of the inner hemispheres. Quite how it manages the trick of storing everything from the smell of your mum to the moons of Jupiter and riding a bicycle is still a mystery, but emotion and meaning seem to play a crucial role in the efficiency with which we store things

Bodily sensation

Almost all of your nervous system is running on automatic and is controlled by the primitive parts of the brain. Hardly a fraction of the vast amount of data your body sends to your brain ever reaches your consciousness, unless you need it to. The feeling of your clothes against your shoulders was ignored until you read this. The nervous system is wired to give priority to different information, depending on its relevance to your current situation, but pain is the only form of information that incorporates emotion. You can see or hear or smell things that may be good or bad, but pain almost always comes with displeasure built in

Language

Birds build nests, humans build sentences. This 'language instinct' is one of the most amazing things about our brain. Unlike reading, no-one has to teach us how to do it. By making funny noises in our throat as we breathe out, we can convey an infinite amount of information to our fellow beings. This remarkable capacity, has, in only about fifty thousand years, led to civilisation, science, religion and has – for better or worse – allowed us to begin to free our species of the natural forces that have dominated our life on this planet for millions of years. How it works is only poorly understood, but it is a safe bet that a language 'template' is buried somewhere in the neurons of the lower, outer regions of the temporal cortex of the dominant hemisphere. Damage to this area, depending upon its precise location, can cause profound disruption of the way we speak, understand or both

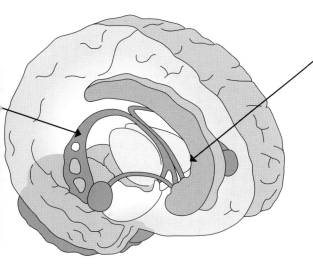

Emotion

No aspect of brain function is as misunderstood as emotion. In spite of our myths about the limbic system, there is no such thing as the 'emotional centre' of the brain. Rather, we have different systems in the brain that serve separate emotions. Some of these, like fear, anger and disgust, are emotions that have changed little since the days of our primate ancestors. The areas of the brain that subserve these functions are intimately connected to learned and automatic behaviours. Other 'higher' emotions, such as sadness, envy and desire, seem to have a much more complex biological basis and impinge on our thoughts and deeds in a more variable way. What emotions do seem to have in common is an intimate association between the upper stem of the brain, and the rest of the body. An important part of our emotional experience involves bodily sensation, our 'gut feeling'. Our upper brain stems are rich in neurons containing the transmitters noradrenaline (norepinephrine) and serotonin. Unsurprisingly, drugs that affect these chemicals have a powerful affect on our mood

Thought

We do it virtually every moment of our life, even when we are asleep, but it is almost impossible to define what it is that we do. We know that it requires a functioning cerebral cortex to do it properly, and that it involves a kind of internal symbolic language, a sort of mentalese, that allows us to perform logical, inferential, probabilistic and woolly operations on a theoretically infinite array of symbols stored in our memory. To do it, we have to burn a lot of glucose and oxygen and, unlike emotion, it is highly private; no one can tell when or why we are doing it. It seems to be a powerful tool for making sense of, i.e. explaining, events in our environment, and so gives rise to the idea of believing. It also seems to be under our conscious control, giving rise to the idea of choice of belief, free will and sense of self. The problem is, no one can say just who, what, why or where the 'me', or 'self' or 'ego' inside our heads actually is

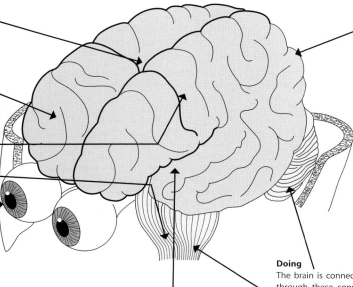

Doing

The brain is connected to every single muscle in the body, and through these connections we carry out every physical act of our lives from breathing and blinking to sex and shopping. Not all of these movements are fully under our conscious control, and intentional movements, as opposed to more automatic ones, seem to arise from different areas of the brain. The initiation of sequences of purposeful movement, otherwise known as 'intentional behaviour', seems to arise from complex connections between the so-called motor cortex, frontal lobes, and coordinating structures deep in the brain known as the basal ganglia. Disturbances of these ganglia, for example, because of the side effects of antipsychotic medication, can give rise to a variety of movement disorders. Our movements are also powerfully influenced by our emotions, and thus our body language can reveal much about our mood. The cerebellum, a large lobe at the rear of the brain, plays an important role in coordination but probably a lot more besides argued over late-night coffee – task of defining what is and what isn't real, being prepared to accept, at least for the practical purposes of clinical work, that the average person can agree that a stone is a stone and that grass is generally green (unless scorched brown in summer). In essence, psychotic patients cannot judge correctly what is going on around them because they cannot perceive correctly and cannot think straight – they are deluded, hallucinated or thought-disordered, or even all three. This may of course be a changeable state, and it will not necessarily stop them doing routine things like eating or drinking or going to the toilet, or even getting to the post office to pick up their benefit money. The Nazi leader Rudolf Hess, Hitler's deputy, despite being psychotically deluded and semi-incoherent, flew a plane quite accurately into wartime Scotland as part of a bizarre and grandiose 'peace mission'. These disorders affect some 1–2% of the population (at some time in their life), are the typical basis for insanity pleas and findings of diminished responsibility in legal, usually murder, trials and, generally, are not difficult to spot. Their presentations often fulfil the public stereotypes of 'mad' or 'lunatic', and their care is mainly provided by specialist psychiatric services.

The neuroses, by contrast, comprise that much larger group of conditions that affect up to 20% of the population at some time in their life (i.e. life prevalence). These patients have a different pattern of symptoms, commonly a mixture of depression and anxiety, but they will be in touch with what is going on and will know that there is something wrong. This insight into their psychological problems makes it much more possible to manage them at the GP's surgery, and the great majority get treated in primary care. Nevertheless, those with more severe and chronic conditions can be just as socially disabled as those with psychoses, and some seem to have just as little, if not less, insight. A typical example would be someone with anorexia nervosa, who refuses to accept what is blindingly obvious to everyone else, that she is deformed in her thinness. Despite these overlaps, the psychotic/neurotic divide is quite useful in classifying and researching mental illnesses, has stood the test of time and has a broad public acceptance.

Table 3.1 ● The symptoms of schizophrenia

Positive	Negative
Delusional beliefs, e.g. delusional perception[a]	Anergia/apathy
Hallucinations, e.g. third-person voices	Anhedonia
Passivity experience	Social withdrawal
Thought disorder (formal)[b]	Poverty of speech
	Flat affect

[a]The specific experience of perceiving something (e.g. traffic lights turning red) out of which a delusion arises (e.g. 'the traffic lights turning red must mean I am the Angel Gabriel – it's a special sign acknowledging this', etc.).
[b]Formal thought disorder includes the experiences of thought block (i.e. your mind going empty), thought withdrawal, broadcast and insertion (i.e. feeling that your thoughts have been taken out of your head, exposed to other people or put into your head from outside). Usually, patients experience only one or two of these, rather than all of them.

Psychoses

1. Schizophrenia and related disorders
2. Manic depressive disorders (also known as bipolar affective disorders)
3. Organic conditions, e.g. dementia, brain tumours

The details of these diagnoses are outlined in Tables 3.1–3.4 and Box 3.3. It should be noted that the symptoms of schizophrenia are generally divided into positive and negative, the former being the distinctive markers of the illness. Having one clear-cut positive symptom is usually taken as diagnostic, provided that there are no other reasons for having it (i.e. a fever). In contrast, it is the collection of symptoms that confirms a manic depressive diagnosis. The organic group is defined simply by an established physical cause with often a ragbag of various (psychotic) symptoms from either the schizophrenic or manic depressive spectrum. There are also a number of associated illnesses, such as acute psychoses (which have lots of different names worldwide) and delusional disorders, which are outlined in Boxes 3.4 and 3.5. Finally, it must be understood that there are two major classification systems in operation, the European-influenced ICD-10, and the *American Diagnostic and Statistical Manual*, now in its fourth edition (DSM-IV). They are generally equivalent in the common diagnoses, with the DSM-IV being perhaps a little stricter (e.g. requiring a 6-month course, at least, to confirm a schizophrenic illness), but they do use different terms for some other disorders, reflecting their differing cultural and academic perspectives.

Table 3.2 ● Diagnostic criteria for schizophrenia[a]

A	B
Thought echo, insertion, withdrawal or broadcasting	Persistent hallucinations of any type, with fleeting delusional/overvalued ideas
Delusional perception or delusions of one's thoughts, feelings or behaviour (including bodily movements) being controlled externally ('passivity experiences')	Interruption in the train of thought causing incoherence or irrelevant speech, or neologisms
Auditory hallucinations ('voices') commenting on or talking about one in the third person	Catatonic behaviours, e.g. mutism, postures, 'waxy flexibility'
Persistent delusions, culturally inappropriate and impossible, e.g. special powers, alien communication	Negative symptoms, e.g. apathy, poverty of speech, blunted affect
	A consistent change in overall behaviour, e.g. aimless, self-absorbed, socially withdrawn

[a]Diagnosis requires one clear symptom (or two 'less clear') from A, or symptoms from *at least* two of the groups in B, all present for *at least 1 month*.

63

Table 3.3 ● The core symptoms of manic depressive psychosis[a]

Manic symptoms	Depressive symptoms
Flight of ideas; pressure of speech	Psychomotor retardation (slowed in speech and movement)
Grandiose ideas leading to delusions	Negative ideas[b] resulting in delusions of poverty/nihilism
Enhanced irritability/impatience	Instability resulting in moodiness/indecisiveness
Euphoria/excessive energy	Tired/low/depressed
Hyperactivity/limited sleep	Loss of drive/insomnia with early morning wakening
Distractible/short attention span	Poor concentration
Spending money/embarrassing behaviour	Social withdrawal/self-blame/suicidal

[a]Patients swing from a manic state ('pole') to a depressive state, over the course of weeks or sometimes days ('rapid-cycling') or vice versa.
[b]Negative ideas can be delusional, e.g. believing that there is no blood in your veins or that you are utterly impoverished.

Table 3.4 ● Diagnostic criteria for manic depressive psychosis (bipolar affective disorder)

1	Repeated episodes of disturbed mood *and* activity
2	Both an elevation (mania) and a lowering (depression) of mood occur during different episodes
3	Usually complete recovery in between episodes
Mania	Elevated mood to elation/excitement
	Increased energy, over-activity and decreased sleep
	Pressure of speech, loud and hard to interrupt
	Disinhibited
	Distractible and disorganised behaviours: grandiose and over-optimistic, often delusional
	Enhanced perceptions, e.g. vivid colours, acute hearing
	Extravagant expenditure, sexually inappropriate behaviour
	Irritable and impatient, sometimes leading to violence
	Persecutory delusions or delusions of special powers/role
	Neglect of meals, sleep, personal hygiene
Depression	Lowered mood and loss of interests/enjoyment
	Reduced concentration, self-esteem, energy
	Impaired sleep, appetite, libido, activity
	Suicidal ideas and/or acts; 'hopeless' outlook
	Sense of guilt, sin and worthlessness (may be delusional)
	Psychomotor retardation; may lead on to stupor
	Hallucinations, e.g. accusing voices or smells of rotting flesh
	Nihilistic delusions, e.g. no blood, no stomach

Box 3.3 Organic psychoses

Require an established physical cause. Common causes include brain tumours/strokes; encephalitis (infection of the central nervous system); human immunodeficiency virus infection (of the brain); severe fevers (e.g. typhoid or malaria); metabolic conditions, e.g. hypothyroidism, Wilson's disease (excess copper deposition); heavy metal poisoning. Rarer causes include general paralysis of the insane (GPI; syphilis of the brain); dementia (whether due to Alzheimer's disease, trauma, e.g. head injury, or vascular accident, e.g. strokes, high blood pressure); chronic alcohol abuse.

Symptoms can be schizophrenia-like (see Table 3.1) or manic depressive in type (see Table 3.3) and are often a mixture of both. There are sometimes odd, isolated symptoms, depending on the part of the brain affected.

May be associated with physical signs, e.g. weakness/loss of movement in a leg or arm and/or epileptic fits. Often their diagnosis also includes a degree of cognitive impairment (i.e. short-term memory loss).

Box 3.4 Acute psychoses (also called reactive/schizo-phreniform/polymorphic)

- Onset within days/weeks and not lasting for more than 1–3 months
- Variable pattern of symptoms – affective/schizophrenic/cognitive – with patients fluctuating between them to varying degrees
- Usually severe in terms of behavioural disturbance/impact of symptoms; patients subsequently showing poor recall of acute phase
- Cause usually *not* clarified; may be drug-induced, secondary to a viral/bacterial infection (i.e. an idiosyncratic reaction) or even puerperal (but puerperal psychoses, i.e. in women after childbirth, are defined as a separate category). Life events preceding them are *not* the norm though may be relevant, e.g. bereavement

Box 3.5 Delusional disorders[a]

- A persistent single delusion, or set of related delusions, without other obvious symptoms
- The delusion usually develops over months or even years, with no initial decline in social/personal behaviour
- Onset is usually in middle age, the context of the delusion and the timing of the emergence tending to reflect a person's life situation
- Delusions vary in content, often being persecutory (e.g. freemasons are ruining your life), grandiose (believing that you have special knowledge) or hypochondriacal (e.g. convinced that your body is misshapen or that you smell)
- Secondary depression and, sometimes, occasional mild tactile or auditory hallucinations may develop and reinforce your belief(s)

[a]Formerly called paranoia or a paranoid state.

Neuroses

1. Depressive disorders
2. Anxiety disorders (generalised, phobic, panic states)
3. Obsessional compulsive disorders
4. Miscellaneous, e.g. somatisation disorders, post-traumatic syndromes (including PTSD), sexual problems, culture-bound syndromes
5. Dependence, especially alcohol/drugs

These conditions are detailed in Tables 3.5–3.7 and Boxes 3.6–3.9, and it will quickly become apparent that there is considerable overlap in the symptom profiles. They are much less clear cut than the psychoses, which probably reflects the fact that they are as much forms of personal reaction to social and/or environmental

Table 3.5 ● Symptoms of depression

Physical	Psychological
Weight loss	Self-blame, leading to guilt
Loss of energy	Hopelessness
Loss of appetite	Helplessness
Loss of libido	Poor concentration
Psychomotor retardation	Irritability
Reduced activity/drive	Feeling low/negative/dysphoric
Poor self-care	Suicidal ideation
Lying in bed	Loss of interests
Impaired sleep (early morning wakening)	Negative cognition[a]

[a]Seeing every situation in a negative light, i.e. dropping something and thinking 'I'm so stupid'.

Table 3.6 ● Common anxiety symptoms

Physical	Psychological
Palpitations and chest pain	Feeling tense/worried
Difficulty breathing	Lacking confidence
Sweats	Avoiding social situations
Stomach churning/cramps	Fear for the future
Legs like jelly	Ruminating over minor concerns
Feeling dizzy/faint	Wanting to run away
Headaches/muscle pain	Depersonalisation/derealisation
Pins and needles	Fears of collapsing/embarrassing oneself/dying
Light-headedness	

difficulties as independent diseases. In fact, most psychiatrists regard them more as provisional descriptions of limited validity, which we have to accept as the going rate in the clinical trenches of the here and now. Research is constantly working towards better definitions for them, the extraction of panic disorder from the loosely assorted anxiety neuroses being the most helpful advance of recent times. However,

Table 3.7 ● Phobic disorders[a]

Agoraphobia	Fear of going out into places where there are lots of people, e.g. shops, markets, public transport. The most common and severe type of phobia, it is often chronic and sufferers may be left housebound
Social phobia	Fear of being scrutinized by other people, in small groups rather than crowds. May be specifically a fear of eating or speaking in public, e.g. addressing a seminar
Specific ('isolated') phobia	A fear limited to one thing, e.g. mice, spiders, heights, needles, flying, car travel. Many people are not too handicapped by these phobias as long as they don't interfere with normal life. They usually start in childhood but may be caused by a specific event (e.g. car accident)

[a]Phobia means an intense fear of something that is not actually dangerous, leading to anxiety (or even panic) and avoidance.

Box 3.6   Panic disorder

- Regular onset of panic that seems unpredictable
- Panic in different situations (but often in closed-in, crowded places)
- Each person has their own set of dominant physical symptoms, e.g. palpitations, choking, dizziness, feeling unreal ('depersonalisation')
- Fear of fainting, losing control, going 'mad' or dying comes on secondarily
- Attacks usually last for only a few minutes
- Overwhelming urge to flee and/or go home, with secondary avoidance
- Usually related to a phobia and 'anticipatory' anxiety

Box 3.7   Obsessional compulsive disorder (OCD)

- Recurring obsessional thoughts and/or compulsive acts[a] (e.g. worrying about dirt and constantly hand washing or constantly checking that things are locked or in the right order)
- Recognition of these as your own thoughts or impulses, not something imposed from outside
- Knowing that the thought/act is pointless or ineffectual but still not being able to resist it
- Thoughts/impulses that are unpleasantly repetitive
- Often accompanied by anxiety and/or depressive symptoms

[a]Recurrent thoughts are also termed 'ruminations' and compulsive acts are called 'rituals'. Some people do one without the other.

Box 3.8   Miscellaneous neurotic conditions[a]

Somatisation	Frequent and variable physical symptoms leading to heavy use of medical services, lots of negative investigations, but refusal to accept reassurance. Personal life is disrupted, and sedatives and/or painkillers are overused
Sexual disorders	In men, the commonest are erectile dysfunction or premature ejaculation. In women, anorgasmia (failure to reach orgasm) is the most typical. The 'paraphilias' are a range of sexual habits indulged in to achieve or enhance orgasm, more often seen in men. They include fetishism (e.g. wearing rubber or leather), voyeurism (watching others have sex), exhibitionism (exposing your genitals to strangers) and sadomasochism (inflicting or receiving pain or humiliation)
Reaction to stress	These include acute stress reactions, adjustment disorders (e.g. following bereavements) and post-traumatic stress disorder (PTSD). They result from a very frightening or life-threatening event (e.g. car crash) and have a mixture of symptoms that include flashbacks, bad dreams, agitation, fearfulness, and feeling 'numbed' and/or jumpy and nervous
Culture-bound syndromes	These are forms of anxiety/depression that are largely seen in one country or region. They include 'koro' (fear of your penis disappearing), 'dhat' (believing that you have lost all your semen), running 'amok' (sudden violent outbursts after a perceived loss/insult) and 'putzwut' (obsessive cleaning behaviour). They are contentious, behavioural presentations rather than specific diagnoses, and demonstrate how different cultures understand illness and its causation

[a]All of these conditions are associated with anxiety and/or depressive symptoms to some degree, which are sometimes the cause of, for example, a depressive reaction and sometimes the 'mask' of the underlying anxiety/depression.

Box 3.9   Drug and alcohol dependence

There are 10 categories of mental and behavioural disorders caused by psychoactive substance use [alcohol, opioids, cannabinoids, sedatives or hypnotics, cocaine, other stimulants (including caffeine), hallucinogens, tobacco, volatile solvents, multiple drug use and others].

Identifying what substance is being used is based on self-report, blood or urine specimens, clinical signs and symptoms, and informed third parties/presence of drugs.

Clinical states caused by substance usage include: acute intoxication, e.g. drunk or 'bad trip'; harmful use, e.g. evidence of damage to health; dependence syndrome, including three or more of the following: overpowering need to use the drug, difficulties controlling use, a physical withdrawal state on stopping/reducing, evidence of tolerance, neglect of other interests/pleasures, carrying on using despite evidence of harm, e.g. liver damage; withdrawal states – symptoms vary depending on the substance, e.g. 'cold turkey' from opiates, 'DTs' (delirium tremens) from alcohol; psychiatric symptoms or disorder – psychosis, hallucinations, amnesia.

they do have some reliability in that clinicians agree on the diagnosis in most cases (some conditions are easier than others in this respect), which is of practical use in treatment. Part of the problem is that symptoms, i.e. the things that patients complain of, tend to predominate in the absence of overt signs (things observable to the outsider, such as bruising or a lump), thus the over-riding importance of a good corroborated history and clinical nous in diagnosing the problem.

It is also true that if you consider, for example, the numerous symptoms associated with depression, one patient could present with an almost entirely different collection of symptoms from another. The effects of age, gender and culture will generate an irritable, self-loathing semi-alcoholic in the case of a 55-year-old middle-class white male but a quiet, withdrawn, somatiser complaining of pain in the case of a 25-year-old Indian woman. The severity of conditions also varies widely, so much so that the ICD-10 has separate categories for mild, moderate and severe forms of the disorder, and it is often difficult to know where the cut-off points are. If someone has only four symptoms rather than the five required for mild depression, is that a real difference? If a diagnosis is important for, say, an invalidity benefit claim or a legal case, you may be tempted to squeeze in 'poor concentration' alongside the insomnia, tiredness, poor appetite and loss of initiative that you have just about managed to extract from a fed-up and not very articulate 'client' pressing for help.

There is no doubt, though, that these disorders do often have a serious impact on people's lives, and such individuals should not just be seen as the 'walking worried', however tempted one may be to use this term. Sometimes, when frustrated by the contrast between a poor, undemanding, lonely schizophrenic man waiting his turn and a well-dressed, partly obsessional professional going on and on about having more twice-weekly therapy, it may seem that such individuals are not really part of your job. However, don't forget that patients with these disorders make up over one-third of a GP's workload, as often as not having what is termed in ICD-10 as 'mixed anxiety and depression'; if they have been referred to a mental health service, it is highly likely that they do have something badly wrong. Often, there will be an underlying problem in terms of their upbringing or personality, and there are also a range of childhood psychiatric disorders that we have not included in this overview of diagnosis. Many of these resolve with growing up (and treatment) but children with conduct disorder and/or attention deficit hyperactivity disorder (ADHD) do tend to have persisting problems in adulthood.

Separate from psychoses and neuroses, but often the basis of hard-to-treat conditions, therefore, are the conditions that are currently known as personality disorders (PDs). These need to be briefly discussed outside the psychotic/neurotic continuum because they really do differ from the illness categories outlined above.

Personality disorders

This troublesome group of presentations (see also Chapter 1) has attracted different labels over time, from the Victorian term 'moral insanity' to the more recent 'psychopathy', as still used in the 1983 Mental Health Act. There continues to be a debate over whether they really are diseases as such, disease (or illness) being defined as a break in the continuity of normal health/wellness, a change for the worse in your physical or psychological functioning (or both). PD does not really constitute a change, rather it describes a continuing 'deeply ingrained, maladaptive pattern of behaviour' that is first seen in childhood or adolescence. These extremes of what might be called character or temperament emerge as one grows up and are persistent traits that define your personality. Without going into the vexed question of how to define personality – what makes you different from others – it is possible to state that there are some people who really do seem to have a different way of dealing with the world. They don't play by the accepted social rules and, as often as not, both they and society suffer because of it. They range from the seriously nasty cold-blooded killer (fortunately quite rare, whatever you might assume from films), who used to be called the 'affectionless psychopath', to the silly, histrionic, overemotional flibbertigibbet, who is forever overreacting to

Table 3.8 ● Personality disorders

Disorder	Symptoms
Paranoid	Suspicious of exploitation, harm or deceit; doubts loyalty of close others; fear of confiding; finds hidden meaning in events; bears grudges; oversensitive to rebuff; often jealous thoughts about partner
Schizoid	Avoids close relationships; chooses solitary activities; avoids sexual relationships with others; few pleasurable activities; lacks confidants; indifferent to praise or criticism; emotionally cold or flat
Schizotypal	Ideas of reference and odd perceptual style; odd beliefs or magical thinking; unconventional thought/speech style; suspicious; restricted or inappropriate affect; eccentric appearance or behaviour; high-level social anxiety with paranoia
Sociopathic	Social non-conformity with repeated unlawful behaviour; deceitful; impulsivity; shows instability and aggression; lack of remorse; irresponsible; disregard for safety of self or others
Borderline personality disorder	Fear of abandonment; unstable attachments to others; disturbance of sense of self/identity; impulsivity; recurrent self harm; labile mood; chronic feelings of emptiness; poor anger control
Histrionic	Needs to be centre of attention; seductive personality; shallow emotional expression; preoccupied with appearance; self-dramatisation; misjudges intimacy in relationships; suggestible
Narcissistic	Grandiose self-importance; fantasies of success, brilliance, beauty, etc.; belief that self is special; need for excessive admiration; sense of entitlement; interpersonally exploitative; lacks empathy; arrogant and envious
Avoidant personality disorder	Avoids activities requiring contact with others; only engages if certain of social acceptance; fear of criticism; feelings of inadequacy in new social situations; oversensitive to embarrassment; perceives self as socially inept
Dependent type	Indecisive; hands responsibility to others; fear of disagreement and confrontation; lacks initiative; excessive need for nurturance; fear of being alone; shifts quickly to new attachment after ending an attachment; preoccupied with fears of abandonment
Obsessive personality disorder	Preoccupied with details and rules; perfectionist; over-conscientious; rejects leisure for work and productivity; hoarding; inability to delegate; miserliness; rigidity and stubbornness

the ups and downs of normal life. The most typical PDs seen in community psy-chiatric practice are the so-called 'borderlines', who tend to repetitively self-harm, who have very changeable moods and who cannot seem to hold down any steady relationships, thus their regular cries for help.

The details of the various PD categories, as outlined in ICD-10, are summarised in Table 3.8. The important point to grasp about this group of patients is that they present with varying degrees of severity, they grow out of their behaviour in time and every team has two or three on the go at any one time. Best considered as hav-ing a kind of impaired emotional intellect, as being children in terms of impulse control despite their apparently adult appearance, they can of course have other illnesses on top of their underlying PD. Recognising them and learning how to cope with their vagaries and presentations is part and parcel of being a competent mental health professional. But remember, it is all too easy to dump anyone that you don't like into the category of PD; it is important, therefore, to ensure that you take a full history and that the facts fit the diagnosis.

A problem with the current classification of PD is that the schemes are too cat-egorical. There is probably too much overlap between the categories to justify their status as separate entities, which seem to resemble horoscopes as much as descrip-tions of individuals. Intuitively, though, they do seem to reflect some recognisable features of human nature. In addition, the scheme does not allow for degrees of disorder, nor does it define a cut-off from reality.

Summary

This chapter has attempted to show that it is possible to understand psychiatric disorder in the light of an understanding of how normal brains work and how people react to personal experience depending on their own environment and background. As outlined at the beginning, such disorders can be very severe (psy-chosis) or at least leave one with a degree of insight (neurosis). Certain symptoms seem to cluster together, resulting in the syndromes used in psychiatry, such as schizophrenia, manic depressive psychosis or anxiety neurosis.

It is accepted that some conditions are more clear-cut whereas others, such as the PDs, are really murky in terms of definition. The defining of these disorders into understandable diagnoses, the working out of effective treatments (whether medical, psychological or even surgical) and the helping of people who suffer from them is the concern of everyone who works in mental illness.

It should also be noted that there is an extraordinarily strong relationship between the way we think or feel and physical disorders. The most obvious example is the way in which sudden sad news can make us cry. People can faint or vomit just at the sight of blood or at an unpleasant smell. More prolonged states of stress and anxiety seem to be strongly associated with stomach ulcers, whereas thyroid disease or Parkinson's disease can cause obvious states of depression or mania. Many drugs, whether illicit or prescribed by doctors, can have a range of effects on both one's physical and men-tal state. The antibiotic that cures an infection can make you feel depressed, whereas the steroid that helps your arthritis can make you feel very happy.

Perhaps most important, however, is the realisation that unusual behaviour is not in itself a mental illness. Behaviour is culturally defined, and just because a young man is running through the streets of London in early January in the middle of the night screaming 'mushrooms, mushrooms, mushrooms', having painted his head with bright blue paint, does not necessarily mean that he is mentally ill. He might be doing it for a dare, it might be a kind of religious ceremony or he might just be drunk. He may even have taken too many magic mushrooms or be upset at the fact that there is unpleasant fungus growing in the bathroom in the rotten house he has been stuck in by some unpleasant landlord. To determine whether he is suffering from mental illness requires him to be assessed and, if there are definite signs or symptoms of an illness in terms of impaired thinking or memory (such as outlined above), for example, then one can call it an illness. Publicly 'mad' behaviour is not the same as having a psychiatric disorder, just as sweating in a crowded room does not generally mean you have a high temperature.

This leads on to the general point that not everything that is strange is necessarily mad. It should also be understood that the word 'mad' is popularly defined. Most 'mad' people do not suffer from mental illness, they just seem unusual or deviant according to the society in which they live. Clarifying the border between such eccentricity and genuine suffering from mental illness is the key task of anyone working in mental health. Although understanding social and cultural perspectives, religious beliefs, family values and personal experience, it is also important not to be fooled by seeing everything as being caused by the environment. If it were, then one would expect everyone in Vietnam or Afghanistan, for example, to be absolutely psychotic given the nightmare experiences that people in these places have been through in the last few decades.

Perhaps the best analogy is the one about fixing the television. If it isn't working properly and given that the aerial is okay, what should you do? You could change the programme, convinced that things would be better on Channel 4 than, say, BBC1. This is a bit like moving a depressed person from what seems like a gloomy flat to a nicer environment. This is all very well and good, but it will not necessarily cure an intrinsic depression, caused by abnormal brain function. The families might feel happier, and they will all thank you for your good intentions, but you have not actually fixed the problem. Identifying the balance between what goes on inside our brains, the influence of the surroundings and how much of an individual's distress is actual illness is difficult but fascinating. You don't have to make a diagnosis of everyone brought to you in distress, but the habit of not trying to do so easily leads into the habit of blaming people for their own problems. Psychiatry has certainly been guilty of peddling its mythologies as certainties, but the evidence of the streets today is that there are thousands of undiagnosed individuals wandering about in states of neglect, and the easiest excuse for not helping them is that 'it must be their own fault'.

If one can understand the ways in which people break down, in terms of their thinking or feeling, it becomes possible to do all sorts of things to assess them and help them. Knowing about the conditions that make up mental illness – psychiatric diagnosis (or call it what you will) – is essential to being an effective community mental health worker. The process of establishing a diagnosis is also somewhat alluring, even addictive. It makes for clarity, decisive action and the wonderful business of getting someone better.

References

Folstein MF, Folstein SE, McHugh PR (1975) 'Mini-mental state.' A practical method for grading the cognitive state of patients for the clinician. *Journal of Psychiatric Research* 12: 189–98.

Rosenhan DL (1973) On being sane in insane places. *Science* 179: 250–8.

Appendix 1 List of categories from the *International Classification of Diseases*, 10th edition (ICD-10)

F00–F09 Organic, including symptomatic, mental disorders

F00   Dementia in Alzheimer's disease
F00.0 Dementia in Alzheimer's disease with early onset
F00.1 Dementia in Alzheimer's disease with late onset
F00.2 Dementia in Alzheimer's disease, atypical or mixed type
F00.9 Dementia in Alzheimer's disease, unspecified

F01   Vascular dementia
F01.0 Vascular dementia of acute onset
F01.1 Multi-infarct dementia
F01.2 Subcortical vascular dementia
F01.3 Mixed cortical and subcortical vascular dementia
F01.8 Other vascular dementia
F01.9 Vascular dementia, unspecified

F02   Dementia in other diseases classified elsewhere
F02.0 Dementia in Pick's disease
F02.1 Dementia in Creutzfeldt – Jakob disease
F02.2 Dementia in Huntington's disease
F02.3 Dementia in Parkinson's disease
F02.4 Dementia in human immunodeficiency virus (HIV) disease
F02.8 Dementia in other specified diseases classified elsewhere

F03   Unspecified dementia
A fifth character may be added to specify dementia in F00 – F03, as follows:
.x0 Without additional symptoms
.x1 Other symptoms, predominantly delusional
.x2 Other symptoms, predominantly hallucinatory
.x3 Other symptoms, predominantly depressive
.x4 Other mixed symptoms

F04   Organic amnesic syndrome, not induced by alcohol and other psychoactive substances

F05   Delirium, not induced by alcohol and other psychoactive substances
F05.0 Delirium, not superimposed on dementia, so described
F05.1 Delirium, superimposed on dementia
F05.8 Other delirium
F05.9 Delirium, unspecified

F06   Other mental disorders due to brain damage and dysfunction and to physical disease
F06.0 Organic hallucinosis
F06.1 Organic catatonic disorder
F06.2 Organic delusional (schizophrenia-like) disorder

F06.3 Organic mood (affective) disorders
  .30 Organic manic disorder
  .31 Organic bipolar affective disorder
  .32 Organic depressive disorder
  .33 Organic mixed affective disorder
F06.4 Organic anxiety disorder
F06.5 Organic dissociative disorder
F06.6 Organic emotionally labile (asthenic) disorder
F06.7 Mild cognitive disorder
F06.8 Other specified mental disorders due to brain damage and dysfunction and to physical disease
F06.9 Unspecified mental disorder due to brain damage and dysfunction and to physical disease

F07 Personality and behavioural disorders due to brain disease, damage and dysfunction
F07.0 Organic personality disorder
F07.1 Postencephalitic syndrome
F07.2 Postconcussional syndrome
F07.8 Other organic personality and behavioural disorders due to brain disease, damage and dysfunction
F07.9 Unspecified organic personality and behavioural disorder due to brain disease, damage and dysfunction

F09 Unspecified organic or symptomatic mental disorder

F10–F19 Mental and behavioural disorders due to psychoactive substance use

F10 Mental and behavioural disorders due to use of alcohol
F11 Mental and behavioural disorders due to use of opioids
F12 Mental and behavioural disorders due to use of cannabinoids
F13 Mental and behavioural disorders due to use of sedatives or hypnotics
F14 Mental and behavioural disorders due to use of cocaine
F15 Mental and behavioural disorders due to use of other stimulants, including caffeine
F16 Mental and behavioural disorders due to use of hallucinogens
F17 Mental and behavioural disorders due to use of tobacco
F18 Mental and behavioural disorders due to use of volatile solvents
F19 Mental and behavioural disorders due to multiple drug use and use of other psychoactive substances
Four- and five-character categories may be used to specify the clinical conditions, as follows:
F1x.0 Acute intoxication
  .00 Uncomplicated
  .01 With trauma or other bodily injury
  .02 With other medical complications
  .03 With delirium

.04 With perceptual distortions
.05 With coma
.06 With convulsions
.07 Pathological intoxication

F1x.1 Harmful use

F1x.2 Dependence syndrome
.20 Currently abstinent
.21 Currently abstinent, but in a protected environment
.22 Currently on a clinically supervised maintenance or replacement regime (controlled dependence)
.23 Currently abstinent, but receiving treatment with aversive or blocking drugs
.24 Currently using the substance (active dependence)
.25 Continuous use
.26 Episodic use (dipsomania)

F1x.3 Withdrawal state
.30 Uncomplicated
.31 With convulsions

F1x.4 Withdrawal state with delirium
.40 Without convulsions
.41 With convulsions

F1x.5 Psychotic disorder
.50 Schizophrenia-like
.51 Predominantly delusional
.52 Predominantly hallucinatory
.53 Predominantly polymorphic
.54 Predominantly depressive symptoms
.55 Predominantly manic symptoms
.56 Mixed

F1x.6 Amnesic syndrome

F1x.7 Residual and late-onset psychotic disorder
.70 Flashbacks
.71 Personality or behaviour disorder
.72 Residual affective disorder
.73 Dementia
.74 Other persisting cognitive impairment
.75 Late-onset psychotic disorder

F1x.8 Other mental and behavioural disorders

F1x.9 Unspecified mental and behavioural disorder

F20–F29 Schizophrenia, schizotypal and delusional disorders

F20 Schizophrenia

F20.0 Paranoid schizophrenia
F20.1 Hebephrenic schizophrenia
F20.2 Catatonic schizophrenia
F20.3 Undifferentiated schizophrenia
F20.4 Post-schizophrenic depression

F20.5 Residual schizophrenia

F20.6 Simple schizophrenia

F20.8 Other schizophrenia

F20.9 Schizophrenia, unspecified

A fifth character may be used to classify course:

      .x0 Continuous

      .x1 Episodic with progressive deficit

      .x2 Episodic with stable deficit

      .x3 Episodic remittent

      .x4 Incomplete remission

      .x5 Complete remission

      .x8 Other

      .x9 Course uncertain, period of observation too short

F21   **Schizotypal disorder**

F22   **Persistent delusional disorders**

F22.0 Delusional disorder

F22.8 Other persistent delusional disorders

F22.9 Persistent delusional disorder, unspecified

F23   **Acute and transient psychotic disorders**

F23.0 Acute polymorphic psychotic disorder without symptoms of schizophrenia

F23.1 Acute polymorphic psychotic disorder with symptoms of schizophrenia

F23.2 Acute schizophrenia-like psychotic disorder

F23.3 Other acute predominantly delusional psychotic disorders

F23.8 Other acute and transient psychotic disorders

F23.9 Acute and transient psychotic disorders unspecified

A fifth character may be used to identify the presence or absence of associated acute stress:

      .x0 Without associated acute stress

      .x1 With associated acute stress

F24   **Induced delusional disorder**

F25   **Schizoaffective disorders**

F25.0 Schizoaffective disorder, manic type

F25.1 Schizoaffective disorder, depressive type

F25.2 Schizoaffective disorder, mixed type

F25.8 Other schizoaffective disorders

F25.9 Schizoaffective disorder, unspecified

F28   **Other nonorganic psychotic disorders**

F29   **Unspecified nonorganic psychosis**

F30–F39 Mood (affective) disorders

F30   **Manic episode**

F30.0 Hypomania

F30.1 Mania without psychotic symptoms

F30.2 Mania with psychotic symptoms

F30.8 Other manic episodes
F30.9 Manic episode, unspecified

F31   Bipolar affective disorder
F31.0 Bipolar affective disorder, current episode hypomanic
F31.1 Bipolar affective disorder, current episode manic without psychotic
    symptoms
F31.2 Bipolar affective disorder, current episode manic with psychotic
    symptoms
F31.3 Bipolar affective disorder, current episode mild or moderate
    depression
        .30 Without somatic syndrome
        .31 With somatic syndrome
F31.4 Bipolar affective disorder, current episode severe depression without
    psychotic symptoms
F31.5 Bipolar affective disorder, current episode severe depression with
    psychotic symptoms
F31.6 Bipolar affective disorder, current episode mixed
F31.7 Bipolar affective disorder, currently in remission
F31.8 Other bipolar affective disorders
F31.9 Bipolar affective disorder, unspecified

F32   Depressive episode
F32.0 Mild depressive episode
        .00 Without somatic syndrome
        .01 With somatic syndrome
F32.1 Moderate depressive episode
        .10 Without somatic syndrome
        .11 With somatic syndrome
F32.2 Severe depressive episode without psychotic symptoms
F32.3 Severe depressive episode with psychotic symptoms
F32.8 Other depressive episodes
F32.9 Depressive episode, unspecified

F33   Recurrent depressive disorder
F33.0 Recurrent depressive disorder, current episode mild
        .00 Without somatic syndrome
        .01 With somatic syndrome
F33.1 Recurrent depressive disorder, current episode moderate
        .10 Without somatic syndrome
        .11 With somatic syndrome
F33.2 Recurrent depressive disorder, current episode severe without
    psychotic symptoms
F33.3 Recurrent depressive disorder, current episode severe with psychotic
    symptoms
F33.4 Recurrent depressive disorder, currently in remission
F33.8 Other recurrent depressive disorders
F33.9 Recurrent depressive disorder, unspecified

F34   Persistent mood (affective) disorders
F34.0 Cyclothymia
F34.1 Dysthymia
F34.8 Other persistent mood (affective) disorders
F34.9 Persistent mood (affective) disorder, unspecified

F38   Other mood (affective) disorders
F38.0 Other single mood (affective) disorders
.00 Mixed affective episode
F38.1 Other recurrent mood (affective) disorders
.10 Recurrent brief depressive disorder
F38.8 Other specified mood (affective) disorders

F39   Unspecified mood (affective) disorder

F40–F48 Neurotic, stress-related and somatoform disorders

F40   Phobic anxiety disorders
F40.0 Agoraphobia
.00 Without panic disorder
.01 With panic disorder
F40.1 Social phobias
F40.2 Specific (isolated) phobias
F40.8 Other phobic anxiety disorders
F40.9 Phobic anxiety disorder, unspecified

F41   Other anxiety disorders
F41.0 Panic disorder (episodic paroxysmal anxiety)
F41.1 Generalized anxiety disorder
F41.2 Mixed anxiety and depressive disorder
F41.3 Other mixed anxiety disorders
F41.8 Other specified anxiety disorders
F41.9 Anxiety disorder, unspecified

F42   Obsessive compulsive disorder
F42.0 Predominantly obsessional thoughts or ruminations
F42.1 Predominantly compulsive acts (obsessional rituals)
F42.2 Mixed obsessional thoughts and acts
F42.8 Other obsessive compulsive disorders
F42.9 Obsessive compulsive disorder, unspecified

F43   Reaction to severe stress and adjustment disorders
F43.0 Acute stress reaction
F43.1 Post-traumatic stress disorder
F43.2 Adjustment disorders
.20 Brief depressive reaction
.21 Prolonged depressive reaction
.22 Mixed anxiety and depressive reaction
.23 With predominant disturbance of other emotions
.24 With predominant disturbance of conduct
.25 With mixed disturbance of emotions and conduct
.28 With other specified predominant symptoms
F43.8 Other reactions to severe stress
F43.9 Reaction to severe stress, unspecified

F44   Dissociative (conversion) disorders
F44.0 Dissociative amnesia
F44.1 Dissociative fugue

F44.2 Dissociative stupor
F44.3 Trance and possession disorders
F44.4 Dissociative motor disorders
F44.5 Dissociative convulsions
F44.6 Dissociative anaesthesia and sensory loss
F44.7 Mixed dissociative (conversion) disorders
F44.8 Other dissociative (conversion) disorders
.80 Ganser syndrome
.81 Multiple personality disorder
.82 Transient dissociative (conversion) disorders occurring in childhood and adolescence
.88 Other specified dissociative (conversion) disorders
F44.9 Dissociative (conversion) disorder, unspecified

F45 Somatoform disorders
F45.0 Somatization disorder
F45.1 Undifferentiated somatoform disorder
F45.2 Hypochondriacal disorder
F45.3 Somatoform autonomic dysfunction
.30 Heart and cardiovascular system
.31 Upper gastrointestinal tract
.32 Lower gastrointestinal tract
.33 Respiratory system
.34 Genitourinary system
.38 Other organ or system
F45.4 Persistent somatoform pain disorder
F45.8 Other somatoform disorders
F45.9 Somatoform disorder, unspecified

F48 Other neurotic disorders
F48.0 Neurasthenia
F48.1 Depersonalization – derealization syndrome
F48.8 Other specified neurotic disorders
F48.9 Neurotic disorder, unspecified

79

F50–F59 Behavioural syndromes associated with physiological disturbances and physical factors

F50 Eating disorders
F50.0 Anorexia nervosa
F50.1 Atypical anorexia nervosa
F50.2 Bulimia nervosa
F50.3 Atypical bulimia nervosa
F50.4 Overeating associated with other psychological disturbances
F50.5 Vomiting associated with other psychological disturbances
F50.8 Other eating disorders
F50.9 Eating disorder, unspecified

F51 Nonorganic sleep disorders
F51.0 Nonorganic insomnia
F51.1 Nonorganic hypersomnia
F51.2 Nonorganic disorder of the sleep-wake schedule

F51.3 Sleepwalking (somnambulism)
F51.4 Sleep terrors (night terrors)
F51.5 Nightmares
F51.8 Other nonorganic sleep disorders
F51.9 Nonorganic sleep disorder, unspecified

F52 **Sexual dysfunction, not caused by organic disorder or disease**
F52.0 Lack or loss of sexual desire
F52.1 Sexual aversion and lack of sexual enjoyment
.10 Sexual aversion
.11 Lack of sexual enjoyment
F52.2 Failure of genital response
F52.3 Orgasmic dysfunction
F52.4 Premature ejaculation
F52.5 Nonorganic vaginismus
F52.6 Nonorganic dyspareunia
F52.7 Excessive sexual drive
F52.8 Other sexual dysfunction, not caused by organic disorders or disease
F52.9 Unspecified sexual dysfunction, not caused by organic disorder or disease

F53 **Mental and behavioural disorders associated with the puerperium, not elsewhere classified**
F53.0 Mild mental and behavioural disorders associated with the puerperium, not elsewhere classified
F53.1 Severe mental and behavioural disorders associated with the puerperium, not elsewhere classified
F53.8 Other mental and behavioural disorders associated with the puerperium, not elsewhere classified
F53.9 Puerperal mental disorder, unspecified

F54 **Psychological and behavioural factors associated with disorders or diseases classified elsewhere**

F55 **Abuse of non-dependence-producing substances**
F55.0 Antidepressants
F55.1 Laxatives
F55.2 Analgesics
F55.3 Antacids
F55.4 Vitamins
F55.5 Steroids or hormones
F55.6 Specific herbal or folk remedies
F55.8 Other substances that do not produce dependence
F55.9 Unspecified

F59 **Unspecified behavioural syndromes associated with physiological disturbances and physical factors**

F60–F69 Disorders of adult personality and behaviour

F60 **Specific personality disorders**
F60.0 Paranoid personality disorder
F60.1 Schizoid personality disorder
F60.2 Dissocial personality disorder

F60.3 Emotionally unstable personality disorder
.30 Impulsive type
.31 Borderline type
F60.4 Histrionic personality disorder
F60.5 Anankastic personality disorder
F60.6 Anxious (avoidant) personality disorder
F60.7 Dependent personality disorder
F60.8 Other specific personality disorders
F60.9 Personality disorder, unspecified

F61   Mixed and other personality disorders
F61.0 Mixed personality disorders
F61.1 Troublesome personality changes

F62   Enduring personality changes, not attributable to brain damage and disease
F62.0 Enduring personality change after catastrophic experience
F62.1 Enduring personality change after psychiatric illness
F62.8 Other enduring personality changes
F62.9 Enduring personality change, unspecified

F63   Habit and impulse disorders
F63.0 Pathological gambling
F63.1 Pathological fire-setting (pyromania)
F63.2 Pathological stealing (kleptomania)
F63.3 Trichotillomania
F63.8 Other habit and impulse disorders
F63.9 Habit and impulse disorder, unspecified

F64   Gender identity disorders
F64.0 Transsexualism
F64.1 Dual-role transvestism
F64.2 Gender identity disorder of childhood
F64.8 Other gender identity disorders
F64.9 Gender identity disorder, unspecified

F65   Disorders of sexual preference
F65.0 Fetishism
F65.1 Fetishistic transvestism
F65.2 Exhibitionism
F65.3 Voyeurism
F65.4 Paedophilia
F65.5 Sadomasochism
F65.6 Multiple disorders of sexual preference
F65.8 Other disorders of sexual preference
F65.9 Disorder of sexual preference, unspecified

F66   Psychological and behavioural disorders associated with sexual development and orientation
F66.0 Sexual maturation disorder
F66.1 Egodystonic sexual orientation
F66.2 Sexual relationship disorder
F66.8 Other psychosexual development disorders
F66.9 Psychosexual development disorder, unspecified

A fifth character may be used to indicate association with:

.x0 Heterosexuality

.x1 Homosexuality

.x2 Bisexuality

.x8 Other, including prepubertal

F68   Other disorders of adult personality and behaviour

F68.0 Elaboration of physical symptoms for psychological reasons

F68.1 Intentional production or feigning of symptoms of disabilities, either physical or psychological (factitious disorder)

F68.8 Other specified disorders of adult personality and behaviour

F69   Unspecified disorder of adult personality and behaviour

F70–F79 Mental retardation

F70   Mild mental retardation

F71   Moderate mental retardation

F72   Severe mental retardation

F73   Profound mental retardation

F78   Other mental retardation

F79   Unspecified mental retardation

A fourth character may be used to specify the extent of associated behavioural impairment:

F7x.0 No, or minimal, impairment of behaviour

F7x.1 Significant impairment of behaviour requiring attention or treatment

F7x.8 Other impairments of behaviour

F7x.9 Without mention of impairment of behaviour

Treatment

4

If this book is about any one thing it is about treatment. It is what practitioners of the healing art *do* to people. Treatment means helping ill people. At some point, especially as we get older, almost all of us will receive it; in fact, we are probably living in a time when more people are being treated, for a greater variety of disorders and over longer treatment periods, than ever before.

What treatment actually involves, whether it works and how it works are questions that many people still regard, rightly or wrongly, as being beyond their understanding, seeing it instead as a rather complex business that is best left in the hands of professionals. On the whole, people prefer not to spend too much time thinking about the unpleasant things in life, so such shirking of knowledge seems forgivable – after all, isn't that what doctors and nurses are paid for? And the medical profession, in spite of having been around for two millennia, has not exactly rushed to explain its business to the general public. Consider Hippocrates' words, written about 2400 years ago (Fig. 4.1):

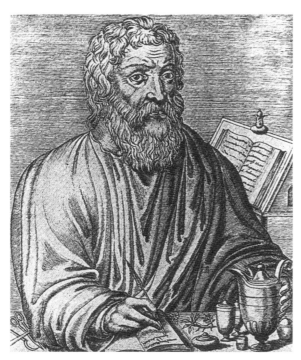

Figure 4.1 ● Hippocrates is portrayed as a bookish figure in this Renaissance engraving.

Life is short, and the Art long, opportunity fleeting, experience treacherous, judgement difficult. The physician must be ready, not only to do his duty himself, but also to secure the co-operation of the patient, the attendants and of externals.

These few lines tell us so much about the meanings of treatment that the first part of this chapter is devoted to them. After highlighting some of the problems that surround treatment, the second part of the chapter will look at specific treatments in turn.

'The art long' but worth it

Treating someone is *always* more complex than we think, but this is not always obvious. Take, for example, a man with a fever and a cough. He visits his GP who prescribes an antibiotic and a few days off work. After this he gets better. What could be more straightforward? But suppose that this man, who is a smoker who works in a chemical factory, has a bathroom cabinet half-full of pills that he has never taken? Can we still be sure that it was the 'treatment' that got him better? And, if so, was it the pills, the rest, both or something else? What if his boyfriend had not persuaded him to take the pills?

To understand how our treatments work and when to apply them, we have to know as much about the world of the individual as possible. The Greek word for knowing everything about a patient comes from 'dia', meaning 'across', and 'gnosis', meaning 'knowledge'. In other words, diagnosis (and its importance is outlined in Chapter 3) and treatment are inextricably interlinked. In medical jargon, $m = d + t$ or management equals diagnosis *and* treatment. As we apply one, so we modify our understanding of the other. Treatment is thus a sort of creative experiment, a permanently changing thing, in constant need of revision as fresh information comes in. And one of the richest sources of such information, not to mention new ideas, will come from a careful evaluation of the effectiveness of treatment so far. To master this art, of treatment as experiment, takes a lot of time – more than a lifetime according to Hippocrates – and a lot of experience.

'Experience treacherous, judgement difficult', so stay sharp

Anyone who claims to have found the perfect treatment for something is wrong. Experience only ever allows us to approach perfection; it never allows us to touch it. This can be hard to swallow if you have been using a treatment for a long time and have built your reputation on it. Being an expert in the treatment of something can carry disadvantages as well as advantages. There is, for example, evidence that some forms of psychotherapy are just as effectively carried out by people with little or no training in the technique. Familiarity can also weaken one's ability to cope with the unexpected or blind one to reason; if I assert that all swans are white, then I may draw on 50 white swans to prove my point. Beyond that, one more white swan does not do a lot for my argument. But all it needs is for one black swan to swim by and my argument sinks. The history of therapeutics is replete with black swans.

The crucial point, therefore, is always to keep an eye out for the unusual and to beware of your own complacency. We need to be constantly vigilant to the danger of getting stuck in our ways. In the first two decades of the 20th century, for example, it was generally held that masturbation or excessive (i.e. non-marital) sex led to depletion of semen, weakness and mental debilitation. It followed, therefore, that vasectomy was a good way of preventing the loss of this precious fluid. Many of the great and good of post-war Europe, including Sigmund Freud himself, signed up for 'Loeffler's operation' (i.e. a vasectomy) before people began to see it for the therapeutic turkey that it was. Over the centuries, this has happened with such diverse practices as bleeding, purging, scarification, injections of monkey glands, removal of 'floating' kidneys, radiotherapy of the thymus, insulin coma therapy, enterovioform tablets and tonsillectomy, to name but a few. Ideas and practices that seem right simply because we have been using them for ages often turn out to be practices well past their use-by date.

'Secure the co-operation of the patient', if you can

As we have already seen, conceptions of just what constitutes an illness are constantly shifting, varying from generation to generation, culture to culture and even person to person. It follows, then, that ideas about who is in need of treatment at any one time will also vary. For community mental health workers, their views of just who *needs* treatment often seem far removed from the general public's view of illness. Does someone running half-naked down the road at 3.00 AM yelling 'mushrooms, mushrooms' need help? Is this despair, drugs and booze, cultural acting out, a student on a rag week stunt or a true psychosis? One of the most important and often underestimated elements of treatment is to try to resolve this confusion, worsened as it is by fear, stigma and simple ignorance. The majority of the lay public still cling to rather unrealistic ideas of what illness – and by this we mean *all* illness, physical and mental – actually involves. A useful way to understand this is by thinking of illness as a way of thinking and behaving. When you are ill, you act in a way that differs from a healthy person. Sociologists sometimes refer to this as 'illness behaviour' or the 'sick role'. In 1952, Talcott Parsons, an American sociologist, defined a set of behaviours and assumptions about being ill (see Box 4.1).

Consider how closely current conceptions about the nature of being ill still agree with his classic definition. Few of us have much difficulty accepting the first condition as an essential part of being ill and, in a sense, treatment begins the moment we sign off from our normal duties. The idea that someone who is ill

85

Box 4.1   The sick role, after Parsons (1952)

1. The sick person is temporarily excused from normal social responsibilities in order to aid recovery

2. The sick person cannot be expected to recover unaided, needing to be 'taken care of'

3. The sick person views their condition as undesirable and wants to recover as quickly as possible

4. The sick person is willing to seek professional help and ready to cooperate in the treatment process to the best of their ability

cannot be expected to cope alone also seems reasonable enough to most people, enshrined as it is in the common suggestion that 'you should see someone'. But most mental health workers will admit that the common idea of illness starts to look a bit patchy when we reach condition number three. As we have observed, not all mentally ill people are willing or even able to see their condition as undesirable. Indeed, when acutely ill, many have difficulty construing anything at all and, even if they could, expediting their recovery may not feature very highly on their list of priorities compared with, for example, finding food and keeping warm. By the time that we reach Parson's fourth condition, the experienced mental health worker will have long since parted from the common idea of behaviours defining the sick role.

The simple truth is that many individuals who end up receiving treatment for a mental health condition are either unable or unwilling to cooperate because of that very same condition. This variation from the neat popular definition of illness leads to all sorts of confusions. One is that if the person does not ask for help then they do not need it. Another is that if they have not got the ability to decide whether or not they need help, they should be given it, regardless of what they may say. A third is that mentally ill people are simply unreasonable and should be avoided at all costs. The public prefers its messages about the worrying things in life, such as wars, life insurance and mental illness, to be straightforward and easily understandable. The fact that there are few simple sound bites for the care of the mentally ill therefore needs to be handled skillfully and acknowledged for what it is, namely a huge challenge for professionals.

In amongst all this uncertainty lies Hippocrates' point: always try to secure the patient's cooperation, get them on your side, even if the reason for this does not always seem obvious at the time. *In the long run*, treatment without the cooperation of the treated achieves little, in some instances it can actually do harm and, as we shall see below when we consider psychological treatments, it may be a complete waste of time. The best way to encourage this cooperation is by communication; always try to take patients' viewpoints into account, even if they do not seem to have one. Displaying patience and calm courtesy to the furious girl with a personality disorder or the dishevelled mute man who seems completely lost inside his own head might not seem like an essential element of treatment at the time, but it cultivates an environment in which a treatment stands the best chance of success.

Much has been written about the importance of cooperation in the therapeutic relationship, but the psychotherapist Jerome Frank provides one of the most useful analyses of how treatment actually works. He boils down the entire process of treating someone into a set of principles, which seem to sum up what it is that works in any treatment and in any culture, regardless of the illness or the patient. Frank argues that, whatever the symptoms, all patients entering treatment are suffering from a state of *demoralisation*. In other words, they are not feeling right, they cannot understand why and they want to get better but do not know what to do about it. Think of how and why a patient presents. Someone complaining of a painful thumb does so not only because of the pain itself but also because of what the pain stops him from doing with his thumb. Thumbs do not become ill, people do. The symptom is stopping him from getting on with his life. This sense of helplessness is even clearer in the major mental illnesses, in which, very often, not getting on with life actually *is* the illness.

All treatments that are truly beneficial to the patient have several things in common. They are aimed at this sense of demoralisation; they should breathe life into the idea that things *can* get better; they should never allow the patient to feel that everything has been tried. The only way to create this hope is via an emotionally charged, confiding relationship. In other words, the carer and the cared for must take each other seriously. For this to happen, both sides must share a language in which to talk about the illness. The process of treatment needs to make sense to both patient and carer. Neither necessarily has to understand every aspect of the treatment – a nurse treating a diabetic patient does not have to be a diabetes expert – but a shared set of symbols and assumptions about the illness and what is going to be done about it are important if the treatment is going to work. These symbols occur in every culture. Today, in the West, we invoke the symbols of science, such as stethoscopes and injections. Elsewhere, people may invoke symbols of demons, cosmic energy or the spirits of ancestors. The setting in which this takes place is also important. In our culture, hospitals and surgeries are seen as places where hope for an end to demoralisation can be aroused. A good care worker should be able to carry this sense of a therapeutic place into someone's front room.

A relationship, a common language and an appropriate setting are thus the ingredients of all successful attempts at treatment, regardless of who or where in the world the therapist is. Be it a tribal healer in a hut in the Kalahari, a Reichian Orgone therapist in his front room in Kalamazoo or a biological psychiatrist at St Bartholomew's Hospital, they all use the same basic therapeutic principles. This explains a curious feature of the treatment business: there is something that works for everyone. This is why we seem to be surrounded by an evergrowing variety of therapies, not all of them necessarily practised with the patient's best interests at heart.

To some degree, all treatments work because of this direct effect of making the patient feel hopeful. The Greek word for 'I please' is *placebo*. Our cynical culture tends to look upon this term as something of a con trick and thereby misses one of the key points about making people better: do everything that you can to make the patient feel happy to be on your side. The act of making the patient feel hopeful explains that well-known phenomenon, the 'placebo effect', whereby one-third of people in a drug trial given a dummy instead of the active medication will still claim significant improvements – and side effects. The care and concern they have received, the reassurance they are getting from 'active' treatment, maybe even a brand-new one, and their own fluctuating symptoms (especially in milder forms of illness) all help to generate the placebo effect. 'We want more of that placebo', cried the crowd in *The Simpsons* when told that an effect was 'just placebo'.

This is not to say, however, that all treatments work as well as each other. Some carry a powerful extra ingredient: they exert a direct physical and biological effect on the disease itself, regardless of the patient's hopes or feelings. It is arguably fair to claim that Western 'allopathic' medicine is the most advanced in this respect, drawing as it does on a body of generally reliable scientific evidence. Many treatment methods that presently find themselves on the borders of mainstream practice, such as acupuncture and homeopathy, are striving to gain acceptance via such empirical legitimacy. It is important to remember, though, that a true biological effect is just one aspect of treatment and, as we have seen, it might not always be necessary.

To describe the entire canon of Western medical achievement as an extra ingredient may seem unjust or plain crazy to some. We do not intend to demean the importance of antibiotics, antipsychotic drugs, keyhole surgery, etc., but we do seek to keep a sense of perspective whenever we ask just what it is about our treatments that really help our patients.

'The attendants' – never forget the network

No one can live in total isolation. Even the most paranoid recluse has to go out for the odd pint of milk or find someone to bring it to them. Humans are uniquely social creatures. No other mammal on earth has such a long period of immature dependency on its parents and, in this long period of pre-adult development, one of the most important things that we learn is how to get on with other people. With few exceptions, other people are necessary to us for our sanity.

This fundamental social need is important to treatment in many ways. The patient's immediate social network may be contributing to the illness process, significantly shaping its course. In some situations, for example drug abuse among the patient's peers, it may even be causing it. Conversely, those who are regularly close to the patient are uniquely well placed to make a positive difference. Such approaches may range from family education in the art of simple understanding and support through to more active involvement in the patient's care, such as encouragement of compliance with drug treatments, behavioural programmes or attendance at day centres, as well as keeping an eye on progress and monitoring for signs of early relapse. Some treatment approaches may even involve a reconstruction of the problem as centring on the family rather than any identified individual. For example, family interventions and education about the illness have been shown to make a significant difference to the course and prognosis of schizophrenia. The involvement of the family is especially important in cases in which the patient's own agreement is inconsistent, such as in chronic psychotic states.

No care plan, therefore, is complete until every effort has been made to understand the role of the patient's broadest social network in his or her life and illness. This network does not begin and end with the family and may extend to a degree that at first can seem bewildering, particularly if the patient is from a different culture. Getting to know the neighbour, the postman, the rabbi, the vicar, the mullah, the milkman, and anyone else you can think of, so often makes such a vast difference to a treatment plan that it becomes difficult to remember how you ever managed without them.

It is also important to remain aware of the fact that, in treating a patient, one also joins their network. Such acceptance must always be seen for what it is: one of the great privileges of working in the caring profession. Few people would let others into their homes and minds with such trust. The power and responsibility that accompany this privilege must never be underestimated or forgotten. A hasty scrawl in a diary may result in what is just a missed appointment to you but, to a vulnerable patient, it may be nearly the final straw before a suicide attempt.

Another common hazard of this privilege is to see oneself as singularly important in the patient's care. Doctors, with the heavy emphasis that their training places on decision-making and initiative, are notorious for this, but many carers at times fall into the trap of 'monopolising' care. Whether or not we like to admit it, many of us choose to go into the caring profession to meet our own needs as well as those of our patients. If left unchecked, these needs can sometimes lead to subtle assumptions of grandiosity and omnipotence, which obstruct rather than enhance the process of treatment. In part, the multidisciplinary team provides a foil to this. By combining the resources and skills of professionals from a variety of disciplines, and sharing the responsibility for care within that team, the pitfalls of therapeutic omnipotence – as well as the despairs of therapeutic impotence when things go wrong – can be watched for, worked through and even avoided.

'And of externals' – time and nature are powerful allies

By now, it should be clear that treatment is a cooperative process. It involves introducing, coordinating and harnessing many factors: the patient's sense of hope, the support of friends and family, the effects of drugs and so on. To this list must finally be added the two most powerful therapeutic agents of all: time and nature. Perhaps because of their obviousness or perhaps because carers prefer to take the credit, these two invaluable allies are often overlooked.

All illnesses, from the nastiest schizophrenia to the commonest cold, have what might be termed a 'natural history', a clear pattern by which they appear, take their course and end. As we have seen, diagnosis is the art of recognising these patterns. A sound understanding of the natural history of an illness is no less crucial to the art of treatment. Someone who is adept at early recognition of a disease will be in the best position to make full use of Ovid's wise words:

> *Principis obsta; sero medicina paratur*
> *Cum mala per longas convaluere moras.*
> *[Stop it at the start, it is difficult to prepare medicine when the disease has grown*
> *strong through delay.]*

This observation is probably truer for mental illnesses than for any other illness. Because the brain is such a subtle and complex organ, with a range of functions influencing everything from sleep pattern to choice of wallpaper, it follows that the way in which its many disorders may emerge will be no less complex, subtle and varied. For example, consider a major depressive episode: a creeping sense of pessimism and despair, weight loss, sleep disturbance, retardation of speech and social withdrawal. By the time that this pattern of features is identified as a discrete morbid process in its own right rather than as an understandable reaction to disappointment at work, a lousy diet or a lot of late nights spent drinking, many of the treatment interventions that might have proved highly effective early on – practical help at work, sensible advice on rest and alcohol, etc. – will simply be inadequate. Starting treatment early means that the patient has the best chance of getting the results that are hoped for.

Apart from the advantage of early intervention, an understanding of the natural course of an established illness – how it is likely to progress over time – is no less helpful to the art of treatment. Will the symptoms fluctuate or remain steady? Is the condition likely to follow an episodic course? Will episodes ever recur? Answers to these questions help treatment in many ways, not least by instilling knowledge and confidence in those asking them.

One of the most remarkable properties of all living things is their natural ability to resist disease. In part, that is what evolution is all about – survival. Over millions of years, our bodies, brains and minds have evolved some astonishingly powerful defences against illness, which we are only slowly beginning to understand. Most living things, given a level playing field, will thus put up a fair fight against disease, which explains why so few diseases succeed in pursuing a steady, unremitting, downward course from onset to end. Physicians have known this for years and have exploited it, not always for the most altruistic of reasons. It is also probably fair to say that the majority of so-called treatments that have been called upon in the name of medicine over the centuries have done little more than act as decoration to the recovery, while time and nature get on with the job. As a famous physician once remarked: 'The duty of the physician is to entertain the patient while the disease takes its course.'

At first glance, this observation may seem unfair to the goodwill of the healer, even cynical. But it reveals several important – and humbling – points about the art of treatment. First, if all one is doing is giving drugs and paying scant attention to the other 80% of the healing process, one is doing it wrong. Second, getting through to the patient is crucial if one is to succeed. Third, the best attempts at treatment always aim to push things as far in Mother Nature's favour as possible. Compared to her abilities, even the finest weapons in the modern medical armoury are feeble.

Knowledge of natural ways and means can often save the care worker a good deal of frustration and disappointment, especially the novice. It is common for the inexperienced, desperate to witness the early fruit of their efforts, to confuse the absence of an early response with no response at all. Optimism often turns to gloom when the florid, distressing, positive symptoms of an acute psychotic state subside to reveal a rather blunted, apathetic and ungrateful person who may want to have very little to do with you. Or when the highly manic individual comes gratifyingly down from a near-disastrous high only to swing into an equally disastrous suicidal depression. Forearmed with this knowledge, we not only avoid these pitfalls but also give off that 'Don't worry, I've seen all this before' manner. Keeping patients and their loved ones entertained and hopeful through the long dark days of a psychotic illness is often more than half the job. On the other hand, it is important not to turn into a guru or a know-all. Troubled families need sensible grown-ups.

Different types of treatment

If all that has been said about treatment so far seems rather detached from a cold depressed patient shivering in an unheated council flat, do not despair. It can be summarised as follows: to work properly, treatment must involve three elements, the biological, the psychological and the social. In this chapter we will take a critical look at each of these elements, to see just how they can help us get better at getting people better.

Psychological therapies

As we have seen, whenever a human being is involved in an attempt to help another, psychological processes always come into play. Therefore, all treatment can, in some sense, be regarded as a form of psychological therapy. In the more modern sense, however, the word 'psychotherapy' has come to refer to a treatment that derives its methods from one or more specific psychological principles or theories. But looking at the sheer complexity of human psychology, as well as the fact that much of it is far from being well-proven science, it soon becomes clear that the field of psychotherapy is anything but straightforward. In fact, the diverse range of therapies often seem to have more in common with religious movements than rational treatments, clinging as they often do to impressive theories advanced by charismatic personalities. Such issues are beyond the scope of this book – indeed, some might argue that too many books have been written about the differences in psychotherapy rather than concentrating on the more sobering questions of whether and how they work, and what their essence is.

Figure 4.2 shows one attempt to identify some coherence among the bewildering array of therapies currently being practised. But before we use it to extract some useful principles and psychotherapeutic rules of thumb from this confusing area, it is helpful to see how psychotherapy got into its present state in the first place.

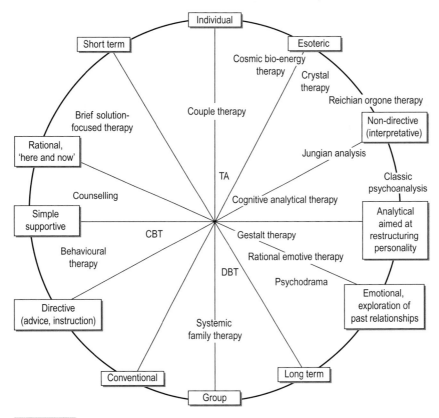

Figure 4.2 ● Making sense of the bewildering complexity of modern psychotherapies. CBT, cognitive behavioural therapy; DBT, dialectical behavioural therapy; TA, transactional analysis.

A brief history of psychotherapy

Psychological treatments have been around for a long time. In Europe, the power of the Roman Catholic confessional, for example, combined with a sense of faith and the ritual invested in the church, has served well to treat many a case of anxiety, depression, guilt or worse over the past 1500 years (Fig. 4.3). But the idea of trying to apply psychological principles to bring about a therapeutic change in someone's physical and mental well-being is a much more recent idea and an essentially European one at that. The Renaissance and the Enlightenment that followed it in the 17th and 18th centuries gave rise to the idea that man might get to know himself better by the reasoned application of experimentation and deduction. In other words, the mind became a legitimate area for scientific enquiry. In the late 18th century, Anton Mesmer proposed that a cosmic theory of 'animal

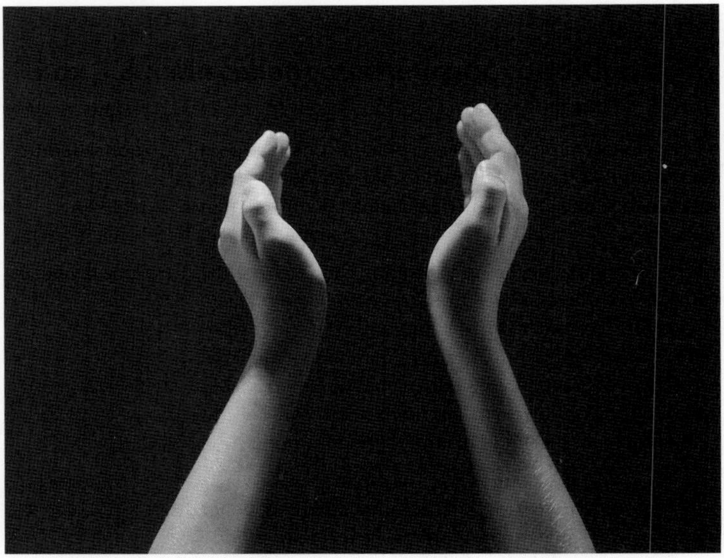

Figure 4.3 ● Prayer: the most established form of psychotherapy.

magnetism' might account, among other things, for changes in thinking, feeling and remembering. Others modified this idea; by the early 19th century, some theorists were explaining 'mesmerism' in terms of a part of the mind of which we were not always consciously aware. Meanwhile, in Britain, James Braid, a true surgeon, stripped the idea of all its psychological connotations, proposing the term 'hypnosis' for an entirely mechanical process in the brain.

Many of the great medical thinkers of the later 19th century, combining ideas of mental processes with the developing theory of an unconscious mind, began to use hypnosis as a therapeutic tool. Among them was the young Sigmund Freud. His early case studies of hypnosis led him to the conclusion that the unconscious mind was dominated by essentially sexual, instinctive drives ('the id') over which the conscious mind ('the ego') constantly struggled to keep control (Fig. 4.4). This struggle was shaped by early life experiences, especially one's relationship with one's parents, who became internalised to varying degrees as a kind of suppressing conscience, the 'superego'. The direction in which a person was propelled by this struggle, he argued, made all the difference to one's mental health. He termed the method for exploring this 'psychoanalysis', a process of unravelling one's primitive 'Oedipal' fears (e.g. of castration) and removing 'fixations' that interfered with one's emotional stability.

After much resistance, even disgust, his ideas became fashionable in Europe and (especially) the USA, keen to understand itself as complex, sophisticated and increasingly individualist. Whatever one thinks about the content of Freud's theories, their impact on the way that we in the West think about thinking and feeling is impossible to overstate. Between the World Wars, his ideas triggered a psychotherapeutic explosion. Some of his associates, in many senses closer to disciples than colleagues, split from Freud's by then established orthodoxy and, borrowing from anthropology here and ethnology there, set up whole new fields of psychotherapy for analysts and patients to roam through. Karl Jung, Alfred Adler and, later, Melanie Klein were the most influential.

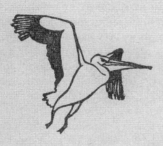

PELICAN BOOKS

TOTEM AND TABOO

RESEMBLANCES BETWEEN THE PSYCHIC LIVES
OF SAVAGES AND NEUROTICS

BY

PROFESSOR SIGMUND FREUD
LL.D.

PUBLISHED BY

PENGUIN BOOKS LIMITED
HARMONDSWORTH   MIDDLESEX   ENGLAND
41 EAST 28TH STREET   NEW YORK   U.S.A.

Figure 4.4 ● Cover of *Totem and Taboo*: psychotherapy meets mysticism?

The problem that few people had considered, in their rush to embrace this exciting new theory, was that Freud's ideas were far from scientific. Rather, they had been based on a series of uncontrolled case studies by an ambitious middle-class European Jewish neurologist, dealing with a group of distressed and impressionable upper-class women. As far as psychoanalysis was concerned, the tradition of doubting enquiry, so emphasised by the great minds of the Enlightenment, didn't get so much as a look in. In the USA, a country not then renowned for its sense of cautious optimism or its tradition of sceptical enquiry, psychoanalytical ideas were taken up with such enthusiasm that they became *the* method by which contemporary psychiatric problems, from communism and homosexuality to depression and schizophrenia, were treated. Before long, much of the Western world had followed suit.

Some psychologists and psychiatrists in the USA, however, were not quite so ready to embrace these ideas. They drew attention to their lack of precision. Just how did you gauge the intensity of 'libidinal cathexis' exactly? To a group of psychologists known as the behaviourists, led by James Watson, measurement was the true gold standard of psychological understanding. If it couldn't be measured, it didn't exist. For the behaviourists, then, this meant that the human head, and all that went on inside it, was a closed black box. In an attempt to counter the perceived woolliness of psychoanalysis – in the scientific sense, at any rate – the behaviourists threw out the baby with the bathwater. It wasn't until the mid-1950s that another school of behaviourism, led by BF Skinner, finally began to suggest that mental phenomena such as thoughts, feelings and impulses (the very stuff we considered in Chapter 3) *could* be regarded as a behaviour, albeit a private one.

Thus was triggered the second major explosion in psychological therapy this century: the so-called cognitive revolution. Slowly, workers began to draw upon the wealth of clinical information on the countless phenomena of mental illness, garnered, in part, through the efforts of many psychoanalysts over the past four decades, and set about establishing rules for a newer, more objectively accountable series of therapies. Some psychoanalysts, such as Beck and Ellis, disenchanted with the post-Freudian camp, defected to the newer schools of thought, bringing with them new ideas about emotion, drive and motivation, creating new hybrid ideas for treatment. Meanwhile, other more humanistic theorists contributed ideas about self-actualisation and self-esteem, and still others brought into the field their knowledge of interpersonal communication, family structure and group dynamics. If, finally, into this motley array of theorists and therapists, we add those whose contribution may be best referred to as 'esoteric', we end up with a rough overall picture of contemporary psychotherapy looking a little like Figure 4.2.

How to make sense of the different types of psychotherapy

As can be seen from the diagram, psychological therapies can be arranged and understood in many ways. Probably the most important classification is the one that has arisen historically, namely the distinction between the so-called rational and psychoanalytic approaches. Rational approaches tend to focus on the present whereas analytical 'dynamic' approaches usually involve more rummaging around in the patient's emotional past. The former sorts of therapy are more readily used in the course of routine work for a number of reasons. By concentrating on the present rather than the past, they tend to help patients face the most pressing issues in the 'here and now' of their life, be they symptoms, practical living difficulties or whatever. They often seek to bring about relatively swift changes over weeks or months rather than focusing on the longer term like the more dynamic therapies. Because they essentially seek to teach patients new tricks for dealing with their symptoms and problems, they are also called the 'educative' therapies, thus they tend to be quite directive. That is, they often involve the giving of advice or practical guidance to the patient or, in the case of cognitive behavioural therapy, they can even involve setting the patient homework.

Psychodynamic treatments, on the other hand, are usually far less directive. Rather, the therapist deliberately seeks to provide a neutral, blank screen on to which the patient is encouraged to project his or her difficulties. By the process of occasional well-aimed interpretations, the patient develops a greater insight into the nature of his or her psychological make up. For this reason, some refer to these approaches as 'reconstructive' psychotherapies. They seek to rearrange no less than the very structure of the patient's personality. Unsurprisingly, such a major undertaking is time consuming (years) and expensive, whereas courses of the more rationally based treatments, aiming to bring about swifter, more modest degrees of improvement, often last much less time (weeks/months). This is by no means a hard and fast rule. In recent years, attention has been paid to 'brief dynamic therapy', with interesting results, whilst arguably the most simple, directive therapy of them all, supportive psychotherapy – otherwise known as care working – may go on for years.

Not all therapies work on a one-to-one basis. Group methods intentionally harness the fact that humans are particularly social creatures and acknowledge that many problems with mental health arise out of the way we deal with others in couples, families and other social groups. They use the group to interpret attitudes and to nurture change. They also have the advantage of helping larger numbers of people at the same time. As we will see later, both clinical work and research have evolved group techniques, which can exert remarkable effects in specific situations. Many of these are highly specialised and involve much practice, but the results that they yield can prove useful and rewarding to the care worker willing to make the investment.

Most psychotherapies, therefore, can be understood as belonging to one of four main types: the simple supportive psychotherapies, the educational psychotherapies, the group psychotherapies and the dynamic psychotherapies. There are, of course, plenty of overlaps and, like any attempt to clarify a foggy subject, some therapies get left out of the classification altogether. Nevertheless, these are the four main areas that care workers are most likely to come across in the course of their careers. Even if they don't end up becoming practitioners themselves, it pays to know a bit about what each can and cannot do, whom it is intended for and how it works. We will therefore consider each of these forms of therapy in turn, while stressing our view that the shared elements of each approach probably outweigh the differences.

The supportive psychotherapies

All health workers are practitioners of simple supportive therapy (Fig. 4.5). Every imaginable piece of casework, from a one-off duty assessment to long-term care work, will benefit from attention paid to this ubiquitous skill. Much of it passes under a variety of names – 'communication skills', 'interviewing technique', 'common sense' or even 'jollying along' – but none of these should detract from a fundamental point: all care work is a form of psychotherapy, just as valuable, effective and unique as any of the supposedly more 'specialised' therapies. For this reason, we will often return to the themes of this therapy throughout the following chapters.

One of the advantages of the supportive approach is that it is suited to everyone. Because its main objective is to make the best of whatever world the patient inhabits, be it an acute crisis or a chronic problem arising from a major mental illness, *it always helps*. It can bolster self-esteem, act as a psychological crutch, challenge pessimism, provide hope or carry patients to a point where they may become fit for work of a more intensive nature.

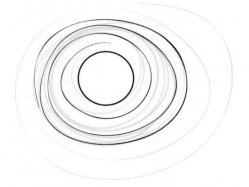

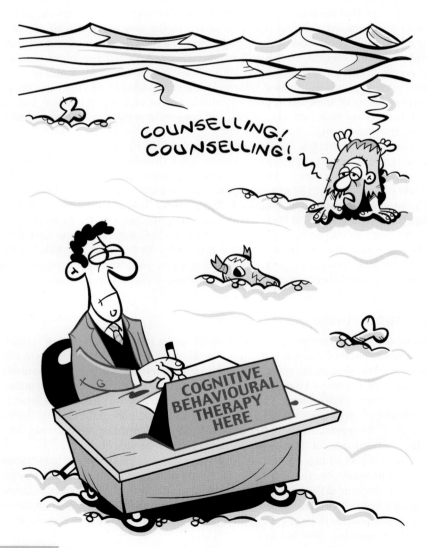

Figure 4.5 ● Between simple supportive psychotherapy and CBT proper there is a desert of unfocused counselling.

The central rule of this approach is deceptively simple: *don't just do something, sit there.* Most of us are brainwashed by the cultural assumption that we are only active when we look active, so we fall into the trap of thinking that listening is a passive process. It is not. The provision of genuine undivided attention by a valued individual, invested with some sense of authority, is one of the most active and powerful therapeutic tools in our kit. In such a setting, listening encourages the ventilation of emotion that can propel psychological recovery. You are helping by the simple act of being there.

Another important element of supportive therapy is reassurance. This often involves a direct refutation of the negative, fearful, hopeless beliefs that patients may hold about themselves, their world or their future, and thereby sustains hope. Some theorists have questioned the wisdom of providing reassurance, pointing to its abilities to induce dependence as well as the dangers of false optimism. Interestingly, most of those who offer such an opinion do so from the comfortable distance of a specialist or academic position, rather than that of a busy front-line worker. For the care worker, the bottom line is often: if in doubt, reassure. Don't be glib or superficial or over-casual but do stay with the positive. If the reassurance turns out to be false, don't worry, just press on. In community care, the glass is always half full, never half empty. There's always something else to be done.

The other important element of the supportive approach is explanation. This explains why a sound background knowledge of diagnosis, natural history and treatment is so important. If you can get your patient to share an understanding of how symptoms arise and how treatment works – even if the understanding isn't quite the full story – this does much to dispel the fear of uncertainty so common in mental illness. Explanation often goes hand in hand with the giving of advice, and several points need to be made about advice. First, our patients are often not in a state where they are likely to remember it. Second, even when it is taken up, it is often translated into something quite at odds with one's original intentions and third, even if it is faithfully absorbed, it is rarely acted upon in the manner hoped for. This often comes as a great source of surprise and frustration, especially to the less experienced worker. Advice, then, is something to be treated with caution. Prepare the ground before giving it and proffer little pieces of it often, rather than occasional didactic dollops. Another knack is to get the patient to feel as if he or she is discovering the advice for themselves. This way, the patient is far more likely to make proper use of information and is more able to take the credit when things start to work out, as well as more willing to shoulder disappointment when things go wrong. Ultimately, trust, respect and patience, rather than information, are the central ingredients of the simple supportive approach. Information, especially when it is tied to a sense of doing something, belongs much more with the educative therapies.

The educative therapies: behavioural and cognitive behavioural

An essential feature of human nature is our ability to learn. By learning, we are able to take information from what's going on around us and use it to modify our actions in thought, belief, word and deed. It follows from this that there is a clear causal relationship between things in our environment and our responses to them. This works both ways: as our environment changes us, we, in turn, change our environment. These systematic ideas of learning, causality (sometimes called 'determinism') and reciprocity, are central to the practice of the two main forms of educative psychotherapy, behavioural therapy (BT) and cognitive behavioural therapy (CBT), and are based on a school of psychology known as 'learning theory'. Through BT and CBT, we identify problematic patterns of behaviour and learn newer, better ones to replace them.

Similarly to simple supportive therapy, these methods can apply to a variety of clinical situations. Because they focus on problems (or symptoms) rather than specific clinical diagnoses, they are highly flexible. CBT, for example, is just as useful for a depressive syndrome occurring in a schizophrenic illness as it is for a depressive episode following bereavement. Another advantage of the educative therapeutic approach is its clarity. Treatment involves clear, methodical progress through a logical sequence of steps (see Fig. 4.6) that define the problem, measure the problem, apply the treatment and re-evaluate it, with incorporation of feedback.

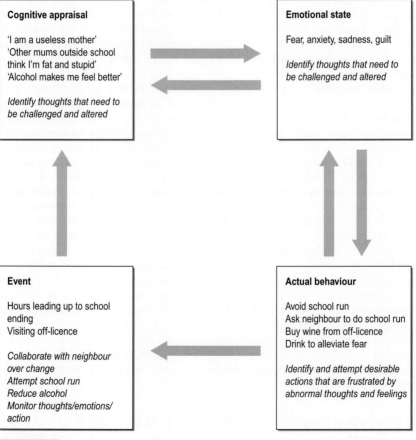

Figure 4.6 ● The logical steps in the process of cognitive behavioural therapy.

Unlike supportive therapy, however, there are limits to this approach. Patients with reasonably clear-cut difficulties, which are more amenable to objective measurement, tend to be more suitable than cases in which problems are multiple, chaotic and highly inter-related. It also helps greatly if the patient has at least a rudimentary understanding of the rationale of treatment itself, even though this may be tailored to the intellectual and abstracting skills of each patient. Generally, behavioural treatments are easier to apply than their cognitive behavioural counterparts. A less easily avoidable problem is motivation. Whereas simple support may work even on those who appear to reject it, educative approaches require willing participation as a necessary precondition for success. Therefore, a considerable part of the initial assessment stage is wisely spent on simple support and persuasion to motivate and secure a willingness to engage. It should also be remembered that things change. A patient for whom behavioural therapy seems pointless today may well be an ideal candidate once other blocks to care have been cleared. A trial session of therapy may also be very illuminating, with any initial change/response generally indicating that it's worth continuing.

BEHAVIOURAL TECHNIQUES Relaxation, breathing exercises and basic social skills training are simple techniques that should form a part of every care worker's toolkit. More complicated techniques are best referred to a specialist, but knowing when to make such a referral is also part of the job. The following description of the main behavioural therapies is focused upon those more relevant to front-line work.

Relaxation This technique is effective for managing anxiety problems in a wide range of settings and manifestations, from primary anxiety neuroses to the anxiety associated with schizophrenia and depression. It is also effective for the many physical presentations and manifestations of anxiety, chronic stress, fatigue or over-arousal, including dyspepsia, tension headache, insomnia, hypertension, muscular spasms and chronic pain. Small surprise, then, that this technique often comes in handy for the community care worker. A simple relaxation technique is described in Box 4.2. It uses three components: visualisation, muscular relaxation and control of breathing. The last component is also a potent technique in its own right for the management of acute anxiety and panic disorder. An important but often

Box 4.2 A simple relaxation technique

- In the surgery, patients are asked to sit or even lie in a relaxed position so that they are feeling as comfortable as possible

- They are then asked to tense up the forearm muscles for 2–20 seconds and then relax them. This should be repeated with the upper arm muscles. They should breathe in when tensing muscles and slowly breathe out when relaxing

- Muscle groups in the abdomen and upper and lower legs should each be tensed and then relaxed in turn, with patients being asked to concentrate entirely on what they are doing, emptying their minds of other thoughts or feelings

- Patients should then be instructed to carry out a similar procedure in a quiet place at home for some 5–10 minutes, several times a day, without any interruptions

- Patients should also be encouraged to adopt just such an approach if they start to feel anxious or panicky in given situations, concentrating entirely on tensing and relaxing their bodily musculature

- This process of distraction helps break the cycle of increasing fear and more pronounced symptoms, and makes it easier to get through the few minutes of a typical panic attack

overlooked element of this treatment is repetition. Very often, cases fail to respond because the patient is not actually using the technique regularly enough.

Systematic desensitisation This method combines relaxation with the psychology of learning theory. It is helpful in a wide range of anxiety-related disorders, particularly when fear (phobia) is associated with a particular place, situation, event or activity. It provides an orderly sequence of steps through which the patient can gradually move towards mastery over the feared situation. First, the patient is taught to relax. Then, through analysis of the particular problem, symptoms and provoking factors are identified. The worker uses this information to help the patient construct a sequence of anxiety-provoking situations, ranging from the innocuous through to the most terrifying. The patient is then exposed to each in turn, moving on only when he or she has mastered the anxiety provoked at each stage. Although every stage is more challenging than the last, at no point is the patient exposed to overwhelming anxiety. Exposure to the feared situation may be imaginary, using filmed material or images visualised mentally through suggestion. Alternatively, exposure may happen in a graded sequence of real-life situations (e.g. travelling on a bus). Both clinical and research experience suggest that the latter is more effective as well as exhibiting more 'stimulus response generalisation', which means that the benefits gained in one setting carry over into other areas of the patient's life.

Flooding This technique uses the desensitisation principle in a non-graded fashion and is otherwise known as 'throwing them in at the deep end'. It tends to be most effective for specific phobic conditions and obsessive compulsive disorders (especially when combined with response prevention) but generally requires that the patient has an otherwise reasonably robust constitution. It is not so well suited to patients with psychotic disorders or those whose personalities operate at borderline levels of integration. Again, exposure may be imagined or real, the latter being more effective. Before exposure, the patient is taught a relaxation technique and an objective measure of anxiety is agreed upon, usually in the form of a self-rating scale.

To work most effectively, the exposure episode should be reasonably prolonged and withdrawal discouraged until the patient's measured anxiety has already clearly begun to decline. Stopping too soon may act as avoidance and actively worsen the problem. At the outset, anxiety is usually intense and unpleasant but, as habituation and adaptation occur (i.e. you get used to it), this invariably declines, providing the patient can stay with the feared situation. A related technique used with obsessive disorders is known as 'mass practice' and involves the patient actively rehearsing the obsession to excess, for example by rehearsing aloud the ruminative thought or listening to a recording of their own voice repeating it aloud. According to learning theory, this 'overlearning' weakens the link between the obsessional thought and the anxiety associated with it.

Response prevention This is effective for the treatment of persistent obsessions or other troublesome habitual behaviours, whether primary or secondary to other disorders. It appears to be particularly effective when the obsessive thinking is accompanied by ritualised repetitive behaviours, termed 'compulsions'. The patient is exposed to a situation that brings on the obsessive response, such as exposure to a 'dirty' object, but is subsequently restrained from carrying out the usual ritual response such as excessive hand washing. It is often helpful if the therapist 'models' the normal behaviour in parallel, for example by eating something immediately after having touched a dirty object and then requiring the patient to do the same. According to learning theory, such a process helps to loosen the causal association between the stimulus (the dirty object) and the response (the obsessional rumination over dirt or the repetitive hand washing).

Social skills training Modelling of ideal behaviours can also form part of social skills training. Many patients with a wide variety of psychiatric problems have difficulty coping with social situations that 'healthy' individuals simply take for granted. Social skills training thus overlaps with many other techniques used in the course of routine care work. The behavioural approach to, say, meeting people allows a patient and therapist to break down the problem into an understandable series of actions. These can be changed gradually by combining reassurance, modelling, response prevention and other behavioural techniques. Social skills training also places emphasis on the non-verbal aspects of social interaction. As social creatures, we are quick to judge others by their immediate appearance and behaviour. Discrepancies between verbal and non-verbal behaviour, apart from being subtle pointers to abnormal mental states, can also powerfully influence, almost automatically, the way we respond to people. By teaching patients to identify and correct such inconsistencies, it is possible to improve their coping abilities in a variety of situations that they might otherwise have avoided. This can, in turn, open up other therapeutic avenues. Social skills training is as easily conducted in group settings as on an individual basis. Such groups often provide valuable support, but care has to be taken to avoid the group reinforcing other maladaptive behaviours.

COGNITIVE BEHAVIOURAL THERAPY One of the drawbacks of simple BT is its emphasis on how you look and what you say at the expense of the inner world of the patient. BT, for example, is known to be less effective in the treatment of obsessional ruminations if they are unaccompanied by external compulsive rituals, such as hand washing. CBT deals with this by explicitly identifying inner mental phenomena as the primary target of change. Because of this focus on what goes on inside our heads, it attaches much more importance to emotion than the purely behavioural approach. The original proponent of modern CBT, Aaron Beck, himself a former psychoanalyst, was aware of the powerful influence of emotion upon cognitive processes. As we saw in Chapter 3, our emotional state acts as a filter that colours the way we see and think about our world and alters the way that we react to it.

Many mental illnesses may be understood in this way. The cognitive approach attempts to identify and modify the 'cognitive distortions' that become habits in our thinking and acting. These distortions tend to recur in a number of recognisable patterns, which can be teased out by systematic analysis of the patient's mental state. Once identified, they are described and measured, just as a behavioural therapist charts problem behaviours. A schedule of exercises to challenge these styles of thought and feeling (e.g. 'alternative thoughts') are then drawn up by the patient and therapist together and put into action. Change in the identified problems over time is taken as an objective measure of the effectiveness of treatment. This approach rarely attempts to address inner mental phenomena in isolation and therapists usually make concurrent use of other behavioural techniques, as described above.

Although the range of applications of CBT is wider than that of simple BT, it is not suited to everyone. Patients need to have a basic ability to itemise their difficulties and need to be willing to consider them in psychological terms. They also need a capacity for introspection. This is easier for some people than others. Individuals who, for whatever reason, have suffered delayed maturation in their capacity for abstract thought and those who display a constitutional tendency towards 'concrete' styles of thinking, as well as individuals with mentally disintegrating psychotic illnesses, are probably not well suited to cognitive interventions. The

101

presence of psychotic symptoms in their own right, however, need not necessarily act as a bar to treatment. Currently, much interesting work is being conducted into the feasibility of cognitive treatments for chronic positive psychotic symptoms, particularly hallucinations and delusions. Such work may eventually open up new combined therapeutic approaches to major mental illness that will be of great use to community care workers.

OTHER EDUCATIVE THERAPIES Not all of the educative psychotherapies place such heavy emphasis upon psychological theories of learning and behaviour. Instead, they draw their inspiration from the 'humanistic' theories of Maslow and Rogers. Central to these approaches is the notion of personal fulfilment, or 'self-actualisation'; those moments in life, usually known only to the person living them, when one feels temporarily but deeply satisfied with something, without any attached sense of self-consciousness or struggle. Rogers based his theories on the clinical observation that human beings seem to have a natural tendency to try to make the best of their individual energies, abilities and talents. He believed that difficulties in achieving this goal of self-fulfilment often gave rise to psychopathology and that this could be identified and overcome by a systematic approach. Maslow mapped out the path to self-actualisation more explicitly, conceiving of human existence as an effort to achieve mastery over a 'hierarchy of needs' (see Fig. 4.7). According to Maslow, the higher needs essential to true mental health could only be achieved once the more basic needs of the human organism had been secured, at least in part.

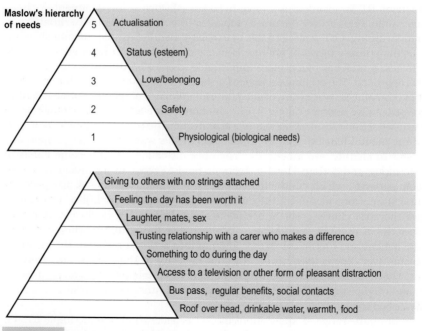

Maslow's hierarchy of needs
5 Actualisation
4 Status (esteem)
3 Love/belonging
2 Safety
1 Physiological (biological needs)

Giving to others with no strings attached
Feeling the day has been worth it
Laughter, mates, sex
Trusting relationship with a carer who makes a difference
Something to do during the day
Access to a television or other form of pleasant distraction
Bus pass, regular benefits, social contacts
Roof over head, drinkable water, warmth, food

Figure 4.7 ● Maslow's hierarchy of needs applied to the real world.

The humanistic approach is attractive for many reasons. The theories make intuitive sense – most of us can recall our own private moments of 'self-actualisation' and how we reached them. Such personal insight can be put to good use helping patients to define, and negotiate towards, their own goals, however modest or ambitious. As we have already seen, to do this successfully the care worker needs to establish a trusting relationship with the patient based upon a sound understanding of just what makes that person tick. Maslow's hierarchy of needs is often depicted as a pyramid consisting of five levels: the four lower levels are grouped together as *deficiency needs* and are associated with physiological needs, whereas the top level is termed *growth needs*, associated with psychological needs (Fig. 4.7). His theory contends that, as humans meet basic needs, they seek to satisfy successively higher needs that occupy a set hierarchy. Similarly, a 'full needs assessment' of a patient can be viewed in the same pyramidal form, with the lower needs having to be met to achieve the higher needs. For example, for a patient to achieve the goal of improved social skills, he may need to attend a group at a day centre. To get to the day centre, he will need cash or a bus pass. To get this, he may need help getting his benefits sorted. Much of the bread and butter of community care involves hard work at the lower levels of the pyramid and this can feel like hard going at times. The humanistic approach helps us to keep our eyes on the stars as we stumble along the gutter.

A comprehensive description of all of the educative therapies is beyond the scope of this book. Only a few of the more common approaches are mentioned here. Some hold closely to the tenets of cognitive and humanistic therapies, whereas others overlap more with psychodynamic ideas. Still others – the so-called 'body' or 'release' therapies – draw upon a variety of dramatic theories and methods, which range from the unusual to the downright spectacular. It is unlikely that any one approach consistently carries any advantages over other methods for most people. With humans fortunately being the individualistic creatures that they are, different approaches are more suited to some than to others. Coming up with a good match – or having some idea of what your patient is getting into – is part of the job.

Rational emotive therapy resembles cognitive therapy in that it is primarily concerned with the beliefs and assumptions that patients hold about reality. It assumes that emotional changes will naturally flow from the identification and challenging of 'irrational' ideas, which the therapist confronts, sometimes quite assertively. It can lead to a lot of shouting, on both sides.

Transactional analysis is an approach based on the work of Eric Berne. This approach focuses extensively on the roles that people adopt when they communicate with each other. According to Berne, each of us has three habitual ways of acting in any relationship, as a 'child', an 'adult' or a 'parent'. Destructive patterns in relationships may emerge when one or both parties adopts an inappropriate role. Our tendency to adopt a particular role in any given situation is tied up with our own unique set of psychological defences, and is reinforced by 'strokes', powerful unconscious emotional responses that we elicit from other people. Therapy employs Berne's symbols to identify, explain and challenge destructive patterns in the way we deal with others, and to encourage healthier alternatives.

Gestalt therapy places less emphasis on cognitions or roles as part of the self and, instead, focuses upon the individual as a whole: mentally, physically and socially. This whole, or gestalt, is kept stable by a process known as 'homeostasis'. The emphasis of treatment here is to create improved awareness and integration of the self. Great attention is paid to emotional expression and posture, which, gestalt therapists argue, reveals subtle but discernible clues to unresolved emotional conflicts. Therapy is usually, but not invariably, conducted in groups. Each person takes turns in a 'hot seat' next to the therapist, who encourages the patient to express or enact ideas and feelings that have been too painful to admit to consciously.

Another therapy that considers cognitive styles along with minute analysis of body and behavioural subtleties is the unfortunately named *neurolinguistic programming* (NLP). This approach focuses upon the various 'preverbal' styles that underlie our habitual ways of thinking and talking. According to practitioners of NLP, we differ in the dominant sensory modality (sounds, images, actions and so on) through which we form beliefs about ourselves and our world. Using a combination of hypnotic suggestion and a set of rules about thinking that are similar to those of CBT, individuals can develop a greater awareness of their habitual responses and be guided towards their alteration.

Other therapies place more emphasis on the process of 'acting out' suppressed emotional material. According to the restructural school of psychotherapy, some emotionally charged thoughts or memories are simply too painful or frightening to hold in our consciousness. They are therefore excluded from our awareness by a process that consumes a lot of mental energy. Such a drain on our mental resources can reveal itself through neurotic symptoms, especially anxiety and depression. The notion of catharsis, familiar to anyone who has ever had the pleasure of clearing a blocked drain or subscribed to the notion of 'getting it off your chest', holds that allowing this emotional material to surface into consciousness may be uncomfortable but is highly therapeutic. Many colourful forms of psychotherapy are based upon this idea, including 'bioenergetic therapy', a method proposed by the charismatic Wilhelm Reich. He believed that patterns of posture and body use could be seen as body armour, which helped to maintain a person's unconscious defences. Reich employed the use of massage, breathing and direct (sometimes quite aggressive) verbal confrontation to overcome these defensive styles, thereby allowing the patient's 'sexual energy' to flow more freely. Reich didn't stop there, however, and went on to propose that an individual's sexual energy could be stored and recalled in his specially designed 'orgone box'. Since his death, others have devised gentler applications of his ideas that make more use of the patient's own actions, emotions and verbalisations.

Another therapy that relies heavily on the notion of catharsis is primal therapy. This was outlined by the analyst Arthur Janov in his book *The Primal Scream*. He believed that emotional events around the moment of birth were of great significance to an individual, and that all neurosis in later life essentially stemmed from incomplete expression of a person's infantile distress. A person could only come to terms with such powerfully dammed-up emotions by regressing to an infant-like state to express that emotion, in the form of a scream. Whether this theory has any scientific merit is anybody's guess, and many have argued that Janov's theory places too much emphasis upon a process that does, after all, happen to all of us, neurotic or otherwise.

Do some therapies work better than others?

Outcome research in psychotherapy is beset by many problems and raises even more questions than it answers. For example, it is very hard to subject a therapy that involves talking to people to the standard scientific test of efficacy, the double-blind placebo-controlled trial. Just how do you keep a patient 'blind' to (i.e. unaware of) the method under study? And just what do you choose as a placebo control? Some studies compare patients on a waiting list, who have yet to get as far as the therapist, with those undergoing treatment, but other studies have shown how even the anticipation of treatment can have a significant effect on someone's mental state, not to mention the simple passing of time. Other studies have compared an active treatment with a more minimal intervention, such as an hour-long chat over a cup of tea with an unqualified person once a week. Still other studies have found that the duration and intensity of treatment are irrelevant; it doesn't matter whether you see the patient for in-depth analysis three times a week or for half an hour each fortnight. All of these studies seem to show very few differences in the results. It seems that it doesn't matter what you do, as long as you do something. This is of no small concern to highly paid psychoanalysts, who have themselves invested the equivalent of a small mortgage in years of personal training therapy. Perhaps unsurprisingly, this group of professionals has recently undergone a neat shift of perspective: 'We no longer ask whether it works, but *how* it works.'

And to some extent, the analysts may be right. Like the giant computer in *The Hitchhiker's Guide to the Galaxy* that answered 42 when asked for the meaning of life, the results of psychotherapy outcome research reveal what happens when you ask a simple question about a complex subject. Simply grouping together and comparing large cohorts of people who have had this or that therapy overlooks the essential individuality of the issue. What is clear is that, regardless of the validity of the often fanciful theories that underlie many of these forms of therapy, many people do experience powerful states of arousal and emotion that can lead to lasting alterations in a person's subjective and objective character. This carries an important message for the care worker. Many patients, who have difficulties living as they might wish because of mental illness or enduring difficulties in their personalities, are easily tempted by the prospect of a psychological 'quick fix'. The market for a bewildering variety of 'new' therapies, practised by all manner of types, from well-meaning hippies and experienced well-trained carers to self-styled New Age gurus and downright charlatans, is probably now larger than ever before. A good care worker should always bear in mind that wisest of adages: 'First, do no harm.'

Group therapies

Some therapies approach the patient not so much as an individual but as a member of a group. As we observed earlier, no one exists in a state of total isolation. The way that we relate to other people influences the sort of person we are, and vice versa. Group therapies attempt to use these beliefs and expectations that we have about other people, and behaviours that we have towards them, to try to bring about enduring psychological change. As with the individual therapies, there is a very wide range of conceptual models and practical methods, coverage of which lies beyond the scope of this book. Some of these techniques lie outside the work of a care worker, whereas others, especially those that relate to the management of more severe mental illness at social and family level, lie at the very heart of the care worker's job.

In its simplest sense, a 'group' means any more than one person. So group therapies may involve couples and parts of or entire families. Alternatively, a group may not consist of people with any previous connection but people who share a common problem or perhaps a wish to share a method of trying to change. Again, the range of groups and methods is very wide, from the 12-step group philosophy of Alcoholics Anonymous to a weekly group run along lines of Jungian psychoanalysis. Still other groups have a more pragmatic purpose, such as the economy of scale that can be achieved by a single skilled worker running a training group in anxiety management, assertiveness or social skills. What all these groups do have in common, however, is that they harness the very powerful effect that other people have upon the way we all think, act and feel.

Couple and family therapies

An important feature of these approaches is that they abandon the central idea of 'the patient' as being the individual with the problem. Rather, all attempts at treatment work on the idea that the problem belongs to the group as a whole. Many trainees who are new to couple and family approaches find it hard to resist the urge to wade in and 'find the one with the problem', which is unsurprising when one considers that much of the basic training for many of the caring professions encourages us to do exactly that. Group and family approaches (the latter being especially useful to help children) take time, patience and proper training before they can be practised effectively, but some of the general principles that these approaches embrace are of relevance to the day-to-day job of the care worker (Fig. 4.8).

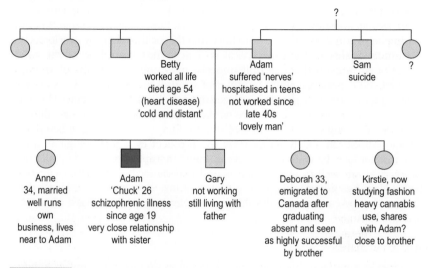

Figure 4.8 ● Geneagrams: a handy way of understanding and recording what happens in a system.

Every member of a family will inevitably have a unique way of seeing the issue, and the skill of the carer lies in trying to understand these various perspectives. It also follows from this that not everyone in a family will necessarily construe the issue as a problem. Consider, for example, a mother in her late 40s. She is unhappily married, her husband apparently preferring to spend his time at a local railway modelling club. She has no friends and her two healthy children have long since left home, leaving her to cope single-handedly with her youngest son, who has chronic severe schizophrenia. When the mother presents with depression and an inability to cope after her son's 10th chaotic admission, just who is 'the patient'? The mother, the son or the reclusive husband? Even this simple vignette illustrates just how widely views on an apparently straightforward issue can vary within a single family. It also helps to explain why not all members of a family may be as keen as others to explore the issues at hand or to actively initiate change. Some family members may, consciously or unconsciously, try to undermine change, preferring the current sorry status quo to the, as yet untested, worry of further change. How freely might this mother cooperate with a care worker for her treatment-resistant son knowing that success might reduce her son's dependence on her, the most important thing left in her world?

In other couples or families, the 'problem' may not be so obvious. Like an iceberg, what is seen above the surface in any given group may only hint at what lies beneath. An apparently straightforward somatic symptom, such as tiredness or headache, may be the earliest signal that power or responsibility is unfairly distributed within a family or that blame, guilt or abuse remain unresolved. An adolescent presenting with episodes of deliberate self-harm may signal discord in the parental relationship as the primary issue rather than adolescent depression. Thus, the notion of a systemic approach is often used by family therapists, working on the *system* of relationships and dependencies rather than focusing on individuals.

Another important aspect of the group approach involves knowing when and when not to use it. A common misconception is that, for a family- or couple-level intervention to work, the participants must necessarily be reasonably intelligent and verbally and emotionally articulate people. This is untrue and, in fact, if individual variations in educational achievement, social disadvantage and communication ability are carefully considered at the outset, even the most complex of problems suffered by the most inarticulate of people may be helped via this method. Nor are extremes of age necessarily a contraindication. Although most family workers are accustomed to working with families with young children, the common misbelief that the elderly are too inflexible to incorporate change into their lives is only slowly shifting and has probably served to prevent many an older family from achieving the changes that they deserve. Generally, there are very few contraindications to the group approach, providing the worker is prepared to act with an appropriate degree of tact and sensitivity from the outset.

There are, however, some people for whom this approach simply does very little. Most care workers, at some time in their practice, will encounter families in which the problems appear so deeply entrenched that they resist even the most intensive efforts to help. Some couples even go so far as to unite against the new common enemy of the therapist, as if the sense of unity and purpose that this creates serves to provide a welcome, if temporary, distraction from the underlying problem. Some, indeed, may appear to thrive on the comforting illusion of being helped and become fixed, disengagement occasionally proving to be a stressful and emotional experience for family and worker alike. A specific 'stuck' situation in which a couple intervention may actually do more harm than good concerns couples for whom the relationship has broken down beyond repair. Although definition of this point of no return is clearly a matter for the couple themselves, therapy can act to delay the moment of decision, sometimes with harmful effects for family members, especially children.

Another group for whom family approaches are probably contraindicated are those individuals who, by virtue of severe personality disorder, are incapable of forming any sustained relationship with others. These individuals very often have a history of extreme difficulties in earlier life, which become quite clearly established as regular patterns of unhealthy behaviours by their mid-teens or early adulthood. Even here, such problems should be considered as a relative rather than an absolute contraindication, given that even the worst of us can change with time and age. But, in cases in which abnormal personality traits, especially of a sociopathic variety, do appear deeply ingrained, wiser workers will usually confine their attempts to simple containment or referral on to more specialist services elsewhere. Remember, for some patients, if they are living at home, are not in hospital and are not in trouble with the law, that is success.

Learning to identify these issues and themes, and successfully negotiating change around them, is very much a matter of time, patience and practice. Many training courses today incorporate group principles into their syllabus.

Some of these are general whereas others may reflect one of the many different theoretical schools of family therapy that have evolved over recent decades. Again, whether any one method consistently has any advantages over the others is unclear and, like the individual psychotherapies, keen adherents to one or other particular model of therapy seem to have about them the air of religious disciples as much as practitioners; however, this should not detract from the central fact that these techniques do succeed in helping many unhappy families, couples and groups explore, confront and change a very wide range of problems.

Other group interventions are structured around specific clinical situations, such as the management of severe anxiety or schizophrenia. An interesting and helpful method that has involved the latter is the Camberwell Family Interview Schedule. This device started out as a research tool used by workers in the late 1970s, who observed that certain types of family attitude, characterised by high or low levels of expressed emotion (EE) towards family members who had schizophrenia, seemed to play a significant role in the outcome of the illness. This work culminated in some reasonably robust findings regarding the influence of families upon the longer-term progress of the illness, which have now been incorporated into sophisticated 'psychoeducation' packages. Training in the theory and use of these models is becoming increasingly available, and many of the central themes are today incorporated into routine community care. We will look at these treatments, more from a social than a family perspective, in Chapter 6.

Physical treatments

Mankind has been using drugs to influence the mind for centuries. Some of the earliest medical treatises, the Hindu Ayurvedas (Fig. 4.9), written around 1500 BC, refer to the useful properties of alcohol, opium, hashish and other interesting herbal preparations. Alcohol and opium were the stock-in-trade of the visiting physician right up to the 20th century but it is really only in the last 50 years that psychopharmacology has become the major player in mental health care that it is today. Before we take a look at the various drug treatments for mental illness, it is helpful to consider how this giant – the pharmaceutical industry – came into existence. Exploring its roots tells us many things about what we can and cannot expect from medications for mental disorders.

The rise and rise of the psychopharmaceutical industry

The two World Wars (1914–18 and 1939–45) changed much more than history, politics and international borders. In particular, they not only altered the way that we treat the mentally ill (especially World War I with 'shell shock') but also stimulated remarkable progress in the pharmaceutical industry. The first antibiotics, the sulphonamides and penicillin, owe their synthesis and mass production to the exigencies of war. By the early 1950s, thousands of new chemicals had been dreamed up and synthesised using methods unheard of in 1914. The problem was that no one knew just what to do with them. Clinically applied pharmacology, therefore, proceeded in an erratic suck-it-and-see fashion, and the big breakthroughs in psychopharmacology of the 1950s owed as much to serendipity as to clever people in white coats.

There was a particular need, for example, for new treatments for tuberculosis (TB). One promising drug, iproniazid, a compound with a three-ringed 'tricyclic' chemical structure, apart from being quite good at zapping TB, seemed to have marked mood-elevating properties. This effect was independent of its antimicrobial properties –

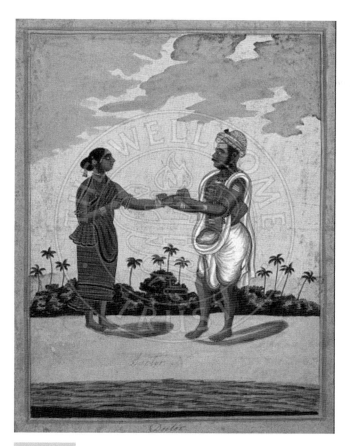

Figure 4.9 ● The earliest reference to psychopharmacology can be found in the ancient Hindu medical tracts, the Ayurvedas.

people on iproniazid cheered up whether or not their TB got better. Thus began the interest in the antidepressant properties of the tricyclic drugs. Soon, a related version of the drug, isoniazid, was developed. Now that the scientists had something to work on, the possible mechanisms of action of this drug were examined in detail.

Isoniazid was found to block the action of an important enzyme in the brain called monoamine oxidase or MAO, and MAO in the human brain was known to be involved in the breakdown of various brain chemicals such as serotonin (5HT), adrenaline (epinephrine) and noradrenaline (norepinephrine). These chemicals, collectively known as the monoamine neurotransmitters, were known to play an important role in the transmission of information between cells in the brain. Therefore, it figured that, if iproniazid could alter mood by inhibiting an enzyme, and this resulted in an increase in the brain levels of, say, noradrenaline, clinical depression might arise from a deficiency of a neurotransmitter in the first place. Thus came about the 'mono-amine hypothesis' of depression, which is still very much in vogue. As we shall see below, antidepressants today are seriously big business. It is no surprise that a recent history of psychiatry was subtitled *From the Era of the Asylum to the Age of Prozac*.

Elsewhere, researchers were studying another group of drugs, the antihistamines, looking at their effects on intestinal worms. One worker noticed a curious effect of a drug called chlorpromazine. Subjects taking this drug displayed a marked loss of interest in and response to their surroundings without any major alteration in their level of consciousness; they remained awake but indifferent. Thus was born the next major class of psychotropic drugs, the 'neuroleptics' or 'major tranquillisers'. In 1953, this drug was tried on people with schizophrenia, with dramatic results. A large number of patients who had for many years been confined to hospital by crippling mental and behavioural problems were suddenly able to lead far more active and independent lives. The word spread. Research into possible mechanisms of action for these fascinating drugs soon followed. In particular, they were found to interfere with the action of another brain neurotransmitter, dopamine. The hypothesis was therefore advanced that abnormalities of this chemical were in some way involved – possibly even responsible for – major mental illnesses such as schizophrenia.

Not all progress came out of the blue. For many years, chemists had sought to improve upon the properties of yet another group of drugs, the barbiturates, which had been extremely popular since the late 19th century. These drugs made excellent tranquillisers and sleeping tablets but tended to be addictive and dangerous in overdose. Marilyn Monroe died from a combination of 'barbs' and alcohol. A related, but safer, group of compounds, the benzodiazepines, was discovered in the late 1950s and rapidly superseded the barbiturates as the world's favourite 'minor tranquillisers' (and made Bayer Pharmaceuticals a major world corporation).

Then something odd happened. Or, rather, didn't happen. For the next 25 years, in spite of vast amounts of money and effort, no new single group of drugs was invented or discovered. Many significant improvements were made to the compounds that already existed, especially regarding their side effects and tolerability, but no really new ground was broken. Hundreds of new compounds came and were hailed as 'breakthroughs' at the time, but none has really had much of an edge on its older cousins. With several key exceptions (see below), it has pretty much stayed that way to the present day.

What has changed over the past 40 years is the attitude of the public to the role and status of psychotropic drugs in everyday life and, indeed, to science itself (Figs 4.10 and 4.11). When the psychopharmacological revolution began in the

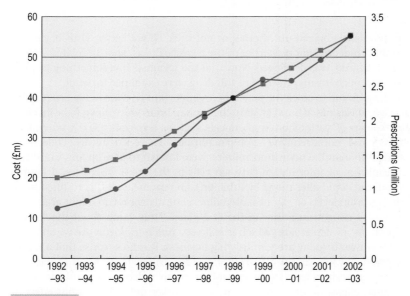

Figure 4.10 ● Increase in the number of prescriptions (grey squares) for antidepressants and the gross ingredient cost (lilac circles) over the past 40 years.

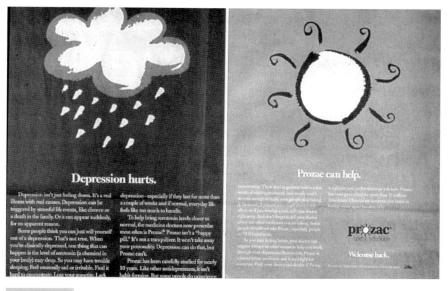

Figure 4.11 ● Blurring the borders of sadness and illness. In the early 1990s the manufacturers of Prozac (fluoxetine) took their campaign directly to the American public, running these advertisements across consecutive pages of 20 consumer magazines.

mid-1950s, the pill-taking public were almost certainly far more trusting and, some would argue, more gullible than they are today. Many people honestly hoped and believed that science would come up with the answers to many of our problems. But by 1969, the growing epidemic of benzodiazepine addiction was teaching the public to be more sceptical about the products – and motives – of the pharmaceutical industry. Box 4.3 summarises some of the great psychopharmacological letdowns of modern times.

The lessons to be learned

THE ROLE OF MEDICATION   There is much in this story of direct relevance to the community care worker. We need to be careful in our claims of what drugs can

---

Box 4.3   Lessons to be learned: some of the great pharmacotherapeutic errors of our time

- Thalidomide: not psychotropic, but the classic case that set the ball rolling
- Purple hearts and mother's little helper
- Benzodiazepines as a 'safe' replacement for barbiturates in the 1960s, ending up with the Roche class action
- Injectable temazepam in liquid capsules
- Suicidal dreams with Halcion (triazolam)
- Zimelidine and Guillian Barré syndrome
- The very late U-turn on thioridazine and droperidol
- Remoxipride, sertindole and the QT interval of the ECG

actually do for our patients. It is a sobering thought that, in spite of more than 50 years of research, we know relatively little about how most of our drugs *really* work on the unbelievably complex organ that is our brain. Drug treatment looks set to remain an empirical business for some time to come, and some humility is helpful. It can stop us from placing undue emphasis on the importance of drug treatment at the expense of the equally important non-chemical aspects of treatment that we have already discussed. In a busy world of high caseloads and crowded clinics, the temptation to fall back on a simple prescription can be very alluring. Psychopharmacological modesty also helps to maintain a sense of proportion in other important ways. Drug treatments are only relevant to a small proportion of the total amount of psychopathology present in the population and are rarely curative in their own right. The unwary care worker, who assumes that a depot injection represents 'the solution' to schizophrenia, runs the risk of making a similar mistake to that made by the Americans in Vietnam. Carpet-bombing an illness with chemicals doesn't necessarily win the battle, you also have to win over hearts and minds.

THE VIEWS OF USERS AND CARERS The attitudes of the public in general, and the patient in particular, to statements about the usefulness of drugs for mental health problems are extremely important. For many, the overoptimism of the 1960s has given way to something much more cynical than healthy scepticism. For some, any attempt to treat mental illness with drugs is seen as a method of social control. Others consider that there is a conspiracy between the medical profession and the giant pharmaceutical companies, each feeding off the other. They reject the idea that it is a genuine effort to try to help sick people. Such ideas are widely expressed in newspaper articles, television programmes and books with titles such as *Toxic Psychiatry*, many of which give quite spectacular emphasis to the side effects of drugs and have probably been produced more to exploit people's uncertainty than to give the facts about drug treatment a fair hearing. Even the Patron of the Royal College of Psychiatrists himself, HRH Prince of Wales, has warned of the menace of 'the liquid cosh'.

The care worker will encounter these ideas in many forms, particularly among those patients and their families who have clear opinions on the political aspects of mental illness and its treatment. A number of co-workers, in the voluntary or local authority sectors, may also be suspicious of pharmacological approaches. Some mental health charities and treatment facilities even have 'no drug' principles written into their constitution. It is important to realise that such views, however forcefully held, should never be regarded – or responded to – as 'wrong', but recognised as a reminder of a need for explanation. When you give a patient a drug, you must always give the patient knowledge at the same time. It is so easy to forget that patients do not share our technical knowledge, in spite of all the information that is available to them from so many sources. These sources, remember, also carry headlines such as 'my date-rape drug hell' or 'miracle drug to cure cancer'. Even the word 'drug' itself has different meanings for different people, illicit drugs such as heroin and cocaine coming top of most people's recognition list.

INFORMATION SOURCES Beware of the sources from which you obtain your own knowledge of drug treatments, especially new ones. Data from pharmaceutical companies should be treated with particular care. In a tough market, where many drugs are more or less equal in what they can offer to patients, it is all too human to put a 'spin' on the advantages of this or that product. Drug reps are also very charming, helpful people, who have access to attractive expense accounts. Cultivate relationships with them but never rely on their product monographs as the only source of knowledge. Regular discussion with your team psychiatrist and reading of up-to-date material from professional sources, as well as the health pages in the press and on the Web, to see what everyone is worrying about this week, will help you stay on top of this vital area of knowledge (see Box 4.4). Two valuable sources of information are the monthly *Drug & Therapeutics Bulletin* (*DTB*; available from every postgraduate centre) and www.mentalhealthnet.com, both of which take a healthily sceptical line on new drug treatments as well as providing regular reviews of established ones.

Box 4.4   Reliable sources of information on psychotropic drugs

- *British National Formulary*: published twice yearly; very comprehensive, practical and easy to follow
- *Drug & Therapeutics Bulletin*: published monthly by *Which*; critical and impartial
- *Maudsley Prescribing Guidelines*
- *NICE Guidelines*

There is a strong and understandable belief among neuropharmacologists that we live in exciting times. For example, we are on the verge of creating new chemicals that can safely reverse many of the nastier symptoms of Alzheimer's dementia. The so-called 'atypical' antipsychotics are likely to turn out to be just the first in a series of 'designer' drugs that will have an ever-increasing specificity for different regions and functions of the central nervous system. Just over the horizon lies the staggering prospect of drugs that are so specific that they can actually 'switch off' genes involved in serious illnesses such as schizophrenia or major depression. And prescribing rights, for so long the exclusive domain of the medical profession, are now being sought by many other professions. Midwives, for example, have been safely using drugs as powerful as diamorphine (heroin) for many years now and this has clearly enhanced the respect given to them by other professionals and the public alike. It is incumbent upon every mental health worker to keep up to date with these changes; the only thing that seems certain is that things will continue to change faster than we can imagine.

The different types of drugs used in psychiatry

Because this is not a textbook of psychopharmacology, the following section seeks only to offer an overview of the main classes of drugs used to treat mental illness at the beginning of the 21st century. Some of the information that it contains may well be out of date even by the time that this book reaches publication. Further details of dosages and other useful information can be found in the sources referred to in Box 4.4. The regularly updated *British National Formulary (BNF)* should always be somewhere within reach.

Psychiatric drug treatments fall into five major categories:

1. drugs to treat psychosis (also known as antipsychotics, major tranquillisers, neuroleptics);

2. drugs to treat anxiety and related disorders (also known as minor tranquillisers, hypnotics, sedatives);
3. drugs to treat depression (antidepressants);
4. drugs to prevent fluctuations in mood (mood stabilisers);
5. drugs to treat problems of substance misuse.

Like any classification, this system is far from perfect as the groups overlap, both in terms of chemistry and usage. For example, antidepressants may often be used to treat symptoms of depression occurring in a schizophrenic illness, whereas chlorpromazine, a well-known antipsychotic drug, can be used at lower doses to treat anxiety or mild insomnia. Sorting this out is largely a question of time and experience, but a useful rule is to try to avoid polypharmacy. By and large, patients should not be on more than one drug from each category.

DRUGS FOR THE TREATMENT OF PSYCHOSIS: ANTIPSYCHOTIC DRUGS, MAJOR TRANQUILLISERS OR NEUROLEPTICS The Ayurvedic physicians of India have been using extracts of the plant *Rauwolfia* to treat disturbed behaviour for over 2000 years. Their potions contain a chemical, reserpine, which disrupts the effects of the brain neurotransmitters serotonin, noradrenaline and, especially, dopamine. All of the modern antipsychotic drugs do something similar and, until recently, 'dopamine-blockade' was thought to be the property essential to their effectiveness.

How do they work? There is a strong relationship between the degree of blockade of dopamine receptors in the human brain and the clinical response to treatment (Fig. 4.12). (Receptors are specially adapted parts of the nerve cell that a specific neurotransmitter locks on to. There are a number of different dopamine receptors, each one shaped slightly differently. The D2 receptor seems, to date, to be the one most involved in psychotic experiences). The greater the affinity of the drug,

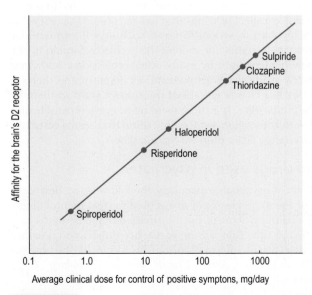

Figure 4.12 ● God's way of telling us we may be on to something. There is a clear linear relationship between the propensity of a chemical to interfere with D2 receptors in the human brain and the clinical effectiveness of antipsychotic drugs.

particularly for D2-type receptors, which are found in the areas of the brain that seem active in organising thinking and feeling and initiating action (Fig. 4.13), the more potent its antipsychotic effect.

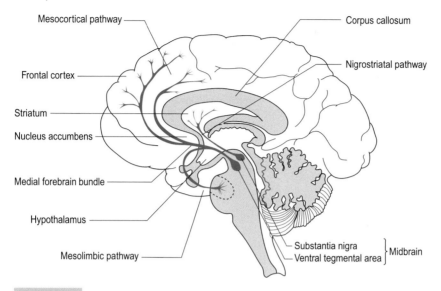

Figure 4.13 ● The main dopaminergic tracts in the human central nervous system.

115

It is a rule of biology that when nature gives you a straight line on a graph, you're usually on to something. The graph in Figure 4.12 forms the basis of current practice in the drug treatment of psychotic symptoms. Once the diagnosis of a psychosis is made, one can start medication and watch how the symptoms change over the next few days or weeks. The graph also contains a great puzzle: although most of the dopamine receptors in the brain are fully blocked within a day or two of starting drug treatment, most patients need several weeks, or even a couple of months, before they start getting better. Any early benefits are usually due to their sedative and, possibly, their movement-slowing properties. Most patients with an acute psychosis, however, suffer not only from the psychotic symptoms themselves but also from unpleasant symptoms of overarousal.

This explains two common observations: why patients often show improvement almost as soon as they reach the ward and why nursing staff prefer to use drugs with sedating as well as antipsychotic properties in the early stages of treatment. Many of the newer antipsychotic drugs are designed to be far less sedating and, thus, often require the additional use of a minor tranquilliser if they are to be used for acute treatment. This distinction between their tranquillising and antipsychotic properties is important, both in managing acute disturbance, when heavy sedation is often useful, and in longer-term maintenance treatment in the community, when it is not. Different stages of an illness will often require different medications.

Positive and negative symptoms Antipsychotics all tend to be far more effective against the positive symptoms of psychosis, such as hallucinations, delusions and thought disorder, than against the so-called negative symptoms, such as social withdrawal, apathy and blunting of mood (see Box 4.5). We say 'so-called' because, to some extent, the negative versus positive symptom dichotomy is an oversimplification. Not all negative symptoms have the same origins. A patient may

Box 4.5   Negative syndromes

Rather than the 'positive' presence of hallucinations, delusions or major mood problems, negative symptoms refer to something missing from the mental state. Thus, negative syndromes involve a diminution in speech, thought, mood and behaviour or a combination of all four. Contrary to popular belief, it is the negative symptoms that constitute the truly awful nature of severe schizophrenia. Voices and crazy beliefs may cause great distress, but they are relatively short-lived and attract attention and even sympathy. Apathetic self-neglect and withdrawal into an emotionally flattened, monosyllabic state is much less interesting and can last a lifetime. It is the negative symptoms of schizophrenia, therefore, that constitute the true burden of the disease for patients, carers and societies. The form and content of positive symptoms changes all over the world and seems, to some extent, to be dependent on culture and local belief. Negative symptoms, on the other hand, seem the same the world over, prompting some to conclude that they comprise the 'true' nature of the illness.

appear withdrawn and apathetic for many reasons; he may, in fact, be profoundly depressed or he may be suffering from a side effect of treatment, such as parkinsonism, that resembles a negative state. Alternatively, he may be suffering from a positive psychotic illness so severe that he has become, so to speak, completely lost inside his own head, to the point where such 'autistic preoccupation' causes him to *appear* to be totally withdrawn and incapable of responding to others. Others may simply be so angry and frustrated by their current situation that their apparently negative state is simply a reflection of their wish to have as little to do with the outside world as possible.

Only when these 'false-negative' symptoms have been eliminated, by careful attention to the patient's mental state or with the use of antidepressants or anti-parkinsonian drugs, can we truly talk of treating the real negative symptoms of schizophrenia. But the extent to which antipsychotics are effective against these primary negative symptoms (with one possible exception that we consider below) remains worryingly unclear.

All antipsychotic drugs are effective against psychotic symptoms, regardless of the underlying diagnosis. They will just as effectively alleviate the hallucinations or delusions encountered in mania as in schizophrenia or, say, an organic cerebral syndrome. This says quite a lot about the shortcomings of the diagnostic system available for disorders arising in something as complex as the human brain, but it also puts paid to the myth that specific antipsychotic agents are the 'drug of choice' for any given condition. There is little hard evidence that any particular drug can be matched to the symptoms of a specific psychotic diagnosis. Some years ago, for example, it was proposed that the drug pimozide was the drug of choice for the treatment of persistent delusions of infestation (Ekbom syndrome). However, subsequent studies have shown equally good results with other antipsychotics. This was probably an example of wishful thinking in an area where our treatments often fall well short of our hopes, but it does show how easily the field of drug treatment can be subject to its own myths and fashions, out of which individuals and companies can build reputations.

Drugs differ widely in many respects, such as their chemical structure, the rate with which they are taken up into the body, their duration of action, etc., but the most important way in which the antipsychotics differ from each other is in terms of their side effects. As with all treatments, side effects of antipsychotic drugs occur when the drug interferes with processes and systems within the body that are beyond the intended target. Some drugs are much 'messier' than others and it is this 'side-effect profile' that defines many of the important clinical characteristics of the drug. One of the first antipsychotic drugs ever synthesised, chlorpromazine, illustrates this point well. The chlorpromazine molecule not only blocks dopamine receptors in the mesolimbic system (see Fig. 4.13), the area thought to be relevant to its clinical effects, but also those in the basal ganglia, giving rise to unwanted motor side effects, and those in the vomit centres of the brainstem, hence its anti-emetic properties. As if this wasn't enough, it also blocks histamine receptors, resulting in sedation, noradrenaline receptors, causing orthostatic hypotension (dizziness on standing, hence 'the liquid cosh'), and acetylcholine receptors, causing dryness of the mouth, urinary hesitancy, irregularities of heart rate and a reduction in the parkinsonism associated with dopamine blockade (it deals with its own side effects!) (see Box 4.6). Chlorpromazine exerts numerous effects on many other tissues of the body as well. These are summarised in Box 4.7. It is a small surprise that the UK trade name for this drug, largactil, echoes these LARGe ACTions. Most of the side effects, particularly those affecting the central nervous system, are 'dose dependent', that is, the higher the dose, the greater both the clinical and the unwanted side effects.

Box 4.6 Neurological side effects of chlorpromazine

- Sedation
- Apathy
- Acute muscle spasms
- Parkinsonian tremor
- Akathesia
- Tardive dyskinesia
- Epileptic fits

Although most of the 'first wave' antipsychotic compounds had many of these unwanted side effects, they revolutionised the practice of psychiatry. Indeed, it is probably fair to say that chlorpromazine and haloperidol were, in part, responsible for the closure of the asylums. Within years of their launch on to the market (mid-1950s, early 1960s respectively), they were in widespread use, transforming the lives of literally thousands of former asylum patients. Unfortunately, popular memory for good news is often short, and soon attention shifted to the more negative aspects of treatment, going on in full view (as they now were) of an increasingly sceptical public. The motor side effects of these agents gave rise to the popular stereotyped belief that antipsychotic drug treatment turned people into mindless shuffling zombies. The cruelty of this perception was doubly unfair: people who had for centuries suffered stigmatisation because of their illness were now suffering because of their treatment. Many people found the drugs unpleasant to take and did not take kindly to the need to take yet other drugs to modify their side effects (see below). They frequently relapsed (some 80% over 2 years) because

Box 4.7   Non-neurological side effects of chlorpromazine

- Dry mouth
- Nasal stuffiness
- Low blood pressure
- Skin rash
- Skin sensitivity to ultraviolet light
- Liver inflammation
- Constipation
- Blurred vision
- Difficulty with micturation
- Weight gain
- Menstrual disturbances
- Gynaecomastia
- Galactorrhoea
- Impotence

of poor compliance with treatment. Worse still, some of the longer-term effects of treatment, which took time to emerge (i.e. a number of years) and were thus named the 'tardive dyskinesias', seemed to be irreversible and difficult to manage.

The pharmaceutical industry went to work to find ways around these problems. In the mid-1960s, dopamine blockers were synthesised in slow-release injectable form, which only needed to be given every 2–4 weeks or so, obviating the need to swallow pills daily. Such drugs proved popular, at least with clinicians and, in the UK, they remain one of the mainstays of treatment to the present day. Over this period, the pharmaceutical industry also kept up its search for newer cleaner compounds with different affinities for various areas of the brain and body. If one could find a drug that blocked the chemical processes related to hallucinations and thought disorders (wherever they might be) whilst sparing those parts of the brain that governed movement, according to theory, one should be able to come up with a much more acceptable treatment. It is testament to man's ingenuity that this theory worked. For the first time, psychotropic compounds were being created through inductive science rather than serendipity (remember, chlorpromazine was first tried out as a treatment for worms!)

The new atypicals During the 1990s, numerous so-called 'atypical' antipsychotics became available. Although they also demonstrate a clear dose–response curve for both antipsychotic and motor effects, they disrupt the latter only at significantly higher doses. Thus, there is effectively a dosage 'window' of opportunity – a range of doses at which many patients may enjoy significant antipsychotic effects without much in the way of parkinsonian and other motor symptoms. Like any new agent, adverse effects will no doubt emerge in time. Already, sedation, weight gain, hyperglycaemia (increased blood sugar) and other odd symptoms such as a stuffy nose are starting to reveal themselves. Whether long-term use of these drugs carries a lower risk of tardive dyskinesia is still unclear.

Many patients certainly do seem to prefer atypicals but, in spite of their advantages, they are only slowly gaining widespread usage. The *National Institute for Clinical Excellence (NICE) Guidelines* (2002) certainly support their use in first-onset psychosis. But old prescribing habits die hard, and the newer agents are still much more expensive than the older ones, some of which are now, in any case, off patent. To protect research costs (which are enormous), pharmaceutical companies are given an exclusive patent over production and sales of a new medication for 5–7 years (varying nationally), after which anyone can sell it. Once off patent, the cost naturally goes down, as with all high-tech products over time. No one should be surprised by the wish of the pharmaceutical industry to make as much money as it can out of its efforts. Nevertheless, it does seem as though these newer agents are a modest 'second revolution' of sorts and that they will be used more and more widely as time passes. Currently, much effort is being put into ways of converting them into long-acting injectable preparations, with the first now being available, namely Risperdal Consta (risperidone).

One particular antipsychotic compound that deserves a special mention is clozapine. This drug differs from all other antipsychotic drugs, typical and atypical, in several ways. It has little or no blocking effect at dopamine receptors but instead exerts a diffuse range of effects at many other sites in the brain. But what is particularly unusual, and useful, about this drug, is its apparently unique effect upon so-called treatment-resistant schizophrenia, that is, symptoms that have failed to respond to other antipsychotic drug treatments. Furthermore, its use carries an extremely low incidence of extrapyramidal side effects (some claim zero). Thus, for many, clozapine is the gold standard of antispychotic drugs and is increasingly becoming the first drug of choice for severe or refractory psychotic illness.

Just how and why it works remains something of a mystery to clinicians and researchers alike, but its benefits come at a price. It is not only the most effective of all antipsychotic drugs but also the most toxic. In up to 2% of cases treated, clozapine causes a dose-independent and potentially fatal agranulocytosis (a loss of white blood cells in the bone marrow), as well as a variety of non-fatal side effects in a much larger number of people. These include somnolence, weight gain, siallorhoea (dribbling), myoclonic jerking and general lowering of the epileptic threshold, rendering the patient vulnerable to epileptic fits. Most of these symptoms are dose sensitive and can be fine-tuned down to a level that is acceptable to the patient by paying close and regular attention to drug dosage, the blood level of the drug (easily measured) and the patient's mental state. For those patients who are unable to achieve this balance, other drugs may be used in addition to control the side effects, for example benzodiazepines to control occasional myoclonus (muscle twitching) or anticonvulsants to modify epileptic problems.

Although clozapine first came on to the market in the late 1970s, well before all the other atypicals, concerns over the agranulocytosis led to its withdrawal. Since its reintroduction, this problem has been simply dealt with by regular (and mandatory) monitoring of the blood of every patient taking it. At the outset, blood samples are taken weekly, and, after an initial all-clear, the dose is titrated upwards slowly, with further blood tests weekly, then fortnightly, then monthly. All samples taken from a patient for the purpose of clozapine monitoring were processed centrally, at the pharmaceutical company's clozaril patient monitoring service (or CPMS). This service came complete with its own forms, result slips and even its own news sheet, keeping the prescriber up-to-date with advances in research into clozapine therapy. Unsurprisingly, the cost of this procedure was reflected in the price of the drug, making it the most expensive drug in the psychiatric pharmacopoeia (costing some £2000–4000 per patient per year or more). More recently mental health trusts have set up their own cheaper systems for monitoring clozapine. Some have suggested that the special aura surrounding these monitoring procedures may somehow have contributed to its apparently greater clinical effect; it has long been recognised that seeing a health professional once every 2 weeks to receive a needle (regardless of whether a drug is given) can exert a powerful effect upon a patient's mental state. However, clinical experience, as well as a handful of studies, do seem to support clozapine's efficacy.

Drugs used to treat the side effects of antipsychotic drugs As we have seen, the drugs commonly used to treat severe mental illness, especially the older ones, are not very 'clean.' They have plenty of unwanted effects, particularly upon the motor nervous system. The acute dystonias seem to affect mainly younger patients, the parkinsonian and akathisia problems can occur at any time, whereas tardive dyskinesia, almost by definition, affects mainly older patients. These effects must be taken seriously, as they can have a very powerful influence on the way that psychiatric treatment is perceived by patient and relative alike; a terrifying episode of acute oculogyric crisis (eyes rolling up uncontrollably) is unlikely to endear the patient to the idea of treatment.

Some of these problems can be alleviated almost totally by the concomitant administration of a group of drugs referred to as the 'anticholinergics'. Their primary action is to interfere with another neurotransmitter, acetylcholine. In the motor part of the brain there is a functional balance between acetylcholine and dopamine. Blocking dopamine in isolation, as the neuroleptics largely do, gives rise to motor problems of stiffness, tremor, rigidity and so on. By blocking acetylcholine as well, the stability of the motor system is somehow restored, with a clear reduction in acute dystonias and Parkinsonian symptoms. These drugs do not have any antipsychotic effect of their own, but at higher doses they can cause a pleasant light-headed sensation that occasionally causes them to be abused. In certain vulnerable individuals, particularly the physically ill or the elderly, they can even cause acute confusional states and so need to be used with care.

Anticholinergics are all short-acting and so should be taken at least twice, if not three times, a day. They are available mainly in oral form, but short-acting intramuscular preparations are occasionally useful, such as when a sudden onset of dystonia causes fear or when the dystonia is of an orofacial distribution that upsets swallowing. These drugs do not seem to work as well against akathisia, which may have its origins in parts of the brain that are not involved in the acetylcholine/dopamine balance. Akathisia also bears a curious relationship to anxiety and may be helped by the short-term use of one of the longer-acting benzodiazepines or by a beta blocker. There is scant evidence, however, that any of these drugs work against tardive dyskinesia, and, if anything, the anticholinergics probably make tardive dyskinesia worse in the longer run.

Given that schizophrenia is such a common illness, forming a large part of the average caseload, it is essential that a care worker is thoroughly familiar with the basic pharmacology of the drugs described here. Knowledge of dose ranges for the most commonly used agents and how to fine-tune doses against symptoms over time, as well as an ability to detect and manage their common and not-so-common side effects, are core skills. A well-thumbed but up-to-date copy of the *BNF* should be on the shelf of every decent community mental health team office.

DRUGS FOR THE TREATMENT OF ANXIETY AND RELATED DISORDERS: THE MINOR TRANQUILLISERS (SEDATIVES, ANXIOLYTICS, HYPNOTICS)

The minor tranquillisers differ in many ways from the major tranquillisers: much more is known about the way that they affect the brain; they are used to treat very different conditions; and they have very different problems associated with their use. Their use is also far more widespread; indeed, they are probably the most widely consumed group of drugs on earth. Over the past hundred years, human beings, having exploited the tranquillising properties of alcohol for centuries, have turned to other drugs to induce sleep, to calm agitated states or to provide relief from various forms of anxiety; these include drugs such as barbiturates, paraldehyde, bromide, chlormethiazole and numerous others. Today, however, most of these drugs have been superseded by another group of compounds, the benzodiazepines, to the extent that (with some recent exceptions) the categories of minor tranquilliser and benzodiazepine are virtually synonymous.

The benzodiazepines work by activating a system in the brain that involves the neurotransmitter GABA (gamma-aminobutyric acid). GABA is one of the main 'brakes' in the human brain; when the GABA system is activated, it serves to dampen down the overall activity of the brain, particularly in the higher regions known as the neocortex. More GABA is found in the neocortex than anywhere else. This explains the ability of these drugs to lower arousal, decrease anxiety and to induce a pleasant state of calm, somnolence and sleep. These are properties that are especially useful in the treatment of anxiety, agitation and insomnia, regardless of cause. If the major tranquillisers are used to treat the psychoses, the benzodiazepines are the drugs used to treat the neuroses. These drugs also seem to lower the outflow of nervous signals to the musculature and so have pronounced relaxant properties that may be of help in reducing painful muscle spasms.

Conversely, relatively few GABA receptors are found in the respiratory area of the brain, and so even at quite high doses, such as that seen in overdose, these drugs cause relatively little depression of respiration, unless taken with large amounts of alcohol. It was because of this low acute toxicity that benzodiazepines so swiftly replaced their more dangerous predecessors, the barbiturates. One pharmacologist, so impressed by the safety profile of these drugs, commented that the only way to die from diazepam was by choking on the lid of the bottle. At the outset, benzodiazepines were used with such enthusiasm that proclamations regarding their absolute safety were taken at face value. This blinded people to other less deadly but significant disadvantages of this new class of compounds, which only became apparent over time.

Although benzodiazepines are very effective in the treatment of anxiety, their use should always be limited to treatment of reasonably short duration. This is because the GABA mechanism adapts quickly to regular exposure to drugs, and so tolerance to the effect of a drug builds up rapidly. In other words, the amount of drug required to obtain the same degree of effect increases quickly. Furthermore, sudden discontinuation of the drug rapidly leads to a state of withdrawal; the GABA mechanism, having adapted to a lower level of activity during repeated dosing of the drug, remains set at low for a while after the tranquilliser is stopped, leading to a period of rebound overactivity of the nervous system. Thus, the 'benzodiazepine withdrawal syndrome' leads to a picture that, at least in the short term, is clinically indistinguishable from anxiety. This is unpleasant for the patient, who may seek to take more of the drug, thereby staving off further withdrawal. In this way, drug use over time may escalate and a dependency pattern may evolve.

The risk of dependency, especially after several weeks of continuous use, is one of the major drawbacks of treatment with this class of compounds. It closely resembles the addictive propensity seen with alcohol, barbiturates and other tranquillisers. Other adverse effects also seem to be related to a disturbance of the brain's basic arousal mechanism, especially with longer-term use. Over time, these drugs can induce lethargy, depression, forgetfulness and often quite subtle disturbances of cognition. Many of these troubles persist long after cessation of exposure to the drug. At higher doses, some of the shorter-acting benzodiazepines can even cause total disruption of memory for short periods. Some, such as triazolam, have been removed from the market because of these quite specific cognitive problems. The status of another short-acting drug, lorazepam, is under review at the time of writing, but its use in acute sedation (even of psychoses) makes it a very useful tranquilliser.

This variation in duration of effect has also been exploited clinically. Different benzodiazepines vary widely in the way that they are metabolised by the body. The longer-acting benzodiazepines, such as diazepam and chlordiazepoxide (which were the first to be introduced in the early 1960s) are broken down into other chemicals, which also exert a tranquillising effect. Thus, a patient may still carry tranquillising products in his or her bloodstream some 72 hours after a single dose of diazepam. This may be ideal if the patient's anxiety causes difficulty during the day, but may be more of a hindrance than a help if the patient also needs to drive or handle a busy job. For such individuals, especially those in whom insomnia dominates the clinical picture, one of the shorter-acting agents is usually preferable.

Several new agents, which are chemically quite distinct from the benzodiazepines, have recently been introduced. Some of these have ultrashort durations of action, so much so that there may be no trace of sedative compound in the body only 3–4 hours after ingestion. Whether these agents really represent an improvement over the short-acting drugs that have been available for many years, such as temazepam, remains to be seen. What we do know is that their capacity to be misused is very similar to that of their predecessors; the problem of benzodiazepine abuse should not be underestimated. It is a sobering fact that virtually all benzodiazepine dependence in the UK is iatrogenic (i.e. induced in a patient by a physician's activity, manner or therapy).

Caution, therefore, is required whenever caring for a patient using benzodiazepines, especially in the longer term. Keep an eye out for sudden inexplicable fluctuations in anxiety, or vague symptoms of lethargy and poor concentration and memory, especially when there do not appear to be other clear reasons for these symptoms. Always enquire about the frequency and duration of prescriptions, and check how quickly a supply is exhausted. The patient's GP, who is usually familiar with the problem of benzodiazepine misuse, will almost always be able to give you helpful information. As a rule, the shorter-acting agents tend to lead to dependency more swiftly than the older compounds. In cases in which you suspect benzodiazepine misuse, do not forget to enquire into the possibility of the parallel use of other minor tranquillisers, particularly chlormethiazole, the newer agents such as zopiclone and zimovane, and alcohol. Interactions with other drugs, especially those that depress the central nervous system, are very important. Although benzodiazepines do not suppress breathing when taken in isolation, they can increase the depressant effects of other drugs and alcohol, with potentially fatal consequences.

If you identify a benzodiazepine dependency syndrome and the patient is willing to participate in an attempt at withdrawal (dependent patients who are not committed to the idea of stopping hardly ever succeed), reduction should always be carried out very gradually, ideally in small steps over months. It is often easier to convert a patient from a short- to a longer-acting agent before embarking upon the withdrawal process, preferably using an agent with which the patient is unfamiliar. The psychological and social state of the patient undergoing withdrawal is as important as the level of drug use itself.

Propranolol This drug is not a benzodiazepine but it is appropriate to mention it here as it is sometimes used in the treatment of anxiety. Propranolol belongs to the beta blockers, a set of compounds that decrease the activity of the sympathetic nervous system by blocking the effects of adrenaline and noradrenaline. Most of this effect takes place in the periphery of the body, outside of the brain. Consequently, propranolol and its relatives exert their greatest effect on the physical manifestations of anxiety: palpitations, nausea, cold sweating, tremor and so on. Although they do not appear to act upon the more psychological manifestations, such as the racing thoughts of panic and catastrophe, the beta blockers nicely demonstrate the close interaction between psyche and soma that is always seen in anxiety states.

By reducing the inflow of somatic anxiety signals to the brain, these drugs reduce the subjective sensation of fear. They tend to be more effective in milder anxiety states or in cases in which a patient dwells unduly upon physical sensations, such as morbid fearful ruminating over a heart attack triggered by panic-related palpitations. This reduction in the somatic element of anxiety does have its drawbacks, however. Beta blockers can cause dizziness, sleep disturbance, tiredness and a lack of mental vitality. An interesting illustration of the lack of mental vitality is the concert violinist who took 20 mg of propranolol to calm performance nerves. Although the reduction in his nervous tremor did wonders for the quality of his *vibrato*, he commented on how emotionally 'flat' he had felt throughout the concert. Bodily sensation is an essential ingredient of emotion, good or bad. Incidentally, propranolol should *never* be given to a patient with asthma or cardiac disease, who may well be relying on his beta-adrenergic nervous system to keep his lungs and heart going.

DRUGS FOR THE TREATMENT OF DEPRESSION: THE ANTIDEPRESSANTS Perhaps no other group of drugs tells us as much about our society as the antidepressants (Fig. 4.14). This heterogeneous group of compounds is one of the fastest growing sections of the lucrative drugs market. Second only to minor tranquillisers and painkillers, every day, millions of people swallow a tablet of fluoxetine, sertraline or one of its cousins. These drugs seem to reflect the growing assumption in our culture that happiness is a normal achievable state, and that any deviation from this is undesirable and should be avoided by any means, preferably chemical. Even the term 'depression' itself has come to take on a wider meaning in recent decades, as ordinary day-to-day unhappiness becomes increasingly construed as an ailment in need of fixing rather than as an understandable reaction to the fact that life is rarely a bed of roses. It is sadly unsurprising that any society quite as absorbed in the 'me first' philosophy as ours should come to talk of Prozac (fluoxetine) as a 'lifestyle' drug or that a busy GP with a crowded waiting room should reach for his prescription pad as an easy end to a consultation with a miserable patient. In the USA, where drug companies advertise directly to the public, full-page advertisements in glossy magazines exhort their readers to 'ask for it by name' and it is a truism that what happens in the USA today happens here tomorrow.

Behind all this fuss about antidepressant drugs lies some simple, much less spectacular, truths. The idea of designer drug-induced happiness is a myth. The antidepressants *do* work, but their effect is far less powerful than many of us would like to believe. Compared, say, with penicillin or even chlorpromazine, their efficacy is quite poor: out of 100 people with a diagnosis of depression who are prescribed antidepressants, only about 50–60% will show much in the way of an effect and, of these, only about one-third will feel the effect to be sufficiently beneficial that they want to keep taking the drug. When one tries to separate out the placebo effect of these drugs from their apparent true chemical effect on the mind (and

123

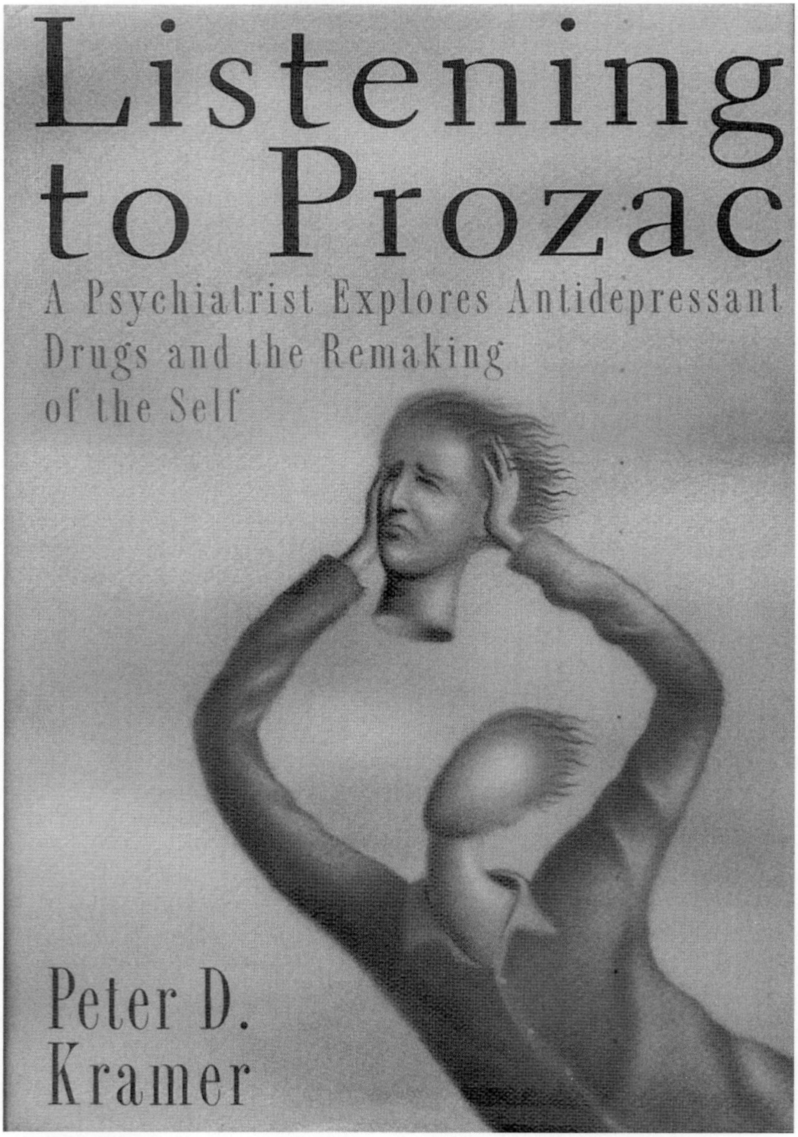

Figure 4.14 ● Pill power: the early 1990s saw a proliferation of books with 'Prozac' in the title. Peter Kramer's 1993 book, *Listening to Prozac*, put the SSRIs at the heart of concern over what became known as 'cosmetic psychopharmacology'.

patients with mood troubles are known to be very sensitive to the placebo effect), their potency seems even weaker. Some studies argue that they have only a 10% greater efficacy than inert sugar tablets. They are certainly not a 'magic bullet' for depression.

What these critics often fail to consider, however, is the design of the studies that come up with these pessimistic findings in the first place. Most involve giving these drugs to people who have been brought together under the common diagnostic heading of 'depressive disorder'. As we saw in Chapter 3, depression is not a homogenous clinical entity. Quite a large number of patients, as any experienced clinician will tell you, do derive quite swift, dramatic benefits from these drugs. The problem is finding out *which* ones these are likely to be. At the present time, our understanding of the emotional part of the brain is so poor that we have no way of doing this. Instead, therefore, we pool together all those patients who apparently have a similar condition. This lumping together of those who respond with those who don't may dilute the observed efficacy of the drug.

There are two clear messages in all this for the care worker. First, if a patient is taking antidepressants, encourage them to do so for long enough and at a high enough dose. At least that way, if the patient is one of those, as yet, biologically unidentifiable responders, he or she stands the best chance of getting a result. Research shows that many of those who fail to respond may simply not have bothered to take the drug in the first place or have taken it for only a short time at a low inadequate dose. The second message is really one of the central themes of this book, namely that if all the patient is doing about their depression is taking a drug, you are not doing your job properly.

How to make sense of the different types of antidepressant Another curious feature of antidepressants is that they all appear to have much the same efficacy as each other, regardless of their chemical structure. The more churlish have taken this as evidence that chemical activity therefore has very little to do with it, although this is hard to square with common clinical experience. What is significant about the differences in chemical structure are the ways in which different compounds carry different side effects. In fact, when it comes to understanding the differences between antidepressants, side effects are *the* most important issue. Despite what the drug companies may say, there is no evidence that, as a direct result of its antidepressant effect, one group of drugs is simply better than any other or any one product is more suited to the treatment of a particular sort of depression. Instead, what usually clinches it are the side effects seen with each preparation.

The earliest antidepressants were potent inhibitors of the brain enzyme monoamine oxidase, hence they became known as the MAOIs. Although reasonably effective as antidepressants, they had a potentially fatal interaction with an important ingredient of some foodstuffs, tyramine. This could lead to dangerous fluctuations in blood pressure, and so patients taking MAOIs were obliged to eat a restricted diet, the most problematic component of which was cheese. These drugs also tended to cause weight gain, fluid retention and tremor, and interacted dangerously with many other common medications (e.g. anaesthetics). They were especially dangerous in overdose, a behaviour not uncommon among people suffering with depression, thus they became difficult to use clinically.

The MAOIs were swiftly superseded by another group of compounds, the tricyclic antidepressants (TCAs). For three decades after their introduction in the late 1950s, these drugs became the accepted standard of antidepressant treatment and many, such as amitriptyline, imipramine, clomipramine and dothiepin, are still prescribed today, particularly by GPs. They lacked the diet-related problems of the MAOIs but were almost equally high risk because of the way that they potentially interfered with the rhythm of the heart. Overdose could easily lead to fatal cardiac arrhythmias. TCAs also carried other less drastic side effects, including drowsiness, constipation, dryness of the mouth, weight gain and a fine tremor. Although feeling drowsy was welcome for some, particularly those suffering with sleep disturbance (and amitriptyline is still used today as a mild, non-addictive hypnotic), these other effects remained troublesome and led many patients to stop

125

taking TCAs altogether. Nevertheless, they continue to have a substantial role in the treatment of both depression and chronic anxiety, especially when patients are non-responsive to SSRIs (selective serotonin reuptake inhibitors; see below).

This dissatisfaction with side effects led to the introduction of many new compounds, with a bewildering variety of shapes and names. Although some were derived from older drugs and were dubbed the 'second generation' tricyclics, many new drugs were derived from completely new formulations. Over the following 20 years, the market exploded. Evidence of this explosion can be found by spending a few minutes browsing through the central nervous system section of the *BNF*.

The early 1980s saw the arrival of a group of compounds that had been refined not only because of their apparently more tolerable side effects but also because they appeared to have a much more focused effect upon specific neurotransmitter systems in the brain. Zimelidine and fluvoxamine were the first of the so-called SSRIs. The drug companies wasted no time in marketing these new agents as a significant breakthrough in the treatment of depression, which by then was accepted as a discrete and legitimate clinical entity, even though the term 'clinical depression' had scarcely been used before 1950. This combination of marketing, cultural change and genuine clinical need seems to have sparked what may be termed an epidemic of interest in antidepressants. Prozac entered the English language, and countless books such as Elizabeth Wurtzel's *Prozac Nation* became best-sellers. But in spite of the enthusiasm for these new compounds (which echoed the introduction of the benzodiazepines in the 1960s), they still carried no real advantage over their predecessors in terms of efficacy against depression. Their side effects, however, do seem less troublesome than those of the TCAs in that they are safe in overdose and tend to cause disruption of gut rather than cardiac function, causing nausea, loss of appetite and diarrhoea in 5–30% of cases. Like their predecessors, they also cause a number of sexual side effects, which are only slowly coming to light, but it is really only their relative safety that truly justifies their use in preference to the older agents.

There is a small amount of evidence that SSRIs may be better at treating some forms of anxiety disorder than the older more problematic compounds, and the evidence that SSRIs may be of help in obsessive compulsive disorder is stronger still; however, against simple clinical depression, the condition for which they are still most often prescribed, unequivocal evidence of superiority is non-existent. Nor is there necessarily anything new about the idea of specificity for brain serotonin. Clomipramine has been shown to be a potent and specific inhibitor of serotonin, even though it is a TCA, and its use in the treatment of obsessive compulsive disorder was recognised long before fluoxetine was promoted for this.

All of this has not stemmed the flood of new compounds on to the market. Selective noradrenergic reuptake inhibitors and all sorts of other acronymous groups continue to appear: NASSAs, RIMAs, etc. None is significantly better than the rest. Some are sedative, others less so. Some companies claim that the less-sedating agents, such as venlafaxine or paroxetine, carry activating properties that may help patients with diminished energy, whereas other agents such as mirtazapine are better for more agitated cases. Other companies claim that their drug works more quickly than the rest. But for every individual whose response seems to justify these claims, there are many more for whom it may cause the opposite effect. If the antidepressants tell us anything, they tell us how little we know about the brain.

DRUGS FOR THE PREVENTION OF FLUCTUATIONS IN MOOD: MOOD STABILISERS A variety of compounds are often prescribed for patients who, when unwell, display marked changes of mood. Mood swings are not necessarily confined to oscillations between elation and depression, but also include irritability, anger, impulsivity and other emotional states. Some drugs can decrease both the intensity and the frequency of these swings, for reasons that remain unknown. These drugs include lithium, as well as certain preparations with anticonvulsant properties, such as carbamazepine, sodium valproate and lamotrigine. These are usually used for patients with more severe forms of mental illness, including manic depressive disorder (bipolar affective disorder; BPAD), treatment-resistant depression and schizophrenia-like illnesses that are strongly coloured by mood symptoms, sometimes referred to as schizoaffective disorder. They may also be used in cases in which marked changes of mood seem to be part of a more general disorganisation of personality (e.g. cyclothymia).

Lithium The sedating effects of lithium have been recognised for centuries, and the first use of this drug for the regulation of mood disorders in humans reaches back to the late 1940s. Although quite a lot is known about the effect of lithium at the cellular level, no one has any idea how it alters something as complex as human emotion; none of our knowledge about lithium fits in a clear way with the monoamine theory of mood disorder.

Lithium remains in quite widespread use and is a drug with a narrow therapeutic margin, that is, the gap between therapeutic and toxic doses is quite small. It is therefore important for the care worker to know about the details of lithium treatment. It is most commonly prescribed as a prophylactic (i.e. protective) agent in mood disorders, although some psychiatrists still use it as a first-line drug in acute manic states. Lithium affects many systems in the body, most significantly the thyroid gland, the nervous system and the kidney. All patients being considered for lithium treatment should be given a full medical examination and routine investigation of thyroid function, renal function and cardiac function (by means of an electrocardiogram). Only once these tests have proven clear should the first dose of lithium be given. Treatment should begin with small doses over the first few days, and the care worker should watch for side effects that commonly occur at the outset, including diuresis, varying degrees of weight gain, dry mouth, fine tremor and a metallic taste in the mouth that some have likened to a cross between sucking on a tin and garlic. For most patients, these symptoms subside over the first week or two, but for a minority, they prove troublesome, especially weight gain and polyuria.

As the dose is increased, in 200-mg steps over days or weeks, regular blood testing should be performed to determine the level of lithium in the blood. At first, these tests should be performed every few days or so, until a steady level is attained within the therapeutic range of 0.7–1.2 mmol/L. For most patients, this can be achieved with total daily doses of between 800 and 1600 mg of lithium per day. Lithium also comes in a puzzling variety of preparations, of which lithium carbonate is the most common and most practical. Significant differences exist between the active amount of lithium salt contained in each preparation, and it is important to keep an eye not only on the dose but also on the brand of lithium prescribed, especially if there has been a recent change of prescribing doctor. Once a stable state has been attained, it is essential to check the blood level every 3–6 months, no matter how stable the patient may seem.

To obtain a clear measure of the steady level of lithium in the bloodstream, testing should be carried out about 12 hours after the most recent dose. Periodic tests of thyroid and kidney function are also necessary, as is constant vigilance for the signs of possible toxicity: tiredness, excessive thirst, deteriorating tremor, nausea, diarrhoea (which can further compound toxicity), confusion and loss of consciousness. Usually, toxic effects are seen at lithium levels above 1.6–1.8 mmol/L.

127

Patients should be encouraged to keep well hydrated, especially during vigorous exercise or during unusually hot weather. Lithium treatment and monitoring should *always* be carried out under the supervision of a doctor.

Discontinuation of lithium treatment, whether because of side effects or lack of efficacy, should always be carried out carefully and slowly, withdrawing in 200-mg steps over a number of months. Even if the patient has been well for years, there is still a significant risk of withdrawal ('rebound') mania (up to 25%!), which is greater if the reduction is too brisk. Those patients who, for whatever reason, stop and start their lithium treatment, and so experience sharp fluctuations in lithium blood levels, often have a much higher incidence of affective episodes.

Other mood stabilisers Less needs to be said about these agents as they generally tend to be safer than lithium, although carbamazepine is very occasionally associated with suppression of the bone marrow and an eye should always be kept out for signs of infection, particularly sore throats and fevers. Carbamazepine, valproate and other similar drugs are often used after an unsuccessful trial of lithium, and it is becoming increasingly common for them to be used singly or together, particularly in cases in which relapses have been multiple and frequent. They often tend to cause a greater degree of drowsiness at therapeutic doses than lithium, although most patients soon become tolerant to this. In situations in which this remains troublesome, the daily dose can usually be divided into two, thereby reducing the 'peaks' achieved shortly after ingestion. One other important point about these drugs is that they stimulate a number of enzymes in the liver and can thereby result in complex changes in the blood levels of other medications that the patient may be taking for other conditions. Regular monitoring of their level in the blood is also necessary and routine, to avoid the potential for toxicity. Unlike the measurement of lithium levels, this is not needed to determine therapeutic dose ranges but merely safety levels. Close medical supervision is always a good idea whenever patients are on combinations of drugs. Very little is known about the way in which these mood stabilisers work in the brain.

Other physical treatments

For many, psychiatry has long been associated with physical treatments other than drugs. This is easier to understand when we consider how different civilisations have dealt with the problem of mental illness over the last thousand years. For most of this time, while ideas and symbols of evil forces and humours dominated our thinking about mental illness, physical methods, especially incarceration, were *the* principal and only effective way of dealing with serious mental illness (Fig. 4.15). Thus, the idea that the mentally ill need putting away or need to have something 'done to them', formed over centuries, is still alive and well today. The humane treatments that have come into widespread use only over the last 50 years still have a long way to go before they erode the memories of strait-jackets, purgatives, spinning chairs, cold showers and all the other forms of mistreatment that once passed in the name of therapy.

Like it or not, psychiatric treatment is still synonymous with torture for many people. Prolonged narcosis therapy with barbiturates was used in the 1950s and 1960s, in spite of the absence of any clear benefit. Insulin coma therapy was last used in the UK in 1970, well after its therapeutic futility was established. The relevance of this to the care worker is more than historical, as the two remaining physical treatments that do confer a genuine therapeutic benefit – electroconvulsive therapy (ECT) and psychosurgery – are still surrounded by this age-old shadow of fear, stigma and pessimism. Any care worker hoping to engage a patient or a

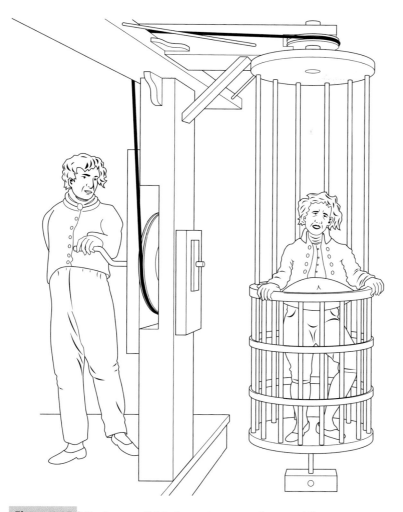

Figure 4.15 ● The horrors of Victorian-era treatments for mental illness.

relative in a meaningful discussion about the pros and cons of these treatments will need to accept that these negative attitudes will tilt the playing field against them from the outset.

ELECTROCONVULSIVE THERAPY If there is one subject in the entire field of mental illness on which almost everybody has an opinion, it is ECT. The merest whisper of these three letters can turn sweet little old ladies and mild-mannered accountants alike into raging polemicists. Very few people are ambivalent about the subject, most seeing it either as a particularly barbaric form of punishment or as a desperate, last-ditch treatment for a life-threatening illness. Type the letters ECT into any search engine and you'll see what we mean. In amongst the high emotions of this debate, the truth is sometimes hard to establish. In spite of many years of high-quality research into the subject, it is still possible to argue for and against ECT. How do they manage without it in Germany, for example?

The truth is probably that ECT is a highly effective, moderately drastic thera-peutic option for severe depression (and catatonia), which should be used only when there is either grave and immediate danger to life or when all other thera-peutic avenues have closed. Much of the anger over ECT doesn't concern whether or not it works, but whether or not it is used indiscriminately. There is plenty of evidence, especially from the 1940s and 1950s, that it was used too often, without other options being considered. This is understandable given that mental services have been undervalued and under-resourced for so long that drug and psychologi-cal alternatives have often not been available. However, as people are becoming much more aware of their entitlement to the best available treatment, this defence is becoming ever weaker. The secret to the appropriate use of ECT, therefore, is to treat all patients as fully as possible before it becomes necessary to use ECT, so that its use, by definition, becomes limited to genuinely resistant illnesses. Sooner or later, most care workers will encounter such a situation, and so it is important to know how it is given, when it is given and what its effects and side effects are.

When to use ECT There are three main psychiatric conditions in which ECT is the unequivocal treatment of choice. Psychotic or major depression with pro-found motor retardation may result in the patient being too ill to hold a cup to his or her lips, leading to potentially life-threatening dehydration. In other cases of major depression, risk of death by suicide may dominate the picture. Catatonic schizophrenia or uncontrollable mania may lead to collapse and coma through exhaustion. The first condition is relatively common, particularly among the elderly, but the other two tend to be rare. There is now a large amount of evidence which shows that ECT is also highly effective against lesser degrees of depression, although less drastic interventions may be equally helpful. The contraindications to ECT are few (only a recent heart attack being an absolute contraindication), and are more likely to be due to the hazards of the anaesthetic that invariably accom-panies the ECT than to the treatment itself. Elderly and physically ill people, par-ticularly those with epilepsy or heart disease, may simply be too unwell to undergo the procedure. This underlines the importance of the involvement of an experi-enced anaesthetist at every session of treatment; decisions regarding the wisdom of anaesthesia should always be left to a medical practitioner.

How it is given ECT should only ever be given at a site adapted for the purpose. The absolute minimum required for any adequate ECT suite includes one of the more mod-ern ECT machines, a trolley with a head-down tilt mechanism (to prevent aspiration of unanticipated vomit), and full anaesthetic and resuscitation equipment, recently tested and stocked; most of this equipment is there to cope with the very rare complications of the procedure. ECT machines themselves have become quite sophisticated in recent years. All of the modern ones now permit an adjustment of the amount of electrical energy that they discharge during any one treatment, allowing a downward titration of the administered current with successive treatments. As we will see, this facility is important in helping to minimise the side effects of treatment. Many machines also incorporate a single-lead electroencephalogram (EEG) facility to confirm that a convul-sion has in fact occurred, something that is not always easy to identify visually if the patient has been fully relaxed by the anaesthetic given beforehand.

Every effort must be taken to put the patient at ease before treatment. When more than one patient is undergoing treatment in the same session, it is prefera-ble for the semiconscious to be allowed to recover in an area away from those still awaiting treatment. No matter how well assured, a profoundly depressed patient is hardly likely to take heart from seeing a fellow patient being wheeled past pros-trate, in a semi-conscious, post-ictal haze.

The actual administration of ECT has changed a lot over the last 50 years. Before the early 1960s, electricity was administered directly to the head of the alert patient. The subsequent unmodified convulsion often led to violent flailing of the limbs, biting, incontinence and, on some occasions, crush fractures of spinal vertebral bones, as the powerful back muscles went into spasm. Two important milestones in the history of ECT were the introduction in the 1960s of short-acting anaesthetics and muscle relaxants, which allowed these dreadful complications to be avoided, and the 1975 release of the film *One Flew Over the Cuckoo's Nest* starring Jack Nicholson, which led most people to think that they still occurred. Modern ECT is now far removed from most people's perception of it. The patient is placed on his or her back and encouraged to breathe oxygen through a face mask whilst a brief anaesthetic is given. Conducting jelly is then applied to two points on the head (see Fig. 4.16) where the electrodes are to be applied. Once in place, the smallest amount of current necessary to induce a convulsion is given, usually via a trigger button situated on the handle of one of the electrodes. The electricity is usually given in the form of a pulsed or square waveform. This leads to a fully blown tonic–clonic generalised convulsion, only perceptible as a tremor of the limbs in the anaesthetised state, which typically lasts for up to a minute. Thereafter, the patient almost always regains consciousness within 5–10 min, but often feels drowsy or disoriented for a short period. Some amnesia for the time around the event is common.

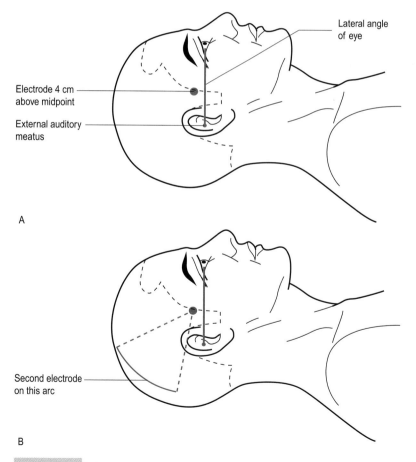

Figure 4.16 ● Placement of electrodes for (A) bilateral (both sides of the head) and (B) unilateral (one side of the head) electroconvulsive therapy.

Although very little is known about the way that ECT exerts its antidepressant effect, some things have been ascertained. For example, we know that it is the convulsion itself, rather than the simple passage of electricity through the delicate tissues of the brain, that is responsible for the mood-altering effect. Convulsions induced by non-electrical means give similar antidepressant results. The degree of amnesia after the treatment correlates with the actual amount of current passed, especially when one considers cumulative dosages of electricity over time. Amnesia can be minimised to some extent by the unilateral application of current to the non-dominant hemisphere (see Fig. 4.16), although this method may be less reliable in initiating a convulsion. Post-treatment loss of memory and the possibility of longer-term brain damage are two of the issues that make ECT such a controversial business. Research shows that ECT does indeed cause memory problems in the longer term, but these usually only become troublesome after multiple courses of treatment, suggesting that some form of cumulative process may be at work. A small minority of individuals, who are sadly impossible to identify beforehand, do seem particularly sensitive to these distressing cognitive side effects, but it should not always be taken for granted that complaints of poor memory or concentration are exclusively the result of ECT. In a treatment that arouses such powerful emotions, amnesia, forgetfulness and muddled thinking can arise from many causes, not least the severe depressive illnesses that require ECT for their resolution.

In spite of all its recent sophistication, the actual sight of ECT being given is still quite a daunting event to witness. Ideas and feelings that have been thousands of years in the making cannot simply be rationalised overnight. It is a good idea for every care worker to visit an ECT clinic to see it first hand. Most hospitals have a consultant who takes a clinical 'lead' in the overall running of the ECT service. They are almost always willing to allow people along for a visit, patient confidentiality allowing. Such a visit will always be a valuable experience when it comes to dealing with the issue of ECT, as is likely in the course of your work.

Summary

Physical treatments, mainly in the form of medication, are an integral part of modern psychiatric practice. They are not by any means a panacea, although their success rates are as good as, if not better than, many of the treatments given in other branches of medicine. They have also made it possible to cope much better with the dreadful handicaps of mental illness, in particular the psychotic states such as schizophrenia that tended to confine people to large mental hospital for half a lifetime or more. In this sense, and despite the understandable concerns about 'drugging patients up' and pharmaceutical company exploitation, it is in many ways modern medications that have both enabled a community care approach and given voice to the increasingly vociferous 'user' movement. By enabling patients who were previously mute and incarcerated to have a say in their treatment needs, medications can be said to have profoundly altered many people's lives. Knowing their place in continuing care, their benefits, problems, dosages and side effects, is a must for anyone working in this field. Likewise, keeping up to date with research and innovation in this area, maintaining a healthy scepticism and a keen critical eye, and always keeping the patient's best interests to the fore are core aspects of modern psychiatric community care.

Going home

5

Introduction

Perhaps the very title of this chapter is a paradox, as it assumes that community care has failed. The fact that a patient has to prepare for 'going home' indicates that they have an illness that is severe enough to have required hospital placement. Given the increasing investment in crisis response teams with their home-based treatment programmes, one might think that there would be a *reduced* demand for hospital beds. Sadly, although such teams and programmes do exist, they often (up to now, at least) reflect short-term, research-led interventions, which can hold things for a year or two but which increasingly end up resorting to inpatient care 5 years down the track. No one disagrees that, especially in stable suburban communities, many fewer beds are required than in the past. However, the fact remains that community care workers will regularly be faced with helping a patient return home from a hospital admission.

The process of getting someone out of hospital and into a stable home, or home-like environment, is the most demanding and fulfilling task of the community care worker. If it is done successfully much else falls into place, because the transitional phase, the first few days and weeks after discharge, is a known risk period for suicide. It is now even a routine requirement for contact to be made within a week of discharge for all patients deemed vulnerable in any way (see below). The discharge process can also colour a patient's whole future if not handled properly. It means understanding the role of the hospital, the problems of being in hospital and the versions of 'home' that are available locally. It means talking through with the patient just what you can and can't do. It means being routinely realistic without being negative and taking on the role of the 'care coordinator', particularly in the context of the Care Programme Approach (CPA). It means being aware that the classic, headline-grabbing, untoward incident occurs at the ward/community interface. It means knowing the personal meaning of 'home', the worries, memories, people and relationships that the patient will be facing.

What do hospitals do?

Many people have no idea what happens in hospital, especially a psychiatric hospital, despite the burgeoning number of television medical soaps. It is worth clarifying this because getting someone home means enabling them to live without the complex – and often quite dependence-inducing – support provided by modern psychiatric wards. Although there are arguments as to the usefulness of doing (apparently) very little, watching television and sitting around in an institutional lounge, it is often amazing how helpful this process can be. This is not to say that active groups, occupational therapy (OT) and personal counselling sessions should not be encouraged, but just 'chilling' can, in itself, be a form of respite for anxious, frightened patients. There seem to us to be at least six key features of psychiatric inpatient care.

A safe environment

A safe environment can be seen as the sanctuary role for which the asylums were originally envisaged in the 18th century. That is, the day-to-day regime is structured, predictable and reassuring. By and large, wards are designed with security in mind, in terms of sight lines for the nursing staff, safety in windows and doors (usually unlocked), and rounded edges to furniture. Regular environmental checks should be carried out to ensure that there are no ligature points (e.g. hooks to hang oneself from) or hidden/potential weapons. However, there should also be spaces for privacy and quiet alongside group areas for meetings, watching television or even playing games. Both night and day, the rhythm of the unit, centred around meal times, changing nursing shifts, ward rounds and community meetings, provides a pattern of regular events (often unappreciated by outsiders) that is intrinsically reassuring to an individual confused by hallucinations, depressive fears or other distressing symptoms.

Getting the balance right between careful support and an overcontrolling regime is the continuing dilemma for all psychiatric ward staff. Delivering observation, advice, practical help and private counselling alongside an insistence on basic ground rules, acceptable behaviours and compliance with medication takes great skill. Ensuring that an acute psychiatric ward remains smart, clean and welcoming also takes top-class management skills, from pushing the health authority or trust into providing replacement equipment, fresh paint or new carpets to keeping the nursing team enthusiastic, well-trained and in good morale.

The role of nurses

The skills of psychiatric nurses, as mentioned above, are often less obvious than those of their uniformed colleagues putting up drips and measuring physiological indices in high-tech units. Nevertheless, the simple ability to talk to someone who is confused, without condescension and without irritation, is a vital skill. The ability to stay calm and to listen, perhaps to the same story repeated again and again, or to cope with repetitive and at-risk behaviours (sometimes quite frighteningly assaultative) takes maturity and courage. Nurses are there to carry out all nursing functions; these include measuring blood pressures and pulses, weighing people, ensuring that medication is taken regularly and safely, and protecting individuals from often severely suicidal beliefs and impulses. In this regard, one of the most difficult nursing jobs is 'special' observations on a one-to-one basis. This may require being within a metre or two of an individual and literally watching over them day and night. The process can be intrusive and distressing for watcher and watched, but can also be vital in holding someone's hand through, so to speak, their darkest hour.

Apart from the practical tasks, such as ensuring that patients wash regularly and eat appropriately, escorting them on walks out of the hospital at the beginning of leave periods and writing up observational notes in the ward records, psychiatric nurses are trained to understand the psychology of individual distress.

This involves recognising symptoms, explaining them to patients, their relatives or other relevant professionals, and evaluating the effects of treatment programmes, whether psychological or pharmacological. The reason why acute psychiatric wards can cope with many forms of distress is because they are staffed by trained nurses. It is not uncommon, therefore, for patients to be admitted 'in crisis' from a residential hostel, to show no particular difference in their initial behaviour on the ward, but to settle down quickly because of their sense of reassurance that people are aware of their distress and know how to deal with it. The 'nursing process' is an amazingly effective way of caring for those in need.

Essential skills for working on a psychiatric ward include the ability to empathise, an awareness of cognitive processes, expertise in de-escalation and, sadly, training in 'control and restraint' (C&R). The first two have been described in Chapter 4. They involve techniques for getting patients to open up about their symptoms or fears, and ways of providing positive alternatives (i.e. different ways of thinking about their problems), subtle corrections and a sense of hope. Calming down angry and agitated patients (de-escalation) also requires adopting the right tone and posture, keeping patients talking, and offering mini-rewards for good behaviour (a cigarette, a cup of tea), yet making clear the boundaries of the acceptable. If these are breached, C&R, making sure (beforehand ideally) that there are enough nurses around and safely restraining, medicating and making the patient safe, are the key elements of good quality care. (More information on the management of aggression can be found in Chapter 8.)

All psychiatric units should have a 'crash team' to deal with such emergencies – just like a cardiac crash team in a general hospital – which is appropriately trained and organised to minimise any at-risk behaviours. Likewise, a psychiatric intensive care unit (PICU), usually with 10–15 beds, locked and with extra staff, is a great asset in supporting the front line, taking patients for agreed periods during their admission when they are too agitated for an 'open' ward.

The Mental Health Act

Part of the reason for being in hospital is that the 1983 Mental Health Act (MHA) uses the phrase 'and requires treatment in hospital' for people being treated against their will. This may seem anomalous in the age of community care, but nevertheless remains a statutory requirement. Thus, if it is felt that a patient requires treatment, for example because they are so manic that they can't sleep or because they are rushing around the streets shouting at people, dominated by the belief that toxic rays are controlling their brain, then the risks to their and other people's health may obviously require inpatient care. By definition, they need to be removed from the home and public environment. Others, of course, may not be so obviously 'at risk'. The older woman sitting quietly at home, overwhelmed by hallucinations but not apparently causing trouble, may only be at risk to her own health because of self-neglect or suicidal ideas. You may want to treat her at home; however, this is currently impossible unless she willingly agrees to accept medication, for example antipsychotic drugs.

Hospital units, therefore, remain central to the initiation of treatment, especially treatment for those who have no insight into their need for medication. It should also be understood that most patients come in voluntarily – about 60–70% overall, although a lesser proportion (sometimes only 20–30%) in some inner-city areas – because they want the help and security that is offered. However, it is

135

still possible to use the MHA if they become too ill to accept necessary treatment or insist on leaving despite their own vulnerabilities. A registered mental health nurse (RMN) in charge of a ward can use Section 5.4 of the MHA, enabling detention of a patient for up to 6 hours pending a medical assessment. Likewise, a doctor [the 'responsible medical officer' (RMO) or the 'nominated deputy', to use the official terms] can detain an inpatient for up to 72 hours pending further review under Section 5.2 (see Chapter 9 for details). These powers again reflect the role of the psychiatric ward as an integral part of patient care.

Diagnosis

It is often forgotten that working out what is best for those with a psychiatric illness can be quite difficult. It is hard to reach a technical diagnosis without actually knowing whether someone is sleeping badly, coping with day-to-day tasks or able to look after themselves, and so time spent in hospital can be very fruitful in understanding what is *really* going on. This works both ways. Patients complaining of all sorts of considerable difficulties may come into hospital and settle down quickly, and the ward and community team can be reassured that home care is perfectly feasible. Alternatively, symptoms hidden from the community team can emerge in hospital, because, for example, the patient's tendency to talk to his voices throughout half the night will become noisily apparent to all and sundry. Consecutive mental-state examinations and more formal psychological testing can elicit problems that remain hidden in the limited overview available from occasional visiting at home.

A ward can also establish a clearer insight into patients' social skills. Do they talk to others at all? Do they partake in any kind of group – whether an OT art group or just a game of scrabble? Do they establish any kind of friendships or do they just hide away in their rooms, trapped inside negative symptoms or paranoid beliefs? How good are they at handling their money? Are they easily exploited by other patients? What about washing, looking after their room and their clothes, and communicating with family and/or friends? These social observations will be vital in seeing what help is needed, what improvements may be required and how a patient will cope independently.

Treatment approaches

Putting someone on medication is a significant decision. The use of major tranquillisers or antidepressants does come with risks and side effects, and starting such treatments under observation on a psychiatric ward is both practical and informative. Side effects, for example sedation or unpleasant muscle spasms, can be observed and dealt with quickly. A patient's response to medication can be monitored and even charted. Standard assessments such as the Brief Psychiatric Rating Scale (BPRS) can be very helpful in monitoring improvement. More urgent treatments, such as electroconvulsive therapy (ECT) for the severer forms of depression, probably always require inpatient admission. In a sense, each patient's response to treatment can be seen as a research trial, ensuring that one only goes on with effective treatments, that patients are comfortable and have insight, and that the pitfalls of non-compliance can be avoided. Never forget that some 50% of all the pills prescribed in general practice end up time-expired in bathroom cabinets, and close vigilance is also needed in hospital. It is not uncommon for patients to suddenly start improving when switched from pills, for example, to a syrup or a liquid preparation.

A modern approach to treatment, and in particular to medication, involves detailed insight training. This can be delivered very effectively in a ward because of the levels of observation available. It requires some training but essentially uses a cognitive approach to get the patients to be aware of their symptoms and how they affect their lives. 'If you keep getting hauled back into hospital whenever the voices get so loud, why not try and keep them damped down (with the medication)?' This can go on to them weighing up the pros and cons of medication, and (hopefully) choosing to go on using what seems to keep them well. Subtle adjustments in dose or type of drug can enhance their sense of having control over how they feel.

Respite care

Part of the reason for going in to hospital is that it gives relief to those at home. This should *not* be undervalued. Research into carers' attitudes and problems usually shows that they undertake enormous responsibilities, have often dealt with violence or abuse, and are embarrassed to ask for help. The emotional response of families to patients, especially those with schizophrenia, can be a vital therapeutic factor in ensuring that they stay well. If put under too much stress, however, families themselves become counter-therapeutic or even 'toxic'. The classic research into 'expressed emotion' (EE) indicates that properly supported families, aware of their emotional responses and knowledgeable about the illness, can be helpful in preventing relapse by keeping the EE low.

Linking hospital admission with family work can be most fruitful by not only helping the carers and the patients but also reducing the long-term need for repeated admission. Families are often mightily relieved by the admission of their relatives (although they might not wish to say it openly), which is why the process of going home needs delicate negotiation with them. Even the most successful home treatment teams do not exclude respite admissions as part of ongoing care. The true 'burden of care', often changing but rarely diminishing, can often be fully appreciated only by assessing patients in the hospital setting.

Hospital wards – the problem

Although being in hospital should be therapeutic, admission can create problems in itself. Modern units, particularly in urban areas, tend to accumulate literally the 'maddest' people of the community, and 15–20 psychotic individuals in one place can produce a frightening scenario. Behaviours can be infectious, symptoms can be magnified and the effect can be more than the sum of its parts. As a result, one can get tawdry 'madhouse-type' surroundings, food can be institutional and regimes too rigid. This loss of individuality can affect both patients and nurses, and there is sadly a high burnout rate for nurses working on some acute inner-city wards. The mix of genders, classes and ethnicities readily creates further tensions, and illness behaviour can even be reinforced in vulnerable people. Control rather than care becomes the dominant style.

For example, those with personality disorders, a tendency to somatoform presentations (i.e. what used to be called hysteria), and drug or alcohol dependence will somehow absorb and react to the atmosphere. They will act out or stir up trouble, or simply collapse into extreme states of dependence. Staff may become cynical, detached and uncaring, taking on the role of stroppy house servant or even 'school bully'. The cynical visitor's comment, so typical of such units, would be: 'I can't work out who is the patient and who is the nurse'. People can also be in hospital for all the wrong reasons (for example police or court insistence, lack of money, social isolation in the community) and so moving them will be actively resisted. Never underestimate this strange, perverse appeal of the acute psychiatric ward to some folk. Getting them discharged can be like pulling Mr Blobby out of quicksand – you can't work out where you are supposed to get hold of them and every attempt seems to result in their becoming even more stuck.

Getting out

Given this background, and let's hope that the ward environment is something positive, any move-on plan must clarify the reason for admission in the first place. Was it voluntary or involuntary? Was neglect or even abuse at home a significant factor? Have there been previous discharges, particularly in the last year or two, understanding the pattern of which could help in getting things sorted out this time? Are there difficult neighbours who will object? Are there supportive ones who can help? Most important of all, does the patient wish to leave hospital? Some do, some don't, and some are quite ambivalent. They really do not know what to do.

All these issues need to be borne in mind when planning a return home and, of course, the best time to start planning this is as soon after admission as possible. Getting a flat repaired or benefit documents sorted out within the first week or two (or at least clarifying what needs to be done), rather than waiting for someone to 'get better', makes a lot of sense. Many of these issues are taken on board, of course, in the CPA documentation. This document is so essential that a typical CPA form is shown in an appendix to this chapter. Nevertheless, what is the CPA?

The CPA (Care Programme Approach)

The CPA has become the gold standard of appropriate community care although it has tended somehow to overawe people, not least because of the language involved and the paperwork required for its implementation. One commentator has called it a combination of 'good clinical sense ... and administrative absurdity'. Do not be put off by this because the heart of the matter is extremely simple. The original reference to the CPA comes from the Department of Health (1990) and is entitled *A Care Programme Approach for People with a Mental Illness Referred to Specialist Psychiatric Services* (joint Department of Health/Social Services circular HC(90)23/LASSL(90)11, HMSO, London). It is one of a number of documents published by the Department of Health outlining the needs and priorities in mental illness; one of the more recent documents to be published was *The Spectrum of Care: Local Services for People with Mental Health Problems* (1996). The debate over the CPA is summed up in Table 5.1.

Table 5.1 ● CPA – the pros and cons

Pros	Cons
Coordination of care – patient/family/GP/CMHT	Excessive paperwork required to document needs/meetings/plans
Multidisciplinary input – medical/nursing/social/OT/psychological/voluntary	Patients dislike large meetings discussing their personal details
Bridging the ward/community team interface	Changing personnel can make process formal/impersonal/stressful
Defined responsibilities and agreed review mechanism	Promotes organisational process over personal contact time
Clearly documented care plan, regularly updated (including crisis response)	Documentation tends to repeat what is written in medical notes
Appointment of a key worker/care coordinator responsible for coordination	GPs very rarely have time to attend and there are time pressures on RMOs
Effective targeting of resources to SMI on a graded basis	Possible increased time in hospital due to administrative delays
Full needs assessment in terms of housing/social/psychiatric problems	Needs assessment cannot necessarily deliver what is asked for (i.e. false optimism engendered by 'ideal situation' scenarios)
Can be audited/evaluated to assess activity (and funding requirements?)	Danger of substituting form filling and box ticking for dealing with emotional needs
Tool for quantitative (+/− qualitative) clarification of local health needs	Number crunching for DoH rather than reinforcing empathy and care

CMHT, community mental health team; DoH, Department of Health; OT, occupational therapist; RMO, responsible medical officer; SMI, seriously mentally ill.

For those not so keen on reading these thoughtful but somewhat opaque government publications, there is a useful summary in the appendix at the end of this chapter. Used as a tool and for organising information, coordinating care and documenting for health authorities that things really are being done, CPA should be an effective flag-waver for mental health in general. It should also not be confused with terms such as 'case management' or 'care management', essentially the model derived from practice in the USA, whereby people being discharged from mental hospitals had support arranged by a kind of middle man, agent or 'broker'. This individual did not actually help with the patients directly, for example in terms of counselling or filling out forms, but merely organised the services. The effectiveness and the costs of this model have been called into question, and the modern thrust is for care workers to become directly involved in helping their patient/client/user/customer.

The practicalities of CPA are quite simple. It outlines who does what, what is to be done, how follow-up will be arranged and how closely a patient will be monitored. Its three core features, therefore, are: (i) the provision of a care coordinator; (ii) a needs assessment; and (iii) agreeing who is going to meet those needs. The term care coordinator means that member of the community care team who is going to take responsibility for that particular patient. It will be his or her job to fill out the forms, see the patient regularly, arrange the next meeting, and bring into play any other specialist or resource that might be helpful. The care coordinator is, so to speak, the spider at the centre of the complex web of community networks and, in terms of local knowledge, knowing who to contact and how to contact them is a vital part of taking on this role. This means, of course, that as the care coordinator, you don't just need to know the number of the housing department but probably need to take time out every now and again to wander around the local area, check out the cafes and local restaurants, see what's happening in terms of local sports and leisure facilities, and keep an eye on the local press for new initiatives. A good care coordinator knows the patch and enjoys being there.

In terms of that troubling phrase 'needs assessment', do not be overawed. Anybody's basic 'needs' can probably be boiled down to three big questions. That is, what do you do during the day, where do you sleep at night (i.e. live), and who do you need to have regular contact with in terms of social and therapeutic input (i.e. counselling, medication, support)? Daytime activity is generally covered by work or not work and, if the latter (as is sadly often the case), a care coordinator should think about day centres, drop-in facilities, local college training initiatives, voluntary networks or even organising activities themselves. For example, taking a few patients on a trip to the seaside (on a nice summer's day) can be refreshing, a break from routine and give insight into how they are coping.

With regard to where a person should live, this is outlined in detail below (What is a home?); it means working out whether an individual can look after themself. With help, in fact, most people can, although some of us may have to ditch our more house-proud tendencies. With regard to the third need, namely therapeutic and social contacts, it's worth listing the people actually seen by a patient in the course of an average week. Sometimes this can be depressing, with it being perhaps just oneself and the local shopkeeper, but, not uncommonly, friendships with other patients, obscure relatives or even cheerful neighbours can emerge. If medication is involved, particularly depot medication, the community psychiatric nurse (CPN) will be involved. She or he may visit the patient at home, be based at the GP surgery or work in a specified depot clinic (and you may in fact be the CPN!). Medication is often the glue that ensures a person's social situation remains stable, in terms of where they live, what they do and whom they see, and should probably be considered as the fourth need in the core list.

Having established a care coordinator and worked out the needs, the final step of a CPA is deciding and defining who is responsible for what. Thus, you may want to enlist a psychologist to do some bereavement counselling, an OT to help with some practical skills and training or even, for example, a dance therapist to help with posture and physical exercise. Imposing activities on someone who is a little bit shy and withdrawn is probably unfair though, and there is no point in being too critical about patients who like sitting around and doing nothing. Many of us love sitting around doing nothing. In fact, when you consider many of the formalities of meetings and ward rounds, sitting around and doing virtually nothing is sometimes called work (especially in the higher echelons of the NHS).

Modern CPA also demands some acknowledgement of risk assessment and, therefore, a crisis plan to cover possible relapse. The terms used to decide the intensity of post-discharge care – or continuing community care – are 'enhanced CPA' and 'standard CPA'. The former involves more frequent contacts, for example weekly, or perhaps more often in times of crisis; earlier intervention if the patient seems to be becoming unwell; and more people being closely involved (e.g. the consultant being part of a regular review). Standard CPA applies to those who are quite settled, who are known to be compliant with medication and who have stable home lives. Occasional contact, for example once a month or even less, might well be sufficient.

A crisis plan should be outlined for all patients, including a checklist of the signs of relapse (a 'relapse signature'), what to do and who to contact, making sure that this is available in the notes/emergency clinic/crisis team records. Some patients will want to draw up their own agreed 'advance directive', which can be most help-ful for carers, crisis teams, acute wards and (of course) themselves. This directive should be negotiated with all those involved (family, care coordinator, perhaps the GP) and copies kept by everyone. Typically, it would include the kind of help that patients would like (home support, timing of hospital care, diet and even things to be said), the medications that they would prefer, and who they would like to look after them (if possible and available). Research into advance directives is rather limited, but the very process of negotiating them can be helpful to all concerned.

What is a home?

Getting someone home means having some idea of what one means by 'a home', and establishing whether or not there is one in the first place. The notion of home is almost magical in modern European culture. Thus, phrases such as 'there's no place like home', 'home, sweet home' or 'home is where the heart is' are built into our personal hardwiring. One of the most popular pieces of classical music of the second half of the 20th century was Dvorak's *New World Symphony*, particularly the part entitled 'Going Home'. In the archetypal, asylum-as-a-nightmare, 1948 movie *The Snake Pit*, one of the inmates of the asylum gets up and sings a song to the Dvorak tune that goes as follows: 'Going home, going home, I am going home – all my friends and family waiting at the door.' Although this may seem somewhat sentimental, behind these maudlin phrases lies a very serious problem, namely, the tragedy of people who, for whatever reason, have no home. Mental illness is a com-mon home-breaker and, after several failures at resettlement or reintegration, it is not surprising that many patients start to prefer the ward as home. There, at least, they are accepted, it's warm and there are people around.

The accompanying algorithm tries to make some sense of how one goes about getting people home, however that may be defined. Thus, having answered in the affirmative the question of whether there is a home to go to, the next question is whether the patient is going to live alone or with other people or even with family. By contrast, if there is no home, what are the alternative resources in the com-munity. The answers to the question 'Is there a home?' can be summarised as follows:

1. Yes, with a family.
2. Yes, alone.
3. Yes, family or alone (temporarily).
4. No, provision required.

141

Going home to family

With luck, the family will want – or at least be happy to accept – their relative back. This may be stated overtly, both in public and in private (check this), and if there are no contraindications (for example, the possibility of abuse in any form or exploitation), it should be actively pursued. Best practice involves visiting the family at home beforehand and talking through what has happened in terms of the illness and symptoms. Educating them about the specific illness and medication, whether individually or in carer groups, and looking at their attitudes towards mental illness in general, can clarify what support they will need. Making sure that they attend relevant CPA meetings is vital in helping them understand what care plans are all about and in getting their cooperation. Advising them about financial matters, in particular disability living allowance (DLA) and the criteria for various levels of this, can help ease monetary worries.

Concerns about critical or even hostile attitudes can be helped (and there is good research evidence for this) by psychoeducation, formal programmes of which are available. Ensuring medication compliance, agreeing on signs of relapse (mother often does know best) and making sure that there are daytime activities that will get the patient out of the house should be part of this discussion; simple things, such as a travel or leisure pass, can oil the wheels. Making sure that respite and relief care is available, that they know who to contact and that the GP has been informed of any prescribing needs is all part of the necessary reassurance. Leave them your card, or something similar from the team, with details of phone numbers, addresses, names, etc. If you haven't got an address card, get one! They are simple to produce, look professional and are much less likely to get lost than a torn-off scrap of paper with an illegible number scrawled on it.

Going home alone

This can be a more daunting prospect for a patient, because the solitariness of sitting in a bedsit, perhaps in a rather neutral block of flats, can be discouraging to say the least. Try to remember what it was like when you first left home, for example to go to college or on a training course, and the difficulties of adjusting to a different style of living. If it's an old flat then it is vital to check that all the facilities are there (gas, electricity), that it's secure and warm, and that there is food and basic equipment for cooking. This should all have been done before discharge, of course. The most useful assessment can be the ADL (assessment of daily living), usually carried out by an OT. Using that as a guide, you can work out how often you should visit, whether you should think about an additional care worker going in to help tidy things up once or twice a week, and even whether it is worth considering having a local volunteer or tenant visit on a daily basis.

Perhaps the biggest problem is money. Most of us can't control our money, and people who have been in hospital are often short of money and are unused to having to buy all the regular things that are provided automatically when in hospital. Bills that appear out of the blue are usually quite distressing. In this sense, it is best for people to have a rechargeable key for electricity, for example, and (if possible) to have their money handed out to them on a regular basis. Lump sums tend to disappear horribly quickly, and if cannabis or alcohol (or even worse, crack) are 'regular habits', it can be tempting for many to spend money on these pleasures rather than on baked beans or some spare toilet paper. Negotiating money with your patients can be difficult, though, because most people want to look after their own money. If it's a real problem, however, taking out a guardianship order (although clumsy) can be the only solution. If patients keep coming into hospital because they run out of money, and they resort to stealing or begging and neglect themselves, it seems cruel to allow them to keep doing this. Drug dealers are particularly sharp at preying on vulnerable souls such as those with chronic schizophrenia.

The other aspect of going home alone is the consideration of risk. People on their own get lonely, depressed and may think about harming themselves. Formal risk assessment considers what people have done in the past, what their mental state is when they go home (e.g. are they still a bit paranoid) and what factors in their local environment can make things worse or better. Many symptoms are hidden, and sending home a slightly depressed, possibly paranoid older man with a tendency to drink and a history of impulsive behaviours should be carefully considered. An early home visit, within a week, would be a must. This is just the kind of person who, in a fit of remorse, perhaps over a long weekend when he has seen no one for a few days, will decide that life is not worth living.

Balancing out this risk alongside the need for an individual to be able to make their own 'life choices' can be very difficult. Again, the provision of a regular support worker, coordinating regular visits, and close monitoring of mental state, medication and a person's surroundings can help with getting things right. Best of all, a nice place to live in (rather than a cold, high-rise, semi-bare flat) is a considerable boost to morale. We often underestimate the effects of our surroundings on how we feel and how we live. Even a pet can change a person's sense of isolation or despair. No matter how unrealistic some patients are in wanting their own place, it is often surprising how well some do cope, given the right level of support.

143

No home to go to

If there is no home to go to, you have to consider what is realistically available in your locality, what your patient can cope with, and how to help him or her decide. It may also be difficult to be clear about what the right placement would be. Some people seem to do quite well in hospital, demonstrate good skills with the ADL and insist that they can look after themselves. It is difficult to go against such optimism, and there are a lot of pressures to accept that people can be independent. After all, we all see ourselves as being independent, we all recognise another person's wish to have their own place, and it is very much the spirit and philosophy of community care.

Often, the more naive patients will somehow expect that a nice little house, perhaps with a garden, will be theirs for the asking, given their 'vulnerable' status. It can be somewhat saddening to have to explain that this is unlikely to be the case. Sometimes, new properties, refurbished to good standards by housing associations, do come up, but there are usually delays in getting on to the right list. A regularly updated checklist of what is available and what new projects are coming on to the market, with useful phone numbers of people in the housing business, is vital to a good community health team. In fact, knowing the local housing/hostels/

residential placement scene is probably a more important skill than being able to counsel someone, and certainly more important than having a knowledge of one of the more esoteric forms of 'therapy'.

How does one decide what type of housing to go for? A brief summary of ideas that can be used to help make up your mind is given below, although telling a patient what is best is always a delicate procedure. In the end, you can only try to stay realistic, give the best advice that you can and make sure that there is a safety net available if you think that someone is not going to cope.

Independent living

Independent living is what everyone wants, not least because it seems to give people more money in their pocket in terms of day-to-day expenditure. Knowing how to contact the local homeless action group, how to access the council housing list and fill out the forms and how to get all the 'points' that are necessary to get priority (which may require a doctor's/consultant's letter to corroborate matters) are the essentials of getting such a residence. If you think that someone who is currently in hospital can look after their money well enough, deal with the basic needs of cooking, keep the place clean and sort out the various bills, demands, etc. that come through the door, it is certainly a reasonable option. Potential antisocial habits, such as being noisy or playing loud music at night, leaving on the gas ring or allowing rubbish to accumulate, should be taken seriously. Complaints or harassment from neighbours can precipitate relapse, and the cycle of failure to live independently has a depressing effect on the way that people see themselves.

Supported housing

There are a number of standard descriptions of what is meant by low-dependence, medium-dependence and high-dependence care. In essence, these revolve around the amount of staff input that is required to support people in the tasks of living. A weekly visit, a daily visit, 2–3 hours support a day, all-day support or 24-hour support are the usual options. The last one will probably amount to what have been called '24-hour staffed' residencies, and the government is being pushed to provide money for such placements. The experience of most community mental health workers is that the higher the dependency needs, the more difficult it is to find people somewhere to live. There is also the difficult problem of getting hostels, of whatever dependency, to accept patients who may have had a history of drug abuse, prison or violent behaviours. Trying to cover up their past 'misdeeds', however, is an absolute mistake. It will simply put you at risk, as well as the patient and staff in the hostel, and doesn't do anybody any good. Try to emphasise the current situation, the support you will offer and the improvements made, and agree on a trial period if necessary.

Most hostels, whether voluntary or run by the local social services department, should have a standard admission procedure. This will involve visiting, filling in some forms and, perhaps, an overnight or weekend stay. This can be very off-putting to potential residents, and you may have to spend quite a lot of time explaining what it's all about. Accompanying, encouraging and being positive about how things can pan out are essential to this kind of work. It is also probably reasonable to keep more than one iron in the fire at any one time. This may require a bit of fancy footwork, but delays can accrue, which quickly lower morale. A personal relationship with those working in the hostels is an absolute boon in these circumstances. Regular telephone and written contact, making sure that you get to meetings on time and having a clear idea as to the kind of folk that a particular place does well with are all part of the game.

Other alternatives

This is when things get difficult. If your patient wants to get out and there's no reason to stay in hospital, but there is no home to go to, the council refuses to accept him or her because they have wrecked too many houses already and there's no appropriate hostel place, what do you do? It may be that the situation is unrealistic. You will have spent hours on the phone, filled out far too many forms, tried to persuade your patient to accept a given hostel place, and explained until you are blue in the face the problems of funding and the reason why he/she will have only about £14 a week at Happy Care House. You point out that having the rent/food/light/heating, etc. all included will make life easier to manage, but to no avail.

Meanwhile, the ward is really pushing you because they are short of beds. The nurses on the ward, the tetchy consultant psychiatrist, the relatives that keep well in the background and your community team leader are all getting on your back. You know quite well that wherever you place your beloved punter, he (unfortunately, it is usually a 'he') will be back within a few months. How do you minimise the risks, try to square the circle and at least give him some time in the community, however inadequate you think the place might be? Remember, although this placement may fail (probably *will* fail), it doesn't mean that you've done something wrong or let him down. In fact, it could be a vital learning experience to get him to accept the appropriate place. In our experience, that's how most people do get to the right place in the end, by learning where they can cope and where they can't.

Listed below, in no particular order, are some possible options for alternative placements:

1. Stay with a friend. This might just be another ex-patient, a gullible aunt or a good-hearted evangelist from a local voluntary group. Give it a go and visit regularly, at a time when you know the patient will be in, to see how things are going.
2. Queue up at the local homeless unit. This needs a letter, the right timing (i.e. getting the patient up before 8:30 AM and into the queue) and the right language of 'vulnerability' and 'needs'. The result will be bed and breakfast in an unsavoury hotel, a not very popular flat or (sometimes) quite a nice place. Again, keeping in touch will be vital.
3. The street (all versions thereof). This means that patients have to fend for themselves and turn up at the local Salvation Army or other homelessness hostel. You can give them the address and see how things work out. Sometimes, the outcome is excellent. Sometimes, you get criticism from, for example, the neighbouring borough where they have ended up. You need to make sure that you have done the right risk assessment but never entirely exclude this option.

Adult fostering

If this doesn't exist locally, move on to the next section. If it does, you should have thought about it some time ago. Schemes vary from borough to borough and county to county, but usually involve the same thing as is understood by foster care for children. That is, a patient goes to live in a household, rather like taking up lodgings in the old days. Patients have their own rooms, meals are provided and the carer/householder is aware of the background illness and perhaps helps with things such as shopping, medication, laundry, etc. Often such carers are ex- (or current) nurses who are very happy to supplement their income. Stable, middle-aged patients who just need a bit of 'mothering' (or 'fathering') are most suitable. Female patients do better than male, and it often works out best as a temporary placement before getting something more definite. That is, if all goes well, the patient may want to move on to their own place; if they seem quite dependent, they can be quietly ushered into a continuing-care hostel with regular care workers.

In our view, this kind of placement (a bit like boarding out in 19th century Scotland) is something that needs to be much more available. It does require an active placement team to advertise, regularly review and support the placements available. But the flexibility of care that can be provided is immense. Many people do have a spare room, do need the money and quite enjoy having someone else around. It gets round the classic problem of loneliness and lack of support, while providing a homely atmosphere, one or two hot meals a day, television in the front room and, perhaps, a pet or two to take for a walk. If you don't have such a resource in your area, you and your team should be agitating to get it developed.

CPA meetings

Once you have identified the right kind of home, got the patient to agree, sorted out the relatives and/or residential workers, lined up the benefits and obtained whatever grants might be necessary (e.g. community care grants to provide furniture and fittings), there are still those awful meetings to face. That is, you have to make sure that everyone knows what's going on, that the whole 'package' is accepted and understood, and (most of all) that you have a happy punter. Also, by and large, patients dislike meetings and explaining to them the need to sort things out can be hard.

Meetings are always difficult to arrange. Getting the time right so that everyone who needs to can attend (and doctors are impossible in this respect), making the atmosphere friendly but efficient, and not intimidating those with limited social skills are all part of the process. Remember, respect everyone's views, don't be evasive when answering questions and be careful not to be seen to overpower people. Be realistic about expectations. Don't, for example, say that you can get the top rate of DLA if you are not certain; this is getting more and more difficult nowadays. Some things may best be said in a one-to-one meeting rather than in the broader group. Meetings that last for more than about half an hour can become stuffy, boring and lose their focus.

Some people also suggest that there can be a kind of therapy in meetings. Remember, in particular, to be aware of unexpected or new information coming out of the blue. Sometimes this can be very helpful. People react with 'Good God,

I never knew that', and there is a degree of enlightenment. Sometimes, sadly, some nice arrangement comes unstuck because, for example, there is a dispute about eating or smoking habits, or because someone's changed their mind. Try to think yourself into the situation of trying to fit into a brand new social grouping, particularly when you don't feel like a particularly clever person. Remember the famous quote of Groucho Marx, that he wouldn't be a member of any club that would have him.

Many patients with relapsing mental illnesses have remarkably low self-esteem, which they find hard to explain, especially when surrounded by bright and competent professionals. Some research into just what support workers should do and what they should talk about showed us that money, housing and medication comprise 90% of the important topics. Concentrate on these in the meeting, keep a record of what is discussed (or even better, get someone to take notes for you) and write it up as soon as possible afterwards. Ideally, write it up straight away, even if it means staying on after the meeting. If you can learn to use a dictaphone, you will be on the front line of modern voice technology. How else do you think this got written?

What should a care coordinator do? (see also Chapter 7)

In terms of getting someone home, the important thing is to remember that this is a transitional phase. Be clear in your mind how often you should see someone, particularly in the first few days and weeks, and where you should see them. This may be a mandatory duty. Keep a notebook or card listing the kind of things that you want to talk about and any particular or personal details that might need checking up on. As well as money and how things are going in terms of the flat or house, keep discussing ideas about leisure, sport, local training colleges, etc. Don't forget also that drug dealers, loan sharks and the advertisements in tabloids that you and I laugh at can be much more alluring to some of your patients. A little bit of street wisdom, around music, art, the local cafes and dance clubs, doesn't go amiss. In the early days of going home, problem times tend to be weekends, particularly holiday weekends, so think about what support can be offered. Is there a duty CPN who can visit? Is there a church or voluntary group event going on that you can take them to? Advice about the simplest of things, such as where the mains water tap is in the case of a leak or how to 'bleed' a radiator, can be really useful.

One thing that most patients will *not* want to talk about is their sexual situation. This is embarrassing, personal and often a problem if they are on medication. It's also probably very dangerous to start talking about sex if you are, for example, a heterosexual male looking after a female patient or vice versa. Visiting patients at home, on your own, could be seen as exploitative, and if you have any concerns about this, *always go accompanied*. However, advice on what's safe, the possible symptoms of sexually transmitted diseases and where to buy condoms may be genuinely helpful. For example, advising your less pernickety male patients that washing regularly and smelling nice can help with their sexual advances can work wonders for enhancing self-care. In more enlightened areas, it may even be possible to 'advise' patients that they can obtain sexual services cheaply and safely, but this is probably best not documented.

147

If there are any basic rules about being a care coordinator in terms of finding people a home, they probably centre around the following core themes:

1. If in doubt, write a note and make sure that it is clear and dated.
2. Keep the GP informed about what you are doing.
3. Provide support but be careful about companionship. Key workers move on, and the task is to link people in with a social network, not be their only companion.
4. Remember 'transition fear'. Things are always more difficult in the first few weeks, and one or two relapses doesn't mean that things are working out badly.
5. It may often seem as if things are in semi-chaos. Bed demands, money, paradoxical injunctions, a change in the weather, difficult neighbours, all of these might screw things up.
6. Remember, for some patients, the fact that they are not in jail or on the street but are in contact with someone is a remarkable success.
7. Don't let the work intrude into *your* home. That is a separate, private place and you should *not* be in the phone book.

Summary

Getting someone home can be frustrating, complicated and boring, and will often get you criticised. It can also be wonderful, rewarding and bring tears to your eyes. Like most procedures, and a medical example might be useful to understand this, the greater the preparation, the easier the task. Thus, a lumbar puncture – sticking a special needle in between two vertebrae in the backbone until it enters the spinal cord space – is rather a nerve-wracking procedure. However, if you reassure the patient, get them in exactly the right position, even if it takes 10–20 minutes, have everything lined up beforehand and laid out, and generally act like a clucking hen, the act itself is a cinch. The same goes with getting people home. Know your patch, expect local opposition, delays and complications, use temporary solutions and keep people informed. Remember the plaintive song of Eliza Doolittle 'All I want is a room somewhere', and that everyone feels like this at some time in their lives.

Appendix 1 Key dates in community care

1959 Mental Health Act
Abolished previous legislation and magistrates' orders; introduced mental health review tribunals.

1962 *A Hospital Plan for England and Wales*

1963 *Health and Welfare: The Development of Community Care* (Ministry of Health)
These outlined plans for restricting hospital services to acute care in the district general hospital while developing local authority services for community care.

1975 *Better Services for the Mentally Ill*
Promoted a continuing shift from hospital to social services care.

1983 Mental Health Act
Introduced 'consent' procedures, the Mental Health Act Commission (MHAC), 'approved' social workers and aftercare responsibilities.

1988 *Community Care: Agenda for Action* (The Griffiths Report)
Community care was 'everyone's distant relative but nobody's baby' – funding needed.

1989 *Caring for People: Community Care in the Next Decade and Beyond: Caring for the 1990s* (Department of Health)
No mental hospital closures unless funded alternatives in place, but little central finance or commitment.

1990 *Care Programme Approach (CPA) for People with a Mental Illness Referred to the Specialist Psychiatric Services* (HC(90)23/LASSL (90)11, Department of Health)
Outline of CPA and its central role in aftercare.

1994 *Guidance on the Discharge of Mentally Disordered People and their Continuing Care in the Community* (HSG(94)27/LASSL(94)4, Department of Health)
Mandatory formal inquiries to be set up for any 'untoward' incidents.

1994 *The Report of the Inquiry into the Care and Treatment of Christopher Clunis* (known as the Ritchie or Clunis Report, NE and SE Thames Regional Health Authorities)
The iconic homicide inquiry that generated the Supervision Register, a Supervised Discharge Order and (in time) more community resources.

1995 *Building Bridges: A Guide to Arrangements for Inter-agency Working for the Care and Protection of Severely Mentally Ill People* (Department of Health)
A response to the 'crisis' generated by the Clunis Report.

2000 *The NHS Plan: A Plan for Investment, A Plan for Reform* (Department of Health)
The outline of new services for mental health, including assertive outreach, crisis intervention and early intervention teams.

2002 *Community Mental Health Teams, Mental Health Policy Implementation Guide* (Department of Health)
Summarising the structure, staffing and role of community mental health teams in line with the NHS Plan additions outlined above.

2006 *Avoidable Deaths*
The 5-year report of the National Confidential Inquiry into Suicide and Homicide by People with Mental Illness. Asks for strengthened observation and CPA procedures, while noting no increase in rate of homicides by the mentally ill over the previous 5-year period.

149

Appendix 2 A sample CPA form

CPA – Care plan

Care plan date _____

Forename		Surname	
NHS No.		Date of birth	
PSA No.		Social services no.	
Main telephone no.		Other telephone	
Address			
CPA level		MHA, legal status	
Diagnoses		ICD-codes	

Name, address, postcode, contact numbers	
General practitioner	
Consultant/RMO	
Care coordinator	
Others (carers, relatives)	

Identified needs		
Accommodation		☐ Yes ☐ No
Employment		☐ Yes ☐ No
Social contacts		☐ Yes ☐ No
Education		☐ Yes ☐ No
Psychological		☐ Yes ☐ No
Medical		☐ Yes ☐ No
Language		☐ Yes ☐ No
Religious, cultural & spiritual		☐ Yes ☐ No

Summary of care plan

All different service options discussed with the service user and carer.
Service user/carer views and preferences, priorities and objectives, reasons for choice of services must be given. List all aspects of the care plan (medication, follow-up, social, psychological and medical interventions)

Agreed action/plan/intervention	Responsible health professional

Contingency and crisis planning

Early warning signs; relapse indicators; triggers; location of any advance statements; whom to contact, service response

Agreed action/plan/intervention	Responsible health professional

Summary: clinical risk assessment and management	
Agreed action/plan/intervention	Responsible health professional

(Non) Attendees/copy of care plan sent to		
Name	Designation	Copy sent?

Next review date		Completed by		
Service user		Designation		Team & locality	
Sign		Sign		Sign	
Date		Date		Date	
Give reason if service user declined to sign			Service user given care plan?	

Staying home, staying alive

6

Imagine the following scenario. It's Friday. You came out of hospital 3 weeks ago after spending 3 months recovering from the worst time of your life. All the fuss surrounding discharge has long settled down. You wake up early – too early – to find yourself in a dingy flat on the fourth floor of a rundown council block built between the wars. It's cold and sparsely furnished – the cheque hasn't come through yet. A weird smell is coming from somewhere. In the first light of dawn you can make out the silhouettes of medication bottles, next to an empty packet of fags on the mantelpiece. You yawn, scratch yourself and wonder about the day ahead. Five quid to last all weekend. No fags. No friends. No one due to visit until next Wednesday, when your social worker comes. You can't work the gas cooker. Nothing to do. Going outside can be tricky because the kids along the balcony take the piss, scrounge fags off you and sometimes throw stones. So what are you going to do today? What are the options? Stay in bed? Masturbate? Turn on the TV? Risk it and go out, maybe down to the phone booth to give your mum a ring? Jobcentre? Kill yourself? Go to the off-licence or the pub where you can score some weed or crack? Go back up to the hospital for a chat? Try and get admitted?

Like it or not, this bleak scenario, or something like it, is a pretty common description of the life faced by many people who find themselves discharged from a psychiatric hospital and trying to square up to the demands of life. And for many people living with major mental illness, the real challenge lies in keeping going and going, on and on, despite the daily grind.

In the last chapter, we saw how going home, if properly planned and executed, is a time of action, attention and vigilance to the possibilities of practical snags and teething problems. Because going home is often such a busy time, it is easy to overlook the all-important question of what happens next. Going home may well carry all sorts of challenges and rewards, but the real challenge lies in staying home and staying alive and staying well.

Helping patients to remain stable and supported in a community, to live to their particular abilities and limitations, is the central task of the care worker. To achieve this, he or she needs to attend to many – arguably countless – aspects of a patient's life. This requires patience, energy, communication skills and, above all, imagination. On top of this, he or she must keep up with paperwork, juggle fresh assessments, do routine clinical chores and keep abreast of new developments in diagnosis, treatment and case management, not to mention local politics. In other words, the successful care coordinator must keep an eye not only on the patient but also on his or her own professional life as well. For this reason, this chapter and the next are devoted to staying alive: helping the patient to survive and helping *you*, the care worker, to survive.

Staying alive: the patient

Many of the principles of successful community care in the longer term have already been touched upon, particularly in the last two chapters. Because of their importance, however, we make no apologies for their repetition here, albeit in a slightly different way. Effective work relies upon the following basic rules (and what they mean in official NHS language):

1. do all you can to build and maintain the relationship (partnership);
2. do all you can to involve the patient as an equal (partnership);
3. always have a long-term (as well as a short-term) plan (flexibility);
4. remember that needs and plans always change with time (flexibility);
5. keep exploring the inner world of the patient (empathy);
6. always share your treatment plan with others (teamwork);
7. never give the patient the impression that you have run out of possible options or that there's no point in trying anything else (recovery).

Building a relationship

For care working to succeed, the patient must be able to feel valued and respected by the person doing it. The word for this is trust. Given that many of our patients live chaotic, isolated lives and often display oddities of manner and behaviour that many find hard to tolerate, this isn't always easy. Anything that can be done, therefore, to cement a sense of trust is a chance to build stability in the longer term.

As in other areas of life, the care worker/patient relationship grows over time, but unlike most other relationships, the care worker will have access to a very large amount of information about the patient from the outset. It is easy for the inexperienced to confuse this wealth of personal knowledge with familiarity. Outside of the caring professions, such privileged access to intimate personal data is gained only slowly – and reciprocally – through countless minor discoveries. During these discoveries, we learn lots of things about someone, things that simply cannot be recorded in a case file or even elicited from an in-depth interview: the funny way a patient has, for example, of clearing his throat when he is upset, or the knowledge that she always wears *that* dress when she is starting to go manic. This kind of awareness builds up far more gradually, but is the sort that, combined with overt clinical information, leads to an effective working relationship.

From this, two useful practice points arise. First, start the relationship as early on as possible. Don't wait for the discharge planning meeting on the ward to introduce yourself to the patient. If you know he or she may be coming on to your caseload and you happen to be on the ward, take a minute or two to shake hands and say 'Hello'. This almost always turns out to be 90 seconds well spent. It also provides a chance to meet outside of the formal, sometimes inhibiting, ward round or clinical meeting, and sends an important signal to the patient that says 'I am a reasonable human being.' As we shall see, coming across as a normal, decent human being lies at the very heart of what is nowadays called 'communication skills'.

Second, less experienced workers find it hard to grow into a relationship gradually. Instead, they race in with all their knowledge on display, eager to take action, offer useful advice and do all sorts of other things that make them appear to be overfamiliar, patronising and overpowering. Although a full needs assessment may have given you the chance to form a good understanding of a patient's difficulties, as well as allowing you to sort out a clear plan for solving them, the patient may still not trust or respect you enough to share your views, let alone act on them. The problems of life only get solved overnight in the movies or on television. So take it gently; time is on your side, and should be.

Learning how to communicate

As you get to know an individual patient, it becomes easier to adopt a particular style of communication, specific to that patient. People vary widely in their abilities to concentrate, take information on board, feel reassured or recognise the boundaries between behaviour that is acceptable and that which is not. Tuning your communication style to the needs of an individual is a fine art that takes many years of practice. Being aware of an unceasing need for sensitivity and flexibility is a sound point from which to start.

For any one patient, different conversations have different purposes at different times. Early on, information gathering comes first, but at these early interviews, progress can also be monitored, trust built (or eroded) and ideas for future plans formulated. Before every meeting with every patient it is a good idea to know which aspect is intended to take precedence. In other words, ask yourself what is the main purpose of the meeting. Is it to find something out? To start a new treatment? To review progress of an established treatment? Or is it just to pop in for a chat and make sure that the new fridge has arrived safely? A preparatory ponder helps an interview to run smoothly.

For many care workers, especially early on, the process of finding out information quickly and in quantity seems to be a daunting skill, its acquisition shrouded in mystery. Clearly, some people are better at it than others and have learned their skill over time, but can it be taught? We contend that effective information gathering skills are a lot easier to acquire than many people think, providing that you do two things: think about it and practise it. This chapter can help with the former, the latter is down to you.

Before starting any face-to-face clinical contact, think of the setting. Is this place suited to a confidential uninterrupted conversation? If you are performing a routine home visit to a well-known patient, such issues are straightforward; however, don't take them for granted. An unannounced visitor may be sitting in the kitchen or a curious builder may be peering in from the scaffolding that has appeared since your last visit. Either way, always check that the patient is happy to talk here and now. Attention to these details shows respect, which can carry all sorts of therapeutic advantages.

If you are carrying a mobile phone or a pager, ask yourself if the interview is one that can bear interruption. Let the patient know if your phone might go off – most won't mind at all especially if forewarned. If you can turn it off, all well and good. Most pagers and mobiles have a silent, vibration mode. If the phone does ring, then no matter how busy you are, always apologise for the interruption and beware of sudden emotional gear changes when speaking to the caller. Leaping from empathic tones of sadness at the death of a beloved cat to delight at the cancellation of an ill-timed meeting does not smack of integrity and sincerity.

Styles of questioning are extremely important. Experienced care workers exploit the difference between open and closed questions, which elicit quite different sorts of information. Open questions are the sort that do not invite any particular category of reply. How are things? What have you been up to since we last met? Open questions get you involved fast and allow patients to feel that they are having their say and being listened to. They usually draw replies that are rich in information, although not all of it is necessarily useful. Open questions are ideal at the outset of a meeting or when moving on to a fresh topic from within an established one. However, they do require the interviewer to keep in control of the meeting, which otherwise descends from an information gathering exercise into a chat. This is not to say, however, that a good chinwag has no place – far from it. Debate over the use of penalty shoot-outs as a way of resolving major football tournaments, for example, can be highly therapeutic and professionally satisfying.

This need for control when using multiple open questions can disconcert the less experienced care worker, who may instead resort to a stream of more closed, directive questions (i.e. the answer is usually 'yes' or 'no'). Have you been going to the day centre? Did you sleep well last night? Closed questions also get you places, but much more slowly and often with an uneasy feeling that you are conducting an interrogation rather than an interview. Another common error made by the inexperienced interviewer is to repeat or rephrase a question before the reply has been given, as if the interviewer lacks confidence in the clarity of his first phrasing, e.g. 'How have things gone since you left hospital, what's it been like?' This can muddle the patient, who may incorrectly feel that he has failed to grasp something, and detract from his confidence in the interviewer.

A helpful way to make progress is by treating every interview of your clinical career as if it was an experiment, aimed at improving your performance at the next one. If you don't feel comfortable with the broad replies that come from open questions, yet feel equally uncomfortable with the grilling of the closed technique, try something in between: 'How have you been sleeping recently?' Expert interviewers use a combination of all these styles but, more importantly, they do it systematically, using a technique known as 'funnelling'. They start open, identify a domain of inquiry, and then close down their questions, homing in on the information that they require. Your preparatory ponder should tell you which funnel to go for in the first place.

Not every word of a clinical conversation, of course, involves a question. If an interview was like a cake, then the questions would only be the currants, embedded in a spongy mix of other words, actions and gestures. These are what make a conversation complete. Thus, in any interview, we may use techniques that clarify, reflect back, invite self-enquiry, facilitate, reinforce, or encourage or discourage an interview from taking a given course. Not all of these techniques are verbal, either. In recent decades, we have come to recognise the important role played by non-verbal cues in carer–patient communication.

The rule here is that establishing a rapport with a patient is as much a function of watching, and sometimes touching, as it is of listening. Pay attention to these non-verbal cues, especially in the moments at the outset of the meeting, before the patient goes into 'interview' mode. The tremor and sweatiness of a handshake or the cheerful bounce of a gait can sometimes give the lie to claims of feeling relaxed or protestations of untreated motor side effects. In some cases, visual and tactile information will be all you have to go by, as, for example, in the not uncommon case of the patient who is so ill as to be largely or totally mute.

As observed earlier, these communication skills are easier to learn from real life than from a textbook, but the following sample, from a clinical conversation with an unhappy patient with a chronic illness, illustrates some of the important techniques:

CW: 'So, what have you been up to since we last met, Barry?' (open question)
B: 'This and that.'
CW: 'For example?' (clarification)
[*Barry is silent, more sullen than usual. He moves his gaze to the floor. CW leans an inch or two closer to Barry.*] (response to non-verbal cue)
CW: 'Been getting out much?' (closed question)
[*Silence*]
CW: 'Well?' (facilitation)
B: 'Yeah, I've been out a bit.'
CW: 'That's good to hear.' (reinforcement) [*Pause*] (Pacing to enhance reinforcement.) 'Where have you been?'
B: 'Been back at the day centre.'
CW: [*pleasantly surprised*] 'Really? That's great. I'm glad you've changed your mind about that place.' (reinforcement) 'How have things been there?' (open question)
B: 'All right.'
CW: 'All right in what way?' (clarification, reflection)
B: 'I seen Steve.'
CW: 'He runs the current affairs group, doesn't he?' [*CW knows this.*] (rapport)
B: 'Yeah.'
CW: 'What is it about that group that you like?' (open question)
B: 'It's the only place where you can have an intelligent conversation.'
CW: [*Pause to show he is considering B's reply.*] 'That's not like you. You're normally ready to argue politics with anyone.' (encouragement) 'What's up?' (open question)
B: 'Not feeling myself lately.'
CW: 'You certainly seem much more fed up than usual.' (empathic reflection) 'Has something happened to upset you?' (closed question)
B: 'Hnnh.'
CW: 'What?'
B: 'They're gonna stop me giro. They want me to go for an interview.'
CW: 'Oh, no.' (empathy) 'Show me the letter.' [*He reads it through.*] 'Hmm. This is just one of those standard computer letters. They still think you're on income support.' (explanation) 'Look, don't you worry about this.' (reassurance) 'You're on top rate DLA, so they can't stop it just like that. When I get back, I'll ring the benefits office. We can get something sorted out.' (affirmation of reassurance) 'We can do them a letter saying you're too unwell to attend. That almost always does the trick. Have you been losing sleep over this one?' (closed question)

Attention to a patient's non-verbal behaviour, combined with well-timed reflection, can often stir up powerful emotions that the patient may be reluctant to disclose, because of stigma, embarrassment or fear of not being taken seriously. A simple description of the patient's appearance such as 'You look very upset at the moment' or 'I see you're really angry about this' can give the patient permission to disclose his or her feelings. Such reflection also signals to the patient that the

157

interviewer has an understanding of his or her feelings and predicament, which is sometimes referred to as 'empathy'.

Empathy is one of the most important ingredients in building trust in the short term and over time. It may be powerfully reinforced by the well-timed use of eye contact, particularly at moments when it *feels* as though the patient has made an emotionally charged disclosure. This raises another important point about communication. Try to be aware of the emotions that the patient arouses in *you*, particularly confusion, sadness and anger. It is a reliable indicator of the emotion experienced by the patients themselves and, of course, the sort of emotion they arouse in others. This can help to promote empathy, as well as help you to understand how others in the patient's social network might react towards the patient.

An important and sometimes overlooked aspect of the use of empathy involves being able to handle the powerful emotional behaviours that it can often release. 'You look as though you're really upset' may make someone start crying and make less experienced workers feel that they are somehow to blame for the distress. It is easy to compound this discomfort with bland platitudes, such as 'you'll feel better in a bit' or 'time is a great healer', utterances which, in truth, serve more to bolster your own mental state than the patient's. A powerful urge to end the meeting and escape the 'scene of the crime' as quickly as possible is another common response.

Such misowned guilt over powerful emotions in our patients also helps to explain why many less experienced carers are reluctant to ask questions about suicide or prevaricate over the breaking of bad news. An open display of strong emotions or a frank discussion of suicidal thoughts almost always does more good than harm, allowing the patient to express thoughts and feelings previously thought to be unmentionable. It is essential that the care worker 'stays with' the patient during this difficult period and keeps control of the interview. The therapeutic relationship will be stronger for it in the longer term. Letting things out, 'getting them off your chest' to use the cliché, really can do some good.

Difficult situations

Handling an angry patient requires a different strategy, particularly if physical aggression seems likely (see Chapter 8). Many people become ill-tempered and intolerant of frustration when in distress, and this can lead to them taking a hostile view of *all* those trying to help. Their anger may arise from many sources. One patient may feel angry because of unrealistic expectations of the treatment, the perceived failure of which means 'it's somebody's fault'. Another patient may feel vulnerable through their illness, and resent the idea of having to ask others for help. Some simply lack the emotional and interpersonal ability to communicate their distress via more cooperative means – a 'complete bastard' or 'a nasty piece of work' might be another way of putting it – but our use of careful psychological language is important here, to clarify the components of why some people are so difficult and how they might be helped. Angry, rejecting responses are very common among people who have experienced abuse (physical and/or sexual) in early life.

Faced with anger, it is important that the care worker resists the all-too-human urge to respond in kind. At half past four on a wet Friday afternoon, this may be more easily said than done, but it is essential for the success of the relationship, and therefore treatment, that you acknowledge the anger and thereafter calmly work to defuse it. Identifying its cause and acknowledging to the patient that something will get done (as a result of its expression) is usually enough to defuse the situation. If this fails, then break the rule of staying with the patient, emotionally and geographically. Leave fast.

Occasionally, an interview is hard to control for other reasons. One common problem is garrulousness, and some people do just talk and talk. It requires patience and skill to keep an interview on track when the patient is circumstantial, vague, pedantic, repetitive or overinclusive (this describes an inability to just give the salient points in a description or line of reasoning – every little aspect is mentioned in unnecessary detail because of an inability to distinguish between what is relevant and what is not; a 'long-winded explanation' might be the layman's term). Again, it is helpful if the care worker has some idea of the reason for this overtalkativeness; some people are constitutionally verbose, whereas others may be anxious and overaroused through nervousness, anxiety, intoxication or serious mental disorder. A valuable knack is knowing how and when to interrupt without appearing to be irritated or unsympathetic. The secret lies in waiting for a pause just large enough to insert a response, and then using a phrase that either echoes the patient's most recent utterance or acknowledges it as significant and an issue to which the interview will return in due course, e.g. 'That's really important, and we'll come back to it, but first I'd ... .'

If patients are allowed to feel that the interruption has not dismissed their concerns or downgraded their status (ideally, it has highlighted something they did want to sort out), they may well be happy to follow the line suggested. Anxious patients may also curb their garrulousness if the interviewer first spends a few moments acknowledging their anxiety and putting them at their ease. Telling them how long they have got (say 20–30 minutes maximum) can also help focus their worries. Keeping control of the constitutionally overtalkative or obsessional patient is less easy and usually requires resort to frequent closed questions with reminders that details considered to be of special importance by the patient will be addressed in due course. A planned bleep or 'urgent' phonecall may be needed to break things up.

Another challenge lies in communicating with a mute or nearly mute patient. The trick here lies in being comfortable with the long periods spent in silence awaiting replies to questions. Write notes, look relaxed and resist the urge to hustle or display the irritability that often accompanies a busy caseload and the feeling that time is not being well spent. It is even more important to form some idea of why a patient is mute than determine, for example, why someone is angry or talkative. A major mental disorder such as severe depression, catatonic schizophrenia or major cerebral pathology may be the underlying cause. The diagnosis can often be made by taking a history from a collateral source and by looking for the characteristic non-verbal signs of each condition (a profoundly depressed patient, for example, may be dressed in black and display a hunched, disconsolate posture, with scant eye contact and signs of self-neglect). Often, the mute patient may be so because he or she is in a state of profound emotional turmoil or anxiety. In such situations, a calm, concerned manner, and the acknowledgement that it is sometimes hard to put thoughts into words, can help the patient begin to explain his or her distress.

Barriers to communication

Other barriers to communication occur because of social and cultural differences. Research demonstrates that 'social distance' (i.e. a perceived gap in social status or class between the interviewer and interviewee) can significantly alter the way in which people express themselves. We all bring a set of values and expectations to each encounter with another person, which act as a kind of template into which we fit our judgements of what we think the other person means. The trust that patients are willing to invest in a relationship with a carer is therefore influenced by age, gender, sexuality, social class, culture and all the beliefs that they carry with them. The care worker also brings his or her own set of stereotypes and pre-conceptions to the relationship. The stage is thus set for potential confusion and misunderstanding; a patient is hardly likely to be honest with someone whom he or she thinks will be critical, condescending or even sexist. This problem, which is inescapable to some degree, can be minimised if you regularly reflect on how your beliefs and prejudices can alter your professional behaviour. There are ways of doing this, which we will explore further in the next chapter, but, in essence, it requires you to cultivate the habit of self-examination, particularly when a patient provokes strong feelings, of whatever variety.

Much the same applies to the more overt issues of culture and language. Many misunderstandings can arise if the patient and the care worker have different cultural backgrounds. Behaviours that are regarded by some as being a sure sign of illness may be regarded elsewhere on the planet as being quite normal. Cultures also differ widely in the thresholds above which discomfort is construed as a symptom in need of attention, as well as the way in which these symptoms are described. For example, transcultural research reveals consistent, wide variations in the tolerance of pain between urban Jewish populations and their Protestant counterparts, whereas the tolerances of rural Chinese labourers are different still. North Americans are likely to present with psychological symptoms of an anxiety neurosis, whereas matching individuals from, say, Turkey or the Middle East will express the same concerns in more somatic terms, for example headache or dizziness.

Similar differences are found in the attitudes of various cultures to the idea of expert help, particularly for psychological issues, as well as the respect with which they regard professionals. Some cultures, such as rural India, continue to view many psychological problems as being either non-existent or a sign of spiritual weakness, whereas North Americans are recognised for the alacrity with which they both seek psychological help and demand full explanations of their treatment. What happens in California often has a habit of happening here 10 years later. The lesson to be learnt from all this is that, when working with a patient from a different culture, it is important to stay vigilant to the possibility that cultural differences – and not just the illness – are playing a part in whatever problem has been encountered.

On a broader level, always be ready to learn about the quirks and rules of a culture that you view as foreign. It takes time (and sometimes a little embarrassment) to learn, say, that an ultra-Orthodox Jewish woman never shakes hands with a man or that one should always offer to remove one's shoes on entering a Hindu household. In Thailand, it is very rude to show people the soles of your feet. Attention to just this sort of detail is the hallmark of a real professional, and can help promote the sense of trust that is so vital to your work.

Language brings these issues into focus even more sharply. Aside from the obvious problems faced by a care worker who does not speak a word of the same language as the patient (a common situation in the inner city), there is much room for misunderstanding when two people differ in the competence with which they speak a common language. If basic linguistic adequacy is in question, it is often better to keep things simple and instead rely more upon the universal human language of emotion and gesture, and to defer any important, fact-based decisions about treatment until an interpreter is available. It is helpful here to recall what Wittgenstein said about language: all language involves people trying to reach an agreement on what a word means and no two people will ever get it exactly right, regardless of linguistic skill. This observation applies particularly to two people who think that they are using the same language, for example two people from the UK and the USA.

Like all professions, mental health has its own dialect, in which quite common words carry very different meanings from those used by the lay public. Thus, terms such as 'hysteria', 'schizophrenia' and 'psychopath' may turn into conversational landmines, easily trodden upon by the unwary care worker. It is also easy to forget that patients and their relatives do not make regular use of medical jargon and, thus, terms such as 'cognitive deficit', 'auditory hallucination' and 'irregular compliance' may be poorly understood and will require careful explanation (see Table 6.1). This problem often occurs in multidisciplinary meetings in which the patient and a relative are present. An unwary care worker will use acronyms and jargon, for example when giving a summary of a patient's clinical progress to a colleague. To be in a room with someone who refers to your 'significant improvement in function since the last CPA [Care Programme Approach], with a marked reduction in antisocial behaviour because of improved compliance with injectable medication' can often leave you feeling more like an insect in a jar than a human being in need of help. We need to use specialist language – it saves a lot of time and confusion – but it is

Table 6.1 ● Psychiatric terms: meanings and misunderstandings

Term	Professional meaning	Possible public meaning
Agoraphobia	Fear of crowded places	Fear of open spaces
Alcoholic	Dependent on alcohol	Street vagrant with a bottle
Aroused/arousal	Agitated and anxious	Sexually turned on
Borderline	Form of personality disorder	On the edge? Nearly dangerous?
Depression	Form of mood disorder	Crying/unhappy
Hallucinations	Abnormal perceptions	Seeing things/on drugs?
Hysteria	Dissociated state	Screaming and shouting
Manic	Form of mood disorder	Bad-tempered busybody
Mental	Non-physical (illness)	Mad/crazy
Mood swings	Bipolar affective disorder	Angry outbursts
Neurosis/otic	Non-psychotic mental illness	Silly and fussy
Obsessional	Struggles with certain thoughts or acts	Can only think of one thing
Paediatrician	Child specialist	Child abuser
Panic state	Form of enhanced anxiety	Out of control
Paranoid	Dominated by delusions	Unfounded persecutory thoughts
Psychopath	Form of personality disorder	Serial killer
Psychotic	Seriously unwell	Very dangerous
Schizophrenia	A form of psychotic illness	In two minds/Jekyll and Hyde

important to keep a watch upon the context. This rule works the other way round, too. Avoid slang, colourful local patois and other colloquialisms unless you are absolutely sure of their meaning. By its very nature, slang changes rapidly. Keep up with it by all means, but be careful of using it; the cool utterances of today very quickly become the naff gaffes of tomorrow.

Another small, but sometimes significant, communication trap involves written notes. Many care workers prefer to devote their efforts to watching and listening to the patient and write up their meetings shortly after the event. This is not always easy, particularly if large amounts of information have been gathered, as at an assessment interview or when a patient has said something that does not seem to make sense. Because our memories rely upon meaning to store information, it is hard to record a verbatim example of faulty logic or formal thought disorder at any time other than when it is uttered. This means that you will occasionally need to make use of written notes during an interview. This needs care, particularly in the presence of a patient who is sensitive to rebuff or who feels persecuted. A quick, well-timed explanation at the outset of the interview – 'Do you mind if I make a few notes as we go along to make sure I get it right?' – usually pre-empts this difficulty.

It will be clear by now that communication skills lie at the heart of successful mental health care work and that they are probably easier learnt than taught, as long as one remains constantly aware of the need to update and improve one's skills and knowledge. A good communicator is valued and respected by colleagues and patients alike. There are many ways, formal and informal, of improving communication skills, which we will consider in the next chapter.

Involving the patient as an equal

All relationships involve status. In even the simplest conversation, the listener may be seen, in one sense, as holding 'low' status, his status reverting to 'high' as he begins his reply. In social situations, we confer status upon people because of particular attributes such as wealth, appearance, birth and so on. Regrettably, serious mental illness still carries a stigma that gives it a low status in our culture; no government has ever put a better deal for the mentally ill near the top (or even the bottom!) of its election manifesto. Status also plays an essential role in the development and survival of the relationship between a care worker and the patient. This is reflected in the language that we use to describe this relationship. Consider the introduction to this book, in which we gave our reasons for using the terms 'patient' and 'care worker'. Others have taken issue with the notions of status that these terms invite. Why use a word such as 'patient', it is argued, when it confers a low status upon an individual, relegating them to passive acceptance of treatment? Why not use terms such as 'client', 'customer', 'user' or even 'survivor', which denote equality and empowerment? These issues, far from being abstract, underline another rule: to be effective, you have to encourage patients to do much of the real work. It is their life, after all. This can be achieved by constantly paying attention to the status of the patient in your relationships with them.

If we are honest about it, most of us go into the caring profession not only out of a genuine desire to help people but also because we like the status (potentially, at least!) in which we are held by both patients and public alike. Acknowledging this fact can help us to be more open and honest with those we are looking after and so improve the treatments that we provide. It can also help us to avoid some major clinical pitfalls. If the patient believes that the care worker is an honest, reliable character who takes the trouble to see things from *his or her* point of view, then the outcome of treatment is likely to be better, both in the short and longer term. As we saw in Chapter 4, patient satisfaction is an important determinant of compliance/adherence with treatment, especially when both patient and care worker share a common model of what is wrong and what they intend to do about it. Working hard to treat the patient as an equal is one way of keeping ourselves focused on this goal. There are many ways to go about it.

Be honest, be reliable

Honesty is crucial and lying is something that most of us do not do very well, so try to be straight and upfront with a patient whenever possible. Diagnosis, prognosis and side effects of treatment are particular areas where it often seems easier to resort to untruths, avoidance or euphemisms. Usually, this only leaves you a hostage to fortune, as something such as illness, which obeys the laws of natural history, always reveals itself in time. Being upfront about the need to take medication for the rest of one's life, for example, is invariably hard for the care worker and the patient alike, but the patient will usually respect you for it, even if he or she disagrees. In any case, the longer term consequences of dishonesty, i.e. mistrust, betrayal, anger, are far worse – unless you leave the job, that is, and make some other unfortunate untangle the mess you have left behind. Likewise, if you think that Barry doesn't stand a chance of getting top rate disability allowance, say so at the outset. It can save hours of filling in application and appeal forms later on.

For really big issues, however, honest, candid disclosures of truth do need to be tempered by tact and are best given slowly, over time. The human capacity for self-deception is truly staggering, and a clearly spoken but unpalatable truth may require many repetitions in different forms before it leads to a change in belief. Just because you have told someone something, do not think that they will take it in or remember it, especially if they don't want to hear it. Part of the impairment of some psychiatric illnesses is just this lack of insight into reality. Write down such statements, send a letter confirming things, copied to the GP, and be prepared to restate things in different ways, over and again, with different people present.

Honesty is also necessary in good times as well as bad. After hours of your hard work have paid off, it is easy to forget to treat the patient as an equal. Consider, for example, the case of a severely psychotic woman. You have been working with her cognitively towards the goals of compliance with drug treatment for her chronic hallucinations. When she gratefully announces at your next session that she has been symptom-free for a fortnight, it is easy to accept praise for your efforts rather than concentrating on hers. By being honest and making it explicitly clear that it was her that did most of the work, rather than the medication, you will enhance her status. This approach fosters a patient's confidence in their own ability to make a difference to their lives and discourages them from becoming excessively dependent upon their relationship with you. It also carries the less cheerful (but useful) advantage that, if a patient later relapses, he or she is less likely to hold you responsible. Being honest with your patients is a rule that you should always try to follow, as there are very few clinical situations that justify breaking it. We will consider some below.

A corollary to being honest is being reliable. If you make an appointment with a patient, keep it. Most patients can tolerate the odd cancellation (they'll do the same to you), sometimes even at the last moment, but the minute they start to identify such behaviour as recurrent, their commitment to the treatment will drop sharply. The same thing goes for promises to write letters, fill in forms, drop off prescriptions and all the thousand and one other things that care work involves. If, for some reason, you fail to deliver, acknowledge it up front and come up with a plausible excuse. This is, perhaps, one of the few areas where scrupulous honesty can give way to truth economics, but make sure that your excuse is straightforward, with valid form and content. A long-promised letter in support of a housing transfer can only spend so long 'in the pipeline', very few secretaries go down with the flu ten times a year and not many reports get eaten by the office gerbil.

When we do let a patient down, it is tempting to try to rationalise the consequences. We may tell ourselves that it was only one occasion, and for a patient who, in any case, seemed to be doing pretty well at the last review. This may well be true, but such solipsism obscures the wider context. By letting a patient down, you are raising the possibility in the patient's mind that it is not only you but also the entire system that is unreliable and uncaring. If the cancelled visit wasn't that necessary, why was it arranged in the first place? Most care workers manage to maintain a high degree of reliability by paying attention to the way that they organise their working week. As we shall see, 'diary husbandry' is an art form in its own right.

Another important advantage of constantly working to treat the patient as an equal (as mentioned earlier) is that it minimises the chances of them forming an overdependent relationship. Few clinical situations are more upsetting to the hard-pressed care worker than the patient who somehow seems to become more and more unable to cope without a high level of purportedly 'therapeutic' attention. It is easy to see how such a situation can arise. For many patients who lack the basic skills to form relationships or to cope with the challenges that most of us consider trivial, the regular arrival of a nice, caring, sympathetic person at the door once a fortnight can actually become the only contact with the world that they require. Unfortunately for some patients, this degree of contact becomes insufficient and, in a manner akin to an addict developing dependence on a soothing drug, they make increasing demands for time and attention.

At first, this may take the form of intense thanks, little notes and even gifts. Early on, the less experienced care worker, possibly flattered by the gratitude, is willing to go along with the happy flow. At this point, the boundaries of a caring clinical relationship often start to become blurred, and the original goals of treatment become lost behind numerous cosy chats. Such reinforcement of dependency may be quite well advanced before alarm bells begin to ring in your head. You now find yourself in the paradoxical position of actually aggravating the very isolation and anxiety that you intended to treat. Methods of disengagement that might have worked a few months ago now lead to far more worrying consequences, such as angry accusations of neglect and rejection, coercive threats of self-harm and, rarely, threats to others. Faced with this situation, it is small wonder that a care worker begins to 'forget' appointments and other agreements, adding legitimacy to the patient's grievances.

Thankfully, few overdependent relationships go so far down this unhappy road. Instead they tend to settle into only a moderately dissatisfying status quo that often remains stable over months and sometimes years. Trying to hold on to the idea of the patient as an equal when working together towards a predetermined goal, with a clear setting of limits (i.e. you are *not* available when off duty), can prevent such relationships from forming at the outset. Another way to keep patients from slipping down the status ladder is by exploring their beliefs about treatment and progress as one goes along, trying to ensure, as it were, that they remain 'on beam'. An advantage of such regular attempts to explore the inner world of the patient, which is often easier said than done in the hurly-burly of daily work, is that it maintains the patient's faith in your regard for them as a human being. Of course, if things can't be stabilised/restored, you may have to withdraw gracefully, handing over to someone else in the team. This happens to everyone now and then, so do not feel that you have failed.

Always have a plan

From what has been discussed in the last section, two further themes of 'staying alive' may be discerned. The first involves reaching an agreement with the patient to work towards a long-term goal, and the second involves trying regularly and systematically to explore the inner world of the patient in a way that encourages them to change. How does one do that?

A well-known psychiatrist once wrote: 'Don't just do something – listen.' This helpful piece of advice isn't quite the full story. Getting patients to do something – in other words, helping them to live their lives to the best of their abilities – is what we are paid for. Much of the fun of being a care worker lies in the often surprising, and sometimes unbelievable, things that our patients end up doing. As they recover from the illness that got them on to your books in the first place, some may end up going places, whereas, for others, simply getting out of bed every morning is a major achievement. Both are equally satisfying in their own way. Within reason, you can help patients to do anything as long as it is *something*, but it is always better if that anything is something that the patients want to do. Otherwise, they might end up not doing much, at least not of the something that you had in mind. What is necessary here is a plan of action, and, using the word 'care' in its broadest imaginable sense, we call this the 'care plan'.

Putting together a care plan can be as complex or as straightforward as you want. It depends on several things: the time and energy that you have available and the mental, physical and social resources of the patient. Because mental illness is so diverse in the ways that it can disrupt people's lives, care plans will vary widely between patients. Some may involve getting the patient back to work or engaging the patient with psychotherapy, whereas others may involve the ongoing acceptance of more chronic illness. Much of the following rests on the assumption that you, the care worker, are likely to find yourself concentrating on patients in the more severe corner of this arena. If you have given some thought to the common sense contained in the last chapter, have got to know something about the patient and his or her world from a 'full needs assessment' and have secured the patient somewhere to live, then you're three-quarters of the way there. The rest really boils down to one question: 'What shall we do today?'

Trying to come up with a universal, textbook answer to this question is a bit like asking: 'What is the meaning of human existence?' Rather than defer to Plato, it seems more sensible to find a more practical, individual answer. It is important to note here that, although it is part of your job to help your patient identify the answer and work towards it, it is ultimately down to the patient and his or her network to achieve it. As a care worker, your job is not to be a companion, home help, day centre, psychotherapist, plumber, GP and close confidante all rolled into one. Sometimes, especially when we find that we quite like a particular patient, it can be hard to avoid this. Having clear, objective goals of what your care is intended to achieve, which are established at the outset and reviewed overtly as you proceed, is one way to keep things on a stable, professional footing.

So, what might these goals be, exactly? For some people, just coping with life in spite of chronic symptoms is a major achievement, whereas, for others, new relationships, creativity and letting go of contact with psychiatric services altogether is the long-term goal. Between these two extremes lies the nitty-gritty of day-to-day life. Box 6.1 provides a checklist of things to consider before and during contact with a patient. Seeing to it that the patient can achieve and manage these things is really the essence of successful care working.

Keep an eye on things

It is extremely difficult for care workers to stay on top of all of the developments in the life of one other human being, let alone the 20 or so others that they might have on their caseload; however, with time, practice and a reasonably unstressed brain, it is surprising how close one can get to this seemingly impossible goal. Apart from looking after yourself, the secret lies in knowing what to keep on the front burner, what to leave on the back burner and what you can safely leave out altogether. By doing this, and having an idea of which issues need to come to the fore before they bubble over, it is usually possible to nip most living problems in the bud.

Issues to do with bricks, mortar and basic equipment rarely go critical overnight. However, pipes freeze, fuses blow and toilets do get blocked occasionally, especially when distressed people put strange things down them. It is helpful to have a list of sympathetic, stigma-free handymen somewhere at the back of your diary and to encourage patients to attend to small things as they occur, rather than resort to 6-monthly blitzes. However, in some cases, handymen may visit at their peril. One author recalls a near-disastrous section assessment of a deluded patient in which the only person at home was a kindly washing-machine engineer, who bore a striking resemblance to the patient. He mistakenly answered 'yes' to a question about the patient's identity, and his belief that he was a washing-machine engineer was clearly seen as evidence of a deluded state. It was not until he arrived on the ward that his alibi was confirmed.

It is a good idea to familiarise yourself with the whereabouts, state and contents of the fridge from time to time, without appearing unduly intrusive. Asking for a cup of tea sometimes helps, so that you can go and get out the milk. Using the lavatory to 'wash your hands' can also clarify sanitary arrangements quite quickly. If required, a small resource bag can then be a real boon. This could have some tea bags, long-life milk, disposable cloths, small bars of soap and disinfectant – ready for instant use, a quick clean-up and refurbishment.

Cash tends to be more mercurial than bricks and mortar, especially if the patient is spending it on something that he or she would rather you did not know about. Although there are no care work courses that offer training in accountancy, budget management is an important skill. It always pays to have a rough idea of a patient's cash flow as well as keeping in touch with the developments on benefits. Housing, sickness and unemployment benefit have always been, and will always be, political footballs and, thus, are likely to be subject to as many cuts, reviews and reconfigurations as the NHS itself. Keeping up with the news and getting to know a local benefits advisor can prove invaluable when one of your patients thinks that he or she is living their own version of the Wall Street Crash. Any half-decent community mental health team should have a qualified benefits worker attached to it. If you detect a gross discrepancy between income and visible outgoings, as well

Box 6.1 Checklist of points to consider before and during contact with a patient

Basic survival

Where does the patient live? Is it warm? Is it weatherproof? Is it hygienic? Is it secure? Is there any light? Is there a water supply? Is there a gas supply? Is there an electricity supply? Is there a fridge? Is there a cooker? Is there a sink? Are there basic cooking and eating implements?

How does the patient eat and drink? Does he cook? Does he always eat out? Where? Who cooks? Who does the shopping? Who does the laundry, the cleaning?

Cash

Does he have a source of income? Does he get a salary/pension? Invalidity benefit? Income support? Does he get cash from any friends/relatives/assets? How does he get his cash? Giro? Cash in hand? Where does he keep his cash? In the home/bank/family? Can he count? Any debts? Any pushy creditors or drug dealers?

Human contact

Does he have a partner? Any mates? Does he have any neighbours? Does he talk to the shopkeeper/postman/gasman/milkman? Does he have/see any family? Drug dealer? Who visits him apart from you? When? How often? Where does he see them? Television? Radio?

Outside world

Does he ever go out? How often? Day or night? How far? Where does he shop? Does he go to any entertainment? Pub? Cinema? Betting shop? Bingo? Park? Any work? Voluntary/paid? Visit family? Walks in the park? A pet?

Contact with caring agencies

GP, psychiatrist, other doctors, OT, day centre, MIND, other mental health charity, drop-in centre, voluntary work, etc?

Sexual relationships

Girlfriend or boyfriend? Partner? Prostitute?

Legal status

Mental Health Act status? Section 117? Section 17 leave? Section 41 'restriction order'?

UK Citizen? Foreign? Asylum status? Leave to remain? Does he have a solicitor?

Medication

Who prescribes, what, when, what taken, how often, how regularly, what route, side effects, beneficial effects? Who monitors? Who encourages? Who discourages?

Symptoms

Does the patient have any ongoing significant physical/psychiatric symptoms? Do they stop him from doing any of the above? How often do you review his symptoms? Is this proving adequate? Does the GP know? Missed hospital appointments? Needs a check-up?

Beliefs/insight

How does the patient think that he is faring? What does the patient think is wrong? How does he get on with you? How does he see the past/present/future?

Faith

Does he know a rabbi/mullah/vicar/pandit/guru?

as a sudden decline in the contents of the fridge, check the television. Also, check the radio and consider drugs or gambling, the paraphernalia of which are usually easy to spot around the house, particularly once the habit is established. Scraps of smoke-stained silver foil, empty plastic bottles with odd holes, torn-off Rizla packets and roaches in the ashtray are the commonest telltale signs.

Because humans are by nature social creatures, a patient's level of interaction (i.e. frequency of contacts, number of friendships) with other people is often one of the most sensitive indicators of mental health. Social withdrawal, especially in a patient who has previously displayed a higher level of interaction, is almost always a sign of anxiety, depression or psychotic relapse. The odd day indoors is one thing, but look out for established changes over days and weeks. Some social relationships are more welcome to the patient than others. Not everyone appreciates cheer-up visits from their mum, and some visitors are frankly unwelcome. As well as drug-dealers, cheap-loan sharks and all the other dodgy characters who make a living preying on vulnerable people, prejudiced neighbours, particularly those belonging to intolerant tenants' associations, and cruel children from along the balcony can often turn a patient's life into a living hell. *Always* take complaints seriously, no matter how deluded or persecuted patients may appear, and weigh their details against the possibility that it might be true. Sometimes people really are out to get you.

Similarly, it always pays to know something about a patient's routine on the occasions that he or she does venture outdoors. For example, the man in the newsagent where he buys his fags (does he ever read the paper?), the launderette assistant (service wash or does his own?), the bloke in the local corner shop (does he live on crisps or can he cook?) and the man in the local cafe may all be able to provide invaluable information in times of concern. Keeping up with this sort of detail isn't quite as hard as it sounds, but the real knack lies in not appearing to be overintrusive or controlling. This requires a delicate balancing act between tact and inquisitiveness – the best guide is the needs of the patient. Only seek out these details if they help you to help your patient. If they don't, then you're just being nosy.

Sexual relationships are a bit trickier, but there are some ways into this delicate area. The first is to have a rough idea of the patient's sexuality and background history, which can often be gleaned from their manner and their medical records, not to mention stuff lying around their home. *Hot Guys* or *Hot Girls* magazines in the toilet speak volumes. If your patient has ever been admitted, he or she has probably been clerked in at some point. In the special setting of a hospital, it is easier to ask delicate questions and, although a lot of routine medical clerkings leave much to be desired, the odds are that precious nuggets relating to sexual history can be unearthed by a careful scouring of the notes.

Second, don't be too shy of approaching the subject, if it seems important. Everyone experiences the desire for sex and companionship (and sometimes both) in some way, and most people don't mind talking about the presence or absence of a significant other in their life. From here, if you don't feel able to approach the matter either sideways or head on, it is usually possible, but not always easy, to infer what is or isn't going on in a patient's sex life. This is one of the rare areas where frankness may be put aside in favour of euphemism ('How's the hydraulics?') and even innuendo. As often as not, once the ice is broken, patients will talk very openly about their problems. It is an area where 'social skills' advice can really hit home, and drug effects on sexual function can be discussed and even sorted out.

Drug treatment in itself also requires close attention. It is incumbent upon every care worker to keep up with exactly what patients have been prescribed, for what particular condition, whether or not they are taking it, how often and by what route. You also need to be totally familiar with the common side effects of all psychotropic drugs, as well as remaining vigilant for the possible occurrence of rarer ones. It will be recalled that some drugs, especially lithium, clozapine and the anticonvulsants, require regular monitoring of blood levels and associated blood indices of physiological function. The ins and outs of drug treatment have already been covered in detail in Chapter 3, but it is worth repeating here that drugs should only ever be seen as a part of treatment, never all of it. If all you talk about when you visit a patient to give a routine depot injection is the depot and its side effects, then your work with that patient is incomplete; seeing the drug treatment as just part of the picture reminds the patient that treatment is about more than symptom control. Some of the earliest signs that drug treatment may be going awry come from the patient's network rather than from the patient. Knowing the details of who collects the prescriptions, how often and in what quantity often turns out to be important when assessing the likelihood of relapse, as well as learning how to reduce the chances of this happening on future occasions.

This is another good reason to share your detailed knowledge of the patient's medication with significant others. Mum is often the first to spot that Barry's wastebasket contains fewer than the usual number of empty blister packets. It is also a good idea to keep a constant eye open for changes in the patient's attitude to medication, especially when it has had bad side effects in the past, where insight into the illness remains poor or where lengthy negotiation was needed to persuade the patient to take it in the first place. Many patients, fearing disapproval, find it hard to be forthcoming with an honest opinion on the value of drug treatment, especially when the treatment is prophylactic (i.e. preventing relapse) and the absence of symptoms seems to obviate the need to swallow pills every day. Patient re-education into the values and principles of drug treatment is often required; however, be careful not to sound slightly bored as you launch into the keep-taking-the-pills routine that you perform five times a week. Spontaneous comments about drug treatment should be examined closely for their explicit and implicit content. 'I hear that there's a much better one out now' may be the first sign that Barry stopped taking his sulpiride 6 weeks ago.

The other important area that requires regular attention is, in some ways, the most obvious: symptoms. Aren't symptoms supposed to be the thing that patients complain about and the thing that we are all supposed to be treating in the first place? Not so. As we have already seen, the art of successful care work lies in treating not so much the symptom as the person attached to it. A symptom that caused such distress when it was first acknowledged may no longer be quite as incapacitating, through familiarity and partial response to treatment, but the absence of complaint does not necessarily signify the absence of symptom. Rather, one patient may feel that there is nothing more that can be done and that he or she will just have to struggle on regardless. Others may now recognise the symptom for what it is and thus be able to manage the fear arising from it, but still experience some equally unpleasant aspects of the illness. Very few treatments – in any field of medicine – are 100% effective; however, it is sometimes hard to acknowledge that some symptoms persist in spite of all our best efforts because this summons up the unpleasant spectre of therapeutic impotence. Faced with this, you may find yourself downplaying the significance of volunteered symptoms with bland assurances ('Oh don't worry, it'll just go away'), which seem to patients to be very much at odds with their own beliefs and concerns.

A better approach to the challenge of ongoing symptoms is to go in search of them pre-emptively and allow the patient to feel that it is all part of your plan, even if it isn't. A good way to create this impression is by appearing to be totally familiar with the clusters of symptoms that go together in the common mental illnesses. Fortunately, the one thing that *all* our patients have in common is that they are human and, consequently, these symptoms, as we saw in Chapter 4, have a tendency to crop up again and again. To a frightened patient, this seen-it-all-before attitude can be quite comforting. Taking time to learn the screening questions listed in Tables 6.2 and 6.3 will always turn out to be time well spent and, providing that you know how to initiate treatment, will tell you what to do next.

Table 6.2 ● Screening questions for anxiety/depressive symptoms[a]

Questions	Answers[b]
Any problem sleeping?	Can't get off to sleep (a) Keep waking/early morning waking (d) Can't get off *and* wake early (a + d)
Feel worried/on edge/nervous much of the time?	Yes (a)
Feel low/tired/down much of the time?	Yes (d)
Panic attacks outside, e.g. crowded shops, Tube, buses?	Yes (a)[c]
Hopeless about the future? Sense of helplessness?	Yes (d + a)
Thoughts and/or plans of suicide?	Yes (d)
Blame yourself?	Yes (d)
Loss of appetite/weight/energy?	Yes (d)
Physical symptoms such as palpitations, headaches, sweating, butterflies in stomach?	Yes (a)

[a] Asking the patient to describe a typical day, from getting up to daytime activities/meals/contacts to evening/bedtime/sleep can helpfully clarify these symptoms and find out how intrusive they are to a given individual.
[b] (a) = anxiety; (d) = depression.
[c] Typical of more severe anxiety leading to agoraphobia and/or panic disorder.

There is, however, an even better way to tackle ongoing symptoms. This method not only guarantees that you almost always look as though you know what you're doing but also gets patients to feel the same way about themselves, too. And, as if that isn't enough, it allows for unanticipated symptoms and other changes in the patient's condition to actually become *part* of the plan. This approach is known as the cognitive behavioural approach, and at the very heart of it lies one simple, central principle: get patients to view the contents of their heads and their lives as processes that require ongoing active involvement and observation.

Table 6.3 ● Screening questions for symptoms of schizophrenia

Delusions/hallucinations	Anything unusual/strange bothering you?
Delusions	Is there something going on that you don't understand?
Paranoid	Do you feel scared to go out sometimes because of the way that people seem to look at you or even talk about you?
Thought interference	Do you ever feel that the television sometimes seems to be talking about you or to be directed at you personally?
Thought broadcast	Do you ever feel that other people know what you're thinking about or can even read your mind?
Thought withdrawal/insertion	Do you ever feel that something's taking away your thoughts or making you think certain things? Is it hard to think straight sometimes?
Hallucinations	Do you ever feel as if there's a voice or voices talking at you, even when no one else seems to be around?
Passivity phenomena	Do you ever feel that your thinking, or even your body, isn't under your control? As if someone else was making you do things or imagine things?

A systematic way of exploring the inner world of the patient

The basic principles of this approach have already been set out in Chapter 4, where they were described in the context of formal cognitive behavioural (psycho)therapy (CBT). For some inexplicable reason, the practice of CBT is still thought by many to be the exclusive domain of clinical psychologists. This is surprising, given that the techniques were first devised by psychiatrists and, in the UK at least, are practised more by nurse specialists than any other professional group. One does not have to be a qualified CBT specialist to put the basic principles of this method to work in the setting of everyday clinical work. This becomes clear when we consider that many of these principles have already been described in this chapter, albeit under a different name – care working!

We can restate them here, in an expanded form that demonstrates how they may be used as a powerful psychological technique for use in day-to-day work:

1. Successful care working involves the patient and the care worker respecting each other and reaching a mutual agreement over how to identify a problem.
2. The best way to reach agreement is by treating the patient as an active participant in treatment and exploring the patient's beliefs about himself, his world, his problems and what he feels he can do about them.
3. A patient's beliefs are a powerful determinant of his mood and behaviour, particularly his interaction with the environment, which in turn can shape his mood and beliefs. This is a two-way process, which can be looked at objectively.
4. Once a set of beliefs, moods and behaviours are identified, they can be stated explicitly, written down and evaluated, and their intensity can be measured.

5. Once their intensity can be measured, they can be followed over time.
6. All beliefs can be challenged by talking and doing things that modify them and/or oppose them.

All of the interventions that use this approach work on the assumption that altering patients' expectations of themselves and their world can lead to change through learning, and that this learning can lead to improved mood and a sense of improved self-efficacy.

Interventions take the form of a cycle with four phases. The first phase is a phase of self-monitoring to identify problematic thoughts and associated behaviours and other symptoms. The second phase is devoted to the acquisition of skills that directly challenge the problems previously identified. This phase will involve debate with the care worker as well as active rehearsal of specific thoughts and behaviours. In the third phase, the newly devised thoughts and behaviours are practised during the day-to-day life of the patient. During this phase, it is important that the patient uses the measuring and recording skills learnt in the previous phase to actively monitor progress. The fourth phase consists of a review by the care worker, in which outcomes and results are discussed and ideas redefined and adjusted, thus modifying the treatment plan. The entire cycle then begins again.

The particular advantage of this approach is that it can be applied to virtually every aspect of the patient's life, from finding the motivation to take the occasional bath or reducing hazardous alcohol intake to coping with the content of distressing auditory hallucinations. Even if the overall complexity of it seems daunting, individual elements can be modified to stand alone. Encouraging patients to keep a diary, for example, can be a very powerful way of helping them to recognise some of the wider consequences of their behaviour and thus alter their willingness to change. Consider a patient, living with his family, who is angry and ambivalent about taking antipsychotic drugs for the treatment of fluctuating, overvalued, persecutory ideas. By getting the patient, in collaboration with his family, to record the number of angry outbursts (behaviour) or the number of times it occurs to him that other people are trying to read his mind (beliefs) when he is either on or off medication – which he also has to record – the care worker is creating a very powerful tool not only to treat the patient's psychosis but also to improve his insight into his illness. In addition, long-standing concerns by his family that there is little they can do to control his outbursts are also addressed.

Diaries can also be used to record negative thoughts and can then be taken back for review and used to devise challenging beliefs and behaviours. Consider the depressed woman who believes that she is a poor mother. She may write: 'I can't cope with this. It feels like it will go on forever. Yesterday I couldn't even make it to collect Jenny from school. I am useless.' With practice, and a little further study into the styles of thinking in depressed patients, it is possible to go though such a record and identify tendencies to overgeneralise, downplay positive attributes and so on, which might, for example, result in a two-pronged piece of homework: reaching the school gate early and use of the statement 'I feel useless, but I have felt more useless than this before and I have improved'. Encouraging the patient to use 'coping statements', based on a more realistic appraisal of the patient's living situation, is another example of a tool that may be borrowed from the cognitive behavioural toolkit.

There are many other advantages of this approach to care working. Its flexibility is such that it allows goals to be varied widely between individual patients, thus avoiding the common pitfall of excessive optimism that can lead to the setting of unrealistic targets. It works equally well for changing socks or enrolling in the Open University. It also provides welcome inoculations against the frustration of very slow progress. It is rare for this approach to have any significant side effects and it leaves the road ahead reassuringly visible to patient, family and care worker alike. Furthermore, it never runs out of ideas for further goals and permutations of goals. If one doesn't work out, try another. The only limitations lie in the imagination of the care worker and the motivation of the patient.

Such an overall approach, combined with good – because you've worked on them – communicative and empathic skills, a sound knowledge of the natural history of the patient's illness and an understanding of the efficacy of drug treatments, as well as the effects of all the other supports and services that you have arranged for your patient, form a very powerful tool for achieving the most important task in your week: keeping the patient alive, in the fullest sense of the word. In the next chapter, we will turn this idea around and see what can be done to keep you, the care worker, alive, in the same sense of the word.

Staying alive – you, the care worker

7

Two young people talk at party. She is pretty and interested.

HER: 'So what do you do for a living, exactly?'
HIM: 'I work in mental health. I look after people with severe mental illness, schizophrenia, manic depression, that kind of thing.'
HER: 'Oh, you must find that *so* depressing.'

Sound familiar? So far, this book has focused on the patient. In this chapter, we turn the tables. It is no exaggeration to say that working with people who suffer from severe mental illness is one of the most exhausting and demanding jobs around. Not only the illnesses themselves but also the stigma of mental illness, the prejudice of the public, the never-ending problem of resources and the constant shake-ups and reorganisations of the health and social services can all create the feeling that one works in a battle zone rather than a community. And, as if that isn't enough, we have to get on with colleagues, be nice to VIPs, cope with paperwork and the ever-increasing complexity of modern technology, juggle an ever-expanding caseload and tolerate ever-unreliable politicians, who keep telling us what to do and how we've never had it so good. Care work is a lot of things, but easy isn't one of them.

The C-zones

It figures, therefore, that if we are going to do a proper job of looking after our patients in this sometimes mean and nasty world, we have to first look after ourselves. One of the best ways to do this is to stay ahead of the game and spot the 'C-zones' of grief before you hit them. In our experience, there are six: chronology, caseload, communication, colleagues, current affairs and consciousness.

Chronology – become a time lord

At work, there are few things as important as time management. Successful working lies in striking the right balance between doing too much and not doing enough. The laws of physics come in handy here. Time always goes forwards at a constant rate, and the amount of energy that you have to expend in that time is always finite. There is no mystery to the fact that all of us have 24 hours in a day and 7 days in a week. What does seem mysterious, however, is how some people seem to cram so much more into this time than others. Two things separate the time lords from the rest of us. First, they always obey the golden rule 'Whatsoever thy hand findeth to do, do it with thy might' (Ecclesiastes 9:10), which translates as 'always give it some welly'. Second, they make the maximum use of *all* time available.

This is not the same as simply doing everything as fast as you can. Many people spend hours of their working week hopping between numerous tasks to which they devote only some, rather than all, of their energy. Hopping itself is an energy-consuming process. Countless precious mental calories are wasted hunting for files or trying to decipher squiggles that seemed so meaningful when they were written. The working week is like a suitcase. You can pack a lot more into it if you think about it before take-off. Overcram it and it will burst open – chaos ensues, and you are overwhelmed.

One way to do this is by structuring your working week. Each week can conveniently be broken down into ten or more 'slots', in other words, mornings and afternoons! This isn't as obvious as it sounds. By keeping the content of any one of these slots reasonably homogenous, you'll get a lot more done. This rule (i) exploits the fact that we tend to get better at something once we've been doing it steadily for a while and (ii) protects us from the common delusion that we can always 'just squeeze this in before we do that'. Sessions can be devoted to anything: visiting, clinics, writing, telephoning, reading, eating, chasing, shopping, painting a wall or searching for a long-lost patient. Just don't try to do too many things in any one slot.

Slots also need to be juggled and arranged to break up the week and keep it interesting. Try and avoid having three consecutive patient-oriented slots. Four is an absolute no-no. The next trick is to keep the slots full, but not too full. Pace yourself, with breathers between patients to allow for essential cups of coffee or time to think about (and write a brief note about) the patient you have just seen or the one you are about to see. Always try to squeeze a light slot in between a couple of heavies. An afternoon spent wrestling over the futility of existence with depressed patients whom you are keeping out of hospital will pass more easily if you have spent the morning at a training course rather than giving depot injections to reluctant patients with schizophrenia.

Most sessions are basically one of five types: face-to-face work with patients; administration; meetings; education and training; or out-and-out fun. The last one is a common cause of guilt in our modern culture, hungover as it is by the Calvinistic notion that for something to be worthwhile it should hurt; sadly, the idea that an happy worker is an effective worker is only slowly gaining ground in our world. In our opinion, there is absolutely nothing wrong with spending a session reading or studying, or out with a colleague or a patient, doing essential research into local markets, cafes, community centres or cinemas, providing it passes one small test: you can justify it to a senior. This situation provides one of those unique opportunities to practise all of your skills of imagination, wit, guile, communication and diplomacy in one go. Phrases like 'groundwork' or 'continuing professional development' can often come in handy here. Every week should have at least one such session.

Working hours is also another area where some flexibility reaps rewards. Slavish devotion to the nine-to-five tradition may be well suited to an office job, but serious mental illness rarely respects timetables. Often, 8 AM is the best time to catch an elusive patient, and it is difficult to simply clock off and go home when your patient has just told you what he or she intends to do with a year's supply of unswallowed amitriptyline. (If you always want to go home on time, resign, join the civil service and sit indoors staring at a monitor for 7.5 hours a day.) People are not machines that can be turned on and off, and being flexible with your time makes for an easier life: you avoid the rush hour; a long day (e.g. an 8 AM visit through to a 7 PM urgent assessment) can be followed by an afternoon off to pick up the kids or do some DIY; more gets done.

Paperwork – get to it before it gets to you

Administration is a beast that must be tamed from the very start. Some people prefer to keep up with their note keeping, phone calls, letter writing, report drafting and so on as they go along, blithely trying to squeeze it in between clinical work. Others leave it and then go for it in manageable dollops. Some simply ignore it altogether and let it grow into terrifying piles that they spend hours staring at, paralysed by the sheer scale of it. This is sometimes known as CPA or 'continuous paper accumulation'. Procrastination, as we shall see later, is an important indicator of our own mental health, but the secret of administrative work is to be pre-emptive. Nobble it before it nobbles you.

There are plenty of ways to achieve this. Technology, as we will see later, can be a great help, but there are a few simple rules, which, if followed painstakingly, will prevent CPA. First, always allocate set times for phone calls and paperwork. Spread this out over the week so that you can react to things as they come up. Keep some time purposely unbooked towards the end of the week – for example part of Friday morning – to catch up on those niggling bits that need sorting out before the weekend. Always fight the urge to put things off, no matter how tempting it may seem. If you are simply too exhausted to start work on an important document, don't agonise over going home and leaving it unwritten, but make sure that you allocate time for it in your next admin slot.

Every now and then you will need to produce a document that is just that little bit more important than usual – a report for a court or for an untoward incident inquiry, for example (such events are considered in more detail in Chapter 8). Here, one or two extra points are important. Before you sit down to prepare your first draft, mull it over and bounce your ideas, thoughts and recollections off a colleague, preferably one with more experience than yourself. Make notes or go over it in your mind as you walk through the park to your next visit. When you do finally get around to that first draft, try to do it early on in the day, when things are quieter and you are feeling fresher. If necessary, come to work a little bit earlier than usual. A letter written before 10 AM is usually 15% shorter than the same letter written after 4 PM, although some people find early evenings are good for brevity.

If those pieces of paper still never seem to leave your desk, in spite of all of your efforts, don't panic. Instead, try out the following handy technique, which we call the 'golden touch method':

STEP 1 Look out of the window, preferably at something green or living.
STEP 2 Go and make the drink of your choice.
STEP 3 Return to your desk with the drink and sit down. Take a slow breath and recite the golden touch rule: *I will touch each piece of paper only once.*
STEP 4 As you drink, identify the whereabouts of the rubbish bin in your office.
STEP 5 Look at the pieces of paper on your desk. *Do not touch them.*
STEP 6 For each document, ask yourself what would really happen if the document suddenly and spontaneously ceased to exist?

STEP 7   For each document, if the answer is 'nothing', go to step 9; if the answer is 'don't know', go to step 10; if the answer is 'something', go to step 8.

STEP 8   Define 'something' in relation to the document and ask yourself: 'Is this something important?' If the answer is yes, go to step 11. If no, go to step 10.

STEP 9   Put it in the bin.

STEP 10   Write 'for filing' on it and give it to someone in the office.

STEP 11   Identify what you need to do in response to the document and *do it straight away, no matter how badly.*

STEP 12   Return to step 5 and start again with the next piece of paper. Continue in this fashion until you have exhausted the pieces of paper.

Some people like to elaborate on this technique, for example by positioning the bin a fair distance from the desk and rolling Step 9 documents into tiny balls for target practice. Others prefer to see how many times they can tear across a single sheet of paper; experts can achieve near shredder-like results. The golden touch rule, however, must be held inviolable; as soon as you have touched a piece of paper, you *must* accept that procrastination is no longer an option and act.

Some people also use the 'red spot' technique. Keep a red pen at your desk, make a red dot or personal squiggle on every sheet that you handle and then act on it. Whenever you come across a document with two dots, bin it or file it. Another handy technique is to move your desk away from the wall. This stops large piles of unanswered paperwork from building up against adjacent walls and allows them to fall on to the floor. Curiously, the most important documents often end up uppermost on the floor. Even on the floor, however, you must still honour the golden touch rule. Remember, also, that if someone else has sent you a document, they will have a copy and so you don't need to keep one.

The noble arts of note keeping and diary husbandry

Two other important things need to be mentioned about paperwork at this point. These involve the two most important pieces of paper in a care worker's armoury: case notes and a diary. Legible, well-kept clinical notes are invaluable, both to patient and worker alike. In the rough and tumble of a day's work, it is easy to forget to record every meeting and every discussion about every patient and just as easy to fall into the trap of thinking that recording your work with a patient isn't quite as important as doing it. In reality, the two are almost equal. Painstaking vigilance here *always* pays off, for many reasons. First, because after a while, conscientious note keeping becomes the norm. Second, because no one cares for patients in isolation, it is a fact that sooner or later, someone else, some-where else, is going to have to rely on your notes to make important decisions about a patient's care. Third, because the case notes are legally admissible documents, there is always the (hopefully rare) chance that one day you may need to rely on your case notes to demonstrate to a court or an inquiry that you did your best. Like it or not, inquiries are unavoidably wise after the event, and usually apply the unforgivingly logical assumption that if you didn't write it down then it wasn't done. We will consider the unpleasant business of inquiries in the following chapter.

Many people find note keeping uncomfortable because it forces them to clarify their views of a difficult problem. Mental health care is an area that is virtually unparalleled in terms of paradoxes, dilemmas, unanswerable questions and all sorts of other conceptual grey areas that seem to defy precise description. People often feel daunted by the task of committing the key issues to paper; instead, they deal with it by writing too little, nothing at all or too much, and end up reading like Marcel Proust. However, there are several things that you can do to maintain a sensible balance. Before you commit yourself to paper, go over the core issues in your head. Jot down rough notes if it is particularly tricky. Before you write anything final, ask yourself: 'What are the really important issues here?' Also, try to avoid writing in conversational style. Instead, try to write like a Dalek. Use lots of short simple statements and numbered points, and avoid long clauses joined by prepositions. Use 'if', 'but', 'because', 'therefore' and 'so on' only sparingly.

Above all, use headings and record the obvious, even if it seems unnecessary at the time. Who was present, where, when and why? In a nutshell, say who said what. If summing up, itemise key happenings since the last meeting. Try to confine it to *news*. People often tend to redescribe the wheel again and again in case notes. If the patient has been admitted or discharged from hospital and there is a referral letter or discharge summary in the notes, then simply write 'see d/c summ. dated ...' and go on to the next bit of *real news*. Do not be afraid of abbreviations either, providing that they make reasonable sense (a list of common case note abbreviations is given in Table 7.1). The other life saver when it comes to note keeping is to make generous use of headings. Headings make you think before you write. The use of terms such as 'recent progress', 'risk', 'impression', 'plan', etc. are a good way of keeping your written records clear and concise, and make it much easier for others to follow. You are writing *notes*, not an essay.

Table 7.1 ● Common case note abbreviations

ADL	Assessment of daily living skills
ASAP	As soon as possible
ASW	Approved social worker
AKA	Also known as
AOS/T	Assertive outreach service/team
ATS	Asked to see
CMHT	Community mental health team
CPA	Care Programme Approach
CPN	Community psychiatric nurse
CRT	Crisis response team
DLA	Disability living allowance
DNA	Did not attend
DOA	Dead on arrival
DSH	Deliberate self-harm
DV	Domiciliary visit
EIS	Early intervention service
FITH	Fucked in the head
FLK	Funny looking kid
FTND	Full-term normal delivery
HPC	History of presenting complaint
IP	Inpatient

(Continued)

Table 7.1 ● (*Continued*)

IV	Interview
I/V	Intravenous
MMSE	Mini-mental state examination (cognitive score out of 30)
NAD	No abnormality detected
O/E	On examination
OP	Outpatient
OT	Occupational therapist
PICU	Psychiatric intensive care unit
STAT	Now, at once
WR	Ward round/review

Formal agencies

CHI	Commission for Health Improvement
DoH	Department of Health
HA	Health authority
MHA	Mental Health Act
MHAC	Mental Health Act Commission
MHRT	Mental health review tribunal
MSU	Medium secure unit
NICE	National Institute for Health and Clinical Excellence
PCT	Primary care trust
SHA	Strategic health authority

Illnesses and symptoms

BPAD	Bipolar affective disorder
Del	Delusion
Dep	Depression
DSPD	Dangerous severe personality disorder
DVM	Diurnal variation (of mood)
EMW	Early morning wakening
Hall	Hallucination
PD	Personality disorder
Scz	Schizophrenia
FTD	Formal thought disorder

Special tests

BSL	Blood sugar level
CT scan	Computerised tomography scan
CXR	Chest X-ray
EEG	Electroencephalogram
FBC	Full blood count
LFTs	Liver function tests
MSSU	Mid-stream specimen of urine
SXR	Skull X-ray
TFTs	Thyroid function tests
U&Es	Urea and electrolytes

The other piece of paper that is essential to a care worker's survival is the diary, but try to avoid keeping more than one. Electronic organisers do not pass the falling down three flights of stairs test half as well as an A5 day-per-page job. Paper does not need batteries and can be read in the Stygian light of a stairwell on the council estate from hell, and pages can be torn out to stick a note under a door. Cultivate the habit of writing everything down – names, times, numbers – and try to avoid illegible hieroglyphics, unless you are sufficiently sure of your own cryptoanalytic skills. Never write down a phone number alone; always note the *name* at the same time. This saves precious hours spent combing through cryptic digits, trying to contact that crucial but half-forgotten support organisation. Diaries can also get lost. As soon as your diary for the coming year arrives, treat yourself to a large white sticker, slap it on the front cover and, in thick black waterproof marker pen, write your name, contact number and 'reward if found' in bold letters.

The diary is an invaluable tool for time management. Time lords can always be recognised by their diary; numerous non-urgent review appointments are spread out exponentially over the weeks ahead, with other sessions clearly 'fenced off' for courses, activities, meetings and so on, as well as space left for a flexible response to inevitable crises. A diary can be used to juggle, arrange and break up the working week to prevent it from becoming humdrum. Above all, pace yourself. Keep the diary full, but not that full.

Once you have got the hang of basic diary husbandry, you can try out some of the more advanced stuff. One technique, often used but rarely acknowledged, is the 'Bunbury', an appointment with a non-existent patient. Admirers of Oscar Wilde's *The Importance of Being Earnest* will recall Algernon's fictional friend, whose difficulties provided a handy reason to be elsewhere from time to time. Every diary should carry an occasional Bunbury. Craft his history skillfully enough and Bunbury can become an invaluable friend in times of need. Also useful is the half-Bunbury, such as the two-till-four planning meeting that you know often ends earlier. In addition, don't forget travel time – ideally include this in the written time slot. However, the core golden rule of having a diary is to *read* it beforehand. Before leaving work, check what you have lined up for tomorrow. At the beginning of the week, have a look and see what will be happening during that week. A quick overview helps to prioritise what will be the highs and the lows, and can prepare you emotionally and organisationally for the future.

Technology – God's gift to communication

Get the hang of technology. Mankind has not spent the last 30000 years banging rocks together for no reason. Apart from the desire to get drunk, one of the things that separates man from the animals is his tendency to use gadgets. Two things about technology seem clear. One is that faxes, computers, e-mails, mobiles, pagers and so on are here to stay. The other is that they are going to get more and more sophisticated. Whether this means that they are also going to become easier to use remains to be seen, but the knack of using technology is to make sure that you are in control and not vice versa.

Many of us still display a Luddite response to the challenge of modern technology, but it pays to resist this defensive reaction. A lot of clever people have spent a long time working out the wiring for this or that little button, which, if pressed, allows you to drink tea while you send a fax or tells you everything that you need to know about the actions of a patient whom you haven't seen for ages. Next time you come across a new gadget that seems annoyingly beyond your ken, don't waste time shouting at it or hitting it. Get out the instruction booklet and spend 15 minutes leafing through the introductory section. Within weeks, you will be able to re-send faxes when lines are busy, enlarge sections of documents using the zoom function of photocopiers, redirect unwanted phone calls to unsuspecting recipients, dial important numbers at the jab of a single button and perform countless other small technological miracles that will nudge up your day-to-day comfort rating. Even better, because so few people actually bother to make use of these details, they will automatically assume that you are a very clever person.

Some devices, however, are more ephemeral than others. In some cases, technological progress even seems to be carrying us backwards rather than forwards. Software viruses, incompatible file formats and funny plugs that don't fit that sort of socket are sadly common features of the modern era, but they should not blind us to the incredible power of the microprocessor. This device is peerless in two areas: gaining rapid access to high-quality clinical information and word processing. In many other areas, papyrus still has the edge.

Familiarise yourself with the operation of your local patient administration software, and get to know what it can and cannot do. A bewildering array of systems are currently in use. Most give access to clinical records, pathological test results and a history of contact with services. Some allow access to clinic booking systems, enabling us to check or create future appointments (but make sure that what it says on the screen matches what is written in your diary). Others even carry standardised encoding of clinical data that enables an at-a-glance assessment of risk or clinical priority. Increasingly, trusts and other organisations are coming to rely upon such data as a way of evaluating clinical activity and efficiency. The implications of this should not be underestimated. In the future, for better or worse, we will probably come to rely upon this sort of information as the least unfair way of allocating ever-scarcer resources. Clearly, the more conscientious and efficient we become at moving data into and out of these systems, the lower the chance of our work being ignored or taken for granted. Most trusts offer training in the principles and practice of the local patient administration system. Go on a course and get to know your local oracle.

Another area where a little learning goes a long way is in the field of word processing. This is one application of the computer that is so useful and so widely employed that it is now hard to recall how we ever managed without it. When was the last time you saw someone using a typewriter? Microsoft Word has all but achieved total domination of the word-processing market, and it pays to know how to create, open, save and edit a file or document in this powerful program. Using the wonderful functions of copy and cut-and-paste, it is now possible to take whole chunks of prose and fashion them into the document of your choice. All at once, a discharge summary can be transformed into a housing report, a handover summary to a colleague or an application for extra benefit, all for the effort of a few altered sentences. Learning to type with all 10 fingers is not as difficult as one might think, and many easy-to-use programs, available on CD, can take the diligent student well beyond the limits of two fingers after only a few weeks of steady practice. Again, many trusts provide training in basic and advanced word-processing skills. Get in touch with your local IT department and see what they have on offer.

If the idea of learning to type seems rather daunting, learn to use a dictating machine. Many people find this device quite off-putting, assuming the need for a fair degree of verbal fluency. In truth, when we have something important to say, most of us waffle on far less than we might think. Before you begin to dictate, go over in your head what you want to say. Who are you writing to? What are the key things that you need to say? How much detail do you need to include? It may help to make a few notes in rough before you begin. Once you start to dictate, try to use short simple sentences and don't forget to say 'stop', 'comma', 'exclamation mark' or 'new paragraph' (although some smart secretaries may prefer to do this themselves). Your secretary will be eternally grateful if you speak slowly and clearly (it doesn't matter how slowly, as there is a go-faster button on the playback machine) and refrain from dictating near noisy people or machines. Practice with a dictaphone makes perfect, but it is pleasantly surprising how quickly most of us lose our verbal hesitancy. Play back what you have said intermittently to check that you are recording – silent tapes of a hard-to-write report can be heartbreaking.

Several other devices have become invaluable in recent years. Mobile phones no longer resemble house bricks and can now go for days on end without the need for recharging. They can also store a lot of useful information. Unfortunately, however, they also have the annoying tendency to ring. Research has proven that the frequency of ringing is proportional to the number of people in possession of your phone number; however, you may not want to talk to many of these people. One small solution to this is to keep the mobile switched off, giving your number to as few people as possible. That way, you can screen all incoming calls, get an idea of their urgency, and reply if and when you want to. This may seem a touch devious, but it can help to protect you from one of the ironies of modern communications technology: the more we are able to communicate with each other, the more we do so unnecessarily and ineffectively. It is becoming ever easier to clog our brains with information that we don't really need or want.

Caseloads

Caseloads are often talked about as though they have a physical existence of their own. Questions such as 'What is the ideal caseload?' or 'What is a manageable caseload?' give rise to the unhelpful illusion that a caseload is a fixed thing, the size of which precisely defines how hard you are working. In fact, size is the only thing about a caseload that should remain reasonably steady. Ideally, everything else within it should be changing. Like a garden, some of its occupants will need cultivation for planting elsewhere, whereas the well-tended, hardy perennials may take longer to grow. Every now and then, a caseload will need vigorous weeding to expel the cases that should never have taken root in the first place.

Keeping one's caseload supple is one of the most important aspects of the job. Its variety and flexibility can exert a powerful effect upon your morale. The feeling that you have too many of the same sort of case, or that difficult cases seem as if they are going to be yours forever, are often two of the clearest signs that you are not controlling your work. There are three main elements to the maintenance of a healthy clinical caseload: (i) maintaining the balance between in and out; (ii) ensuring that the variety (or 'case mix') matches your abilities; and (iii) ensuring that you receive adequate, regular supervision.

Maintaining the balance between in and out

Cases will come into your care from a variety of agencies that will, of course, depend on the type and structure of your team. Most community mental health teams receive their input from hot and cold sources. Not all of these sources may be legitimate. Some cases may have a particular type or severity of problem that, from the outset, is better disposed of by handing on to a more appropriate service. Knowledge of one's local network and geographical boundaries, as well as a confident adherence to one's own acceptance criteria, are obvious but easily overlooked ways of heading off a small but significant amount of work before it arrives.

Acute 'hot' cases are often seen at times and places beyond one's control, for example at a walk-in, at someone's home or at a police station. The process by which someone undergoes the transition from a stable member of the community into someone in need of assessment by a mental health professional is extremely complex and dependent on countless factors. Because of the emotion that psychiatric emergencies can generate, it is often easy, in the heat of the moment, to offer more long-term help than can be realistically provided. As society becomes increasingly more medical in its approach to many problems, it is all too easy for a care worker to be drawn into an assessment and even ongoing care for a problem that only a few years ago would have been regarded as a domestic or social issue. Cold cases, on the other hand, tend to come through telephone or written referral, usually after initial contact with some other service. They can often be dealt with at a more measured pace and so carry less risk of clogging one's caseload.

Severe mental illnesses, almost by definition, are likely to be long term. They usually involve short periods of detailed assessment, after which they may either be passed on or find their way on to your personal caseload. It is important at the outset to draw a clear distinction between assessing a patient's needs and accepting responsibility for doing something about them. A team that does not make this distinction is often poorly organised. Well-organised teams always have some structure in place for fairly distributing all cases on a basis that meets both the needs of the patient and the worker.

There is always a risk that the caseloads of the more enthusiastic or experienced workers will clog up with more severe cases, especially those patients who require higher degrees of multi-agency support. This can be countered by constant reviews of the changing needs of each patient. Almost invariably, after the 'going home' period is over, there is some reduction in the level of monitoring and care required by each patient. There is a fine art to both recognising and responding to this drop in need, either by delegation to another worker within or outside of your own team or by closing the case altogether. When input is reduced rather than ended, responsibility can be reduced to maintaining a care coordination role by convening regular reviews and supporting the designated contact person.

Moving patients on

Whenever your involvement in a case changes, it is up to you to make sure that other people know about it. Again, well-worn grooves of communication are essential. Clear notes of who will be doing what from now on and to whom, and a brief letter to the patient's GP, should be a routine element of care every time patients move in, out or down your caseload. Paying attention to the detail and language of this communication can improve the flow of patients out of your caseload. Only a significant minority of cases coming under the care of a busy mental health team are likely to disengage permanently from all forms of support or the need for contact with caring services. Instead, most are usually passed on to the care of other agencies, re-hospitalised or referred back to their GP or support organisation. Therefore, with every handover there is a small hurdle to overcome if a given patient is to be discharged from your load.

It pays, therefore, to think ahead about the sort of things that the receiving agency will want to know about before they may be willing to consider accepting responsibility for your patient. Being aware of who will want to know what about any given case is more than just a matter of experience. A concise account of the patient's recent progress (or lack of it), significant risk factors and current medication and an assessment of the patient's ability to cope, i.e. an up-to-date occupational therapy (OT) assessment of daily living skills (ADL), will almost always accelerate, or at least lubricate, the handover process. In cases in which there has been a history of risk to self or others there is a legal and professional obligation to pass on this information, usually within a coherent framework such as the Care Programme Approach (CPA). Many organisations now insist on the completion of a form that lays out the minimum required information needed before they will begin their process of acceptance. Sometimes, this may serve the devious function of delaying the procedure, occasionally to the point at which other clinical issues supervene. In a world where pressure on scarce resources seems to rise as fast as the thresholds for admitting people into residential units, such Machiavellian methods seem almost necessary. Standardised forms also carry the inevitable drawback of any mass-produced item, namely a lack of flexibility. No matter how well thought out an application form is, human nature is so varied as to almost always guarantee that something needs to be written in a section of the form that does not appear to exist. The covering letter is the necessary solution to such bureaucratic inflexibility.

Although a crucial basic amount of information should be passed on with any patient moving out of one's care, there is also much to be gained from paying attention to the subtle details of any communication, whether by phone, open letter or standardised form. There is a sort of unwritten etiquette about handing patients on, the central rule of which is always to polish before you push. If possible, try to put more positives than negatives into the opening and closing sections of your handover statements and always avoid the complacent assumption that acceptance is a foregone conclusion. For example, if you were the slightly precious proprietor of the Happy Vale Rest Home for young people with enduring mental illness and had only one remaining vacancy, to which of the following two letters would you respond the most quickly?

'Dear Madam

I am writing to ask if you would be willing to assess this articulate young man with a diagnosis of paranoid schizophrenia, currently in stable remission. He is once again beginning to put down roots in the local community. Although this has in the past been complicated by substance misuse and short-lived episodes of challenging behaviour, he has achieved a sustained reduction in his substance misuse as well as signs of enduring commitment to alter his behaviour for the better.'

or

'Dear Madam

I am writing to ask you to take over the care of this argumentative 'revolving-door' schizophrenic who has recently been discharged from our acute unit after a relapse complicated by polydrug abuse and coercive threats of self-harm. He has taken no further overdoses since discharge and has agreed to see a drug counsellor next week.'

Most acceptance procedures will tolerate, or even expect, a degree of euphemistic truth bending. Erratic bathing patterns or the loud slurping noises that a patient makes when happy may be truthfully economised, but it is important not to lie or omit whoppers from a patient's history, particularly when these relate to risk. Rather, pains should be taken to spell these out as unequivocally as possible.

Another important way to maximise the flow of cases out of one's caseload is simply to know the local network inside out. The more hostels, drop-ins and support organisations that you know about, the more you have room for manoeuvre. New services open all the time and older ones close. If you can find or create time to keep up with this ever-shifting mosaic of care, it will almost certainly help to keep your caseload, as well as your energy levels on a Friday afternoon, at a healthy level.

Clogging of one's caseload can also derive from the powerful attachments that often arise between patient and carer over time. For many patients, the caregiver relationship can be one of the most important relationships in their life – sometimes it is the *only* relationship. This can easily foster a state of dependence, often revealed in the expressed belief that only one person can possibly understand or help a given patient, a view that is often eagerly shared by busy colleagues. Managing the dependent patient is a skill in its own right and an issue that we will consider in the next chapter.

Keeping an eye on the case mix

Ideally, the cases in any one caseload should be almost as varied as one's working week. Of course, the precise composition will depend on your location and the type of team in which you work. For example, more severe degrees of mental illness will often dominate the caseload of a generic adult general team working in a busy inner-city area, at the expense of neurotic or mood disorders. Often, one or two workers within a team, usually those with more experience, tend to build up either an interest or a reputation for managing a particular type of clinical problem. Although this can carry advantages for worker and patient alike (additional skills are useful for the whole team), it brings with it the risk of stagnation.

Caseloads need to be balanced not only between 'hot' and 'cold' cases but also between many other things. Juggling between male and female, happy and sad, psychotic and neurotic, acute and chronic, as well as between routine case work and the never-ending demands of duty work, is far easier to achieve on paper than it is in practice. It is therefore important to have as clear an idea as possible of the case mix that works for you, and to devote your energies and time to achieving it. One important way to achieve this is through the process of supervision.

Getting decent supervision and appraisal

No one should be left to manage a caseload of 15 or more mentally ill people single-handedly. People grow used to each other over time and are often inattentive to things that change either slowly or not at all. Because of this, it is impossible for any of us to correctly judge when to discharge every patient 100% of the time. It is the job of a supervisor to help you achieve this. Apart from seeing patients, supervision of one's clinical and academic work is one of the most important events in the weekly timetable; however, regrettably, it is still one of the most poorly carried out. All too often, especially in the more hard-pressed areas, it doesn't happen at all, usually because other issues are somehow seen to be more important or at least more urgent. This almost always turns out to be a false economy, as a well-planned care process, implemented by competent, well-supervised staff, reduces the chances of urgent distractions in the first place.

There are many important points about supervision, not all of which are obvious. It should always occur at a fixed time and place and last for an agreed period. There is no hard and fast rule about how long one should spend with one's supervisor, but, generally, anything less than half an hour is too short to cover several issues in any useful depth, and anything more than an hour eats too large a hole in the day. If the session does need to be moved occasionally, or even cancelled, this should always be acknowledged and met with an agreement to meet at another time and place.

The relationship between the supervisor and the supervised is just as important as the constancy and timing of the supervision. It helps if the supervisor is older than the person they are supervising, and a greater degree of experience is mandatory. One doesn't necessarily have to like one's supervisor, but respect for that person is essential. It should be clear to all outside agencies that supervision time is a priority that should be interrupted only by serious matters. Bleeps and pagers should be silenced and non-urgent calls either redirected or ignored altogether. If your supervisor is constantly signing letters, nipping out of the room or taking or making the odd call during your allocated time, you can be reasonably sure that he or she is not that interested in your work.

Just what is talked about in these sessions is entirely up to you. Some people like to structure the session, for example 15 minutes spent on clinical cases, 10 minutes spent on case note review and another 15 on other matters, such as professional and personal development. In our experience, it is best left as free as possible, with the content largely determined by the supervised rather than the supervisor. Although this carries the risk of the entire session descending into a cosy chat, it does help to ensure that one of the most important goals of supervision is not overlooked, namely that the session may be a dumping ground for a worker's angst. The world in which all mental health workers operate is far from ideal and it is a virtual certainty that sooner or later, every worker will need to let off steam, confess to a half-baked idea or ask for a spot of compassionate leave.

Once or twice a year, a supervision session should be devoted to appraisal. This involves reviewing what you have done, your timetable, your training needs and your goals for the coming year. Writing these down to help the review is vital. Aiming to do something and realising that you have achieved it gives a good focus to a year's work and your job prospects will benefit.

If, for some reason, supervision does not seem to be happening on a regular basis, it is important to try to identify the reason why. If a supervisor constantly provides a series of apparently plausible reasons why your session has been cancelled several times each month, do not accept this at face value. It is not easy to sit in a room with a junior colleague and listen patiently as he or she grapples with problems that, to you, seem relatively minor. Many supervisors, rather than face up to this discomfort, try to avoid it and may resort to all sorts of means to do so. If you feel that supervision sessions are happening less often than you would like, and if when they are cancelled another session is not promptly issued, do something about it. Otherwise, inactivity or complacency will all too often be taken as a sign that you happy with the arrangement.

Another thing to watch out for in supervision is the occasional reversal of roles. Being a manager or team leader of a busy mental health team is rarely a picnic and occasionally one finds oneself not so much receiving supervision for one's clinical work but, instead, providing a form of supportive psychotherapy for one's supervisor. Such a shift in roles usually creeps in over time, but being aware of this, and being able to mention it, is an effective way of preventing your supervisor from joining your caseload.

Handling colleagues and esprit de corps

Whoever said that liking your colleagues is a bonus was an arrogant, miserable person, but probably right. Mental health work attracts an extremely varied range of professions and personalities, so it is unrealistic to expect that you will become happy comrades-in-arms with all of them all of the time. Because of the demanding nature of the work, however, a degree of mutual support, comradeship and even friendship is important if we are ever going to feel like getting out of bed on a Monday morning. How you function as part of a team and, in particular, the way that you communicate with and respond to the actions of your colleagues, is something that requires thought. Much of this, of course, relates immutably to one's own personality and personal style of communication and, as a smart Irishman once observed, nothing worth knowing can ever be taught. We contend, however, that it can be learnt. Paying attention to the way that you communicate and cooperate as part of a team, and how you deal with conflict, will directly increase the quality of your work as well as the satisfaction of a job well done.

It goes without saying that one should treat all colleagues and patients with politeness and respect at all times, but there are certain members of the team whom it pays to treat like gold dust. Typists, secretaries, administrators and clerks are the unsung heroes of most mental health teams. Although much of what they do seems so uneventful that is taken for granted by many, their memories of names, events, phone numbers and so on can make a major difference to the management of a case. Treat staff who have been in a post for much longer than you with particular respect and take some time out to get to know how they work, as well as identifying their likes and dislikes.

Try to smile at people on at least a semi-regular basis and take time during the hustle and bustle of the day to chat to people for example about their kids or their new hairdo or shirt. Machiavellian perhaps, but if you want a permit for that new controlled parking zone that the council has just installed outside your office, it helps to be on good terms with the person who fills out the application forms. If you think that a piece of work has been well done or made a particular difference to a case, say so – but don't overdo it. Near-American degrees of sharing, hugging and sincerity still don't go down too well in our sceptical, emotionally constrained Anglo-Saxon world. As the Duke of Wellington said when asked on his deathbed if he had any regrets about his life: 'I would have given more praise.'

Handling conflict

Clear communication is important in your dealings with all colleagues. If things are unsatisfactory, make this clear. Handling conflict and disagreement is something that most people do badly. Virtually all of us, to varying degrees, are afraid of appearing weak, of being humiliated or of receiving an angry rebuff. In fact, frustration and disappointment at the consequences of a problem left unaddressed are far more likely to occur. If you are not happy with what is going on, say so, mention it in supervision and get it out in the open. That's what team meetings and teamwork are all about – not letting things fester. Those who are new to a post, or those who are just plain lazy, can easily take silence over a shabby job as tacit admission of acceptance.

The rules for dealing with conflict are similar to those for breaking any bad news. Try to have a clear idea of what it is that concerns you and think about what you want to say and how you intend to say it well beforehand. Find an appropriate time and place, preferably away from gawping colleagues, and make your case clearly, tactfully and calmly. No matter how delicate an issue, there is *always* a tactful way to deal with confrontation without someone bursting into tears and locking themselves in the toilet. Try to pay close attention to your own emotional state, especially if the issue has been bugging you for a while. If you can, try to keep half a mental eye on your breathing and jaw tightness as you speak, and try to keep a calm, even tone to your voice. Whatever you do, never lose your temper, use aggressive gestures or make threats. It may seem like a good idea at the time, but it always goes down badly at industrial tribunals. Having made your point, don't walk off; allow time for the other person to take it in and react. Listen as sympathetically as possible, even if someone is trying to justify their personal responsibility for World War III. Finally, try to reach some sort of clear agreement on what needs to be done next. If all this fails, then that it is exactly what supervision is there for: offload your angst on your supervisor, not on the focus of your irritation.

Because of the pressured, overstretched and (usually) underfunded climate in which we work, team morale is a complex, delicate thing that will always have its ebbs and flows. Try to maintain a feel for the well-being of this delicate creature known as 'the team', but don't get too hung up on the concept. Beware of pointless discussions about 'what the team might think'. To paraphrase one politician, there are no such things as teams, only people. Sooner or later, every team loses a beloved leader or some other solid type upon whom so much seems to depend. At other times, because of the very nature of the work, teams will have to deal with some sort of human catastrophe. Like it or not, violence, self-mutilation, arson, suicide and homicide are inevitable accompaniments of the trade and something that people will need to weather together from time to time. Everyone will play a role in creating the nature and identity of the team, which tends to take on a curiously mutable life of its own. Nowhere is this life more clearly evident than in meetings.

How to chair a meeting

Although they should be avoided if at all possible (or at least carefully rationed), meetings are a particular form of social interaction where all of one's intuitive communication and team-playing skills are brought into play at once. They are events in which the bewildering complexity of human nature is on show for all to see. In fact, meetings are such fertile grounds for psychological exploration that entire libraries have been written about them. Much of what has been written is superfluous to the care worker – if not to the entire human race – but some themes do emerge from this corpus of wisdom that can improve one's ability to manage any sort of meeting, from a care plan review to a trust AGM.

The ability of any group of people to rationally evaluate and deal with an issue is inversely proportional to the number of people in that group (i.e. the fewer there are, the easier it is to agree – and the easier to fix a date to meet). This is not as glib as it sounds when one considers the sheer complexity of the process known as 'discussion'. Even a single phrase, no matter how elementary, has its ambiguities. Consider this statement: 'Time flies like the wind.' To most of us, this well-known phrase simply means that time can pass faster than we think. It metaphorically compares time, an abstract concept, with wind, a more concrete noun with a mercurial quality. This seems fairly comprehensible. However, it is also possible to interpret this statement in other less obvious ways. What if 'time' was an imperative verb rather than a noun, instructing you to measure flies (i.e. small insects) in the same way as you might measure the wind? Or, what if a curious species of insect, the time fly, happened to like windy days?

In the same way, one can ask what is the meaning of the phrase 'We must treat his schizophrenia aggressively'. If one also considers not just an isolated utterance but a full-on discussion of the question 'Is marijuana making my son go schizophrenic?' among a roomful of people, each with their own beliefs and agendas, it becomes easier to understand just how complicated a meeting can become.

It is the job of a decent chairperson to introduce an element of coherence into this potential verbal battle zone, thereby transforming the meeting into an event that not only entails the useful sharing of information but also produces a result that should make a difference to someone, somewhere. Making a difference is the most important point of all. If a meeting doesn't change anything, it should not have happened in the first place. This underscores an important characteristic of a good chairperson: know the agenda inside out. It need not necessarily be written down, or even stated explicitly (although as we will see, this is often helpful), but, as far as possible, the chairperson should have a clear idea of what the meeting is about, who will be present and what can (hopefully) be achieved by going ahead with it. Refreshing oneself with a brief résumé of the story so far and paying particular attention to the ways in which different players in the story might see things can often save a lot of embarrassed wriggling and dodgy moments after kick-off. In fact, the idea of the meeting as a game is useful. The chairperson, as referee, should not also be the main player. Rather, from the very beginning it is down to him or her to keep the rules clear and so draw the best performances from all present.

Make sure that everyone in the room knows who everyone else is, what they do and why they are here. Many of us can recall meetings at which we have bemoaned the absence of anyone with personal knowledge of Harry, only to discover that the quiet lady in the corner who arrived late is in fact Harry's mum. The tradition of asking all those gathered to introduce themselves one by one is well worth keeping to. Attendees should also be invited to say more – but not much more – than their name. People remember things better when a label is served up alongside something meaningful. Less experienced chairs often avoid this, wrongly fearing that the amount of information it generates is either useless or overwhelming to those present. This is not so. To discuss something as important as someone's health without identifying all those present is not only inconsiderate but may also be harmful: you never know when a tabloid journalist may be present.

It is also helpful to establish a few other points at the start of a meeting. Agreeing that all comments go through you, i.e. no one talks unless asked by you, sets a tone of order and non-interruption, and gives everyone a chance to air their views. Denoting your status to the group from the outset is particularly useful when verbal fisticuffs break out and intervention becomes necessary. It is also important to state the purpose of the meeting, what it can realistically hope to achieve and how long it is likely to last. Try to identify those who need to leave early, otherwise they may not be around to contribute to an issue that may later turn out to be crucial. Sometimes, early leavers may be trying to wriggle out of something. Knowing who is coming, going and saying what enables you to ensure that everyone gets a chance to play a role and to guide the meeting towards a result. Early agreement on the date and time of a follow-up meeting, if needed, can also reassure people.

The other essential element of every well-run meeting is a reliable record. The choice of minute taker is more important than seems obvious at first glance.

Choose someone whose skills you feel are reliable and never assign this role to someone who is likely to play a large part in the discussion. A carer who has become the object of a patient's obsessions cannot be relied upon to act as an impartial note taker.

Surprisingly, the position of the minute taker in the room can also be important. Try to keep the recorder in your eyeline (ideally sit close to him or her), as non-verbal communication is often a useful way of ensuring that a point is recorded, particularly when the conversation is too important, or too heated, to interrupt. Often, the solution to a point of particular difficulty seems to arise for just a few fleeting moments. If this seems significant, make a very brief note of your own or find the courage to halt the flow of the meeting and make sure that it gets written down. This is occasionally a helpful way to put gentle pressure on a prevaricating member of the group, from whom clarity (will they help or won't they) can help a patient's care take a significant step forwards.

The rules for handling conflict in meetings are slightly different from those we considered earlier, particularly when patients, carers, relatives and other interested parties are present. A little letting off of steam can even prove therapeutic. How far you allow this steam to rise, however, is a matter of skill, intuition and luck. Don't think that the meeting is going pear shaped just because someone gets angry or upset. Always keep your own cool, but, equally, never be afraid of confronting someone if you feel that things are getting out of hand. Trading of insults, or even actual fisticuffs, although a rich source of entertainment, are completely out of the question. If things do seem to be heading in that direction, never hesitate to invoke your ultimate power as the chairperson and call the meeting to an end. Protagonists may, if they choose, continue their wrestling in the car park.

It is always helpful to keep an overall view of the general direction that a meeting is taking, especially when an emotive topic is under discussion. One of the more useful insights that has emerged from the voluminous literature on group psychology is the idea of 'risky shift'. Individuals who share a strong opinion on an issue (e.g. how best to respond to a violent patient who has recently threatened a colleague) can often reinforce increasingly biased thoughts and decisions. This can lead to an outcome that none of those present would ever have sanctioned had they deliberated on the matter alone. Beware, therefore, of the way that meetings can descend into something out of *Lord of the Flies*. 'Kill the pig' is not a useful management plan for a depressed patient with a history of aggression. It is the job of the chairperson to ask the question of whether the meeting is heading towards a decision that is completely at odds with what is achievable in the world outside.

The emotions that meetings can generate should also be watched for other important effects. Social hierarchies, pecking orders, professional jealousies and long-concealed grievances may often reveal themselves with surprising speed and ugliness. Watch out for the early emergence of blame or scapegoating, particularly of someone who is absent. The 'bad guy' is an archetypal role that is buried deep in our primaeval unconscious and needs careful watching. It can pop up all too easily, particularly when provision of care has been found lacking.

Equally, the emotional states of particular individuals can sometimes distort the decisions reached at a meeting. Watch out for the exhausted prophets of doom, with a 'seen it all before and none of it makes any difference' philosophy. They may occasionally be right, but, more often than not, they are in need of a change, a decent holiday or a kick up the backside. It is the job of the chairperson to stamp out the contagion of despair before it takes hold. If the glass of community care was half empty rather than half full, we'd never get out of bed on a Monday.

Other situations in a meeting can also act as fertile ground for demoralisation. More than one person talking at once should not be tolerated more than once or twice every 15 minutes and is a key test of your chairing skills. Otherwise, things can very quickly deteriorate into something resembling a bad party with no drinks, from which everyone goes home empty handed. Also, keep an ear open for the 'round the houses' trap. This usually crops up when one of the classic dilemmas of community care is being discussed. Should we intervene when the risk is in the history rather than the current mental state? Should we disclose a patient's history to the police? Should we close an impossibly difficult case? Is it madness or badness? No one has a clear answer to any of these questions. A shrewd chairperson will know when to protect the participants from the sinking feeling that they too have failed to clinch the issue. Because of their conundrum-like quality, these debates can easily take on a dispiriting circularity. Once one has gone around the loop three times or more, it is easy to feel as though the discussion is a waste of time, so don't let it get beyond the second loop. Agree a review date, perhaps a simple task and close out the meeting.

This section began with the advice to avoid meetings if at all possible. It ends with a justification of this statement. Increasingly, mental health workers are finding themselves asked to confront problems that have no clear-cut or simple solution. In the present climate of untowardness, litigation and blame, the urge to adopt a defensive, cover-your-own-back working style is becoming ever stronger. All too often, therefore, we find ourselves present at meetings in which the most important issue on the agenda appears to have nothing to do with the well-being of a particular patient or the running of an efficient service. Instead, an ever-increasing number of meetings seem to take place for no clear reason at all other than to provide short-term reassurance to those present, in particular those in senior management positions who want to be seen to have done something, such as hold a meeting.

It is very easy here to confuse form with content; just because we appear to be doing something by holding a meeting, it does not necessarily mean that we are doing something. Never go to a meeting the primary purpose of which is to decide whether or not to have a meeting. There are some good meetings, but only one in ten is actually worth attending. The secret lies in knowing which one, and that knowledge can take years to acquire.

How to take care of yourself

It is often said that doctors and nurses make the worst patients. The reasons for this are varied and interesting, but it is probably something to do with having the sort of personality that becomes drawn into the caring profession in the first place. By nature, most of us seem to enjoy putting others first, or perhaps ourselves last. Another aspect involves mental self-defence – people who spend their working day peering into the abyss of sadness and madness have to develop a frame of mind that enables them to cope. Consider, for example, the popularity of gallows humour in your own team. In order to deal with the assorted negatives that form a routine part of our daily work, we devise all sorts of tricks to help sustain the belief that 'it couldn't happen to us'. One aspect of this is the stigmatising belief that severe mental illness befalls only a weaker race of people, somehow distinct from ourselves. Another involves buying into the myth that we are that little bit tougher or somehow more immune to the knocks of life than our lay brothers and sisters.

Although we know that these ideas are largely untrue, we put a lot of effort into ignoring the evidence against them. We easily misconstrue asking for help as a sign of weakness and often downplay signs and symptoms that would have sent any sensible person running for help a long time ago. It is almost as though we train ourselves to ignore Ovid's advice to nip it in the bud (see page 91). Instead of nipping anything, we laugh it off, swallow a couple of paracetamol, have a cigarette, go to the pub, go out clubbing, stay on a bit later at work or generally do anything to delude ourselves that all will be okay once the weekend comes. It is ironic that, although we spend much of our working week monitoring the mental states of those at risk, we rarely pay this sort of attention to ourselves. Small surprise, then, that so many of us appear exhausted, are off sick or talk of working somewhere else. If we can identify some of the subtle ways in which we put ourselves at risk, we can more easily do something to rectify the situation.

This is not to say that we should avoid taking risks with our health or encourage a whinging, neurotic introspection of Woody Allen proportions. The last thing we need to do is place ourselves on our own caseloads. What we do mean, however, is that monitoring one's own physical and mental state is an essential part of the job. You can't look after other people properly unless you first look after yourself. Cultivating the habit of introspection, and generally listening to what your body and brain are trying to tell you, also has advantages that go well beyond helping you to stay sane. It can actually help you to listen to, understand and help your patients more effectively, especially the more difficult cases on your books, i.e. the ones who elicit strong emotions and behaviours in others. And, as if this isn't enough, it can even help you to live longer and have more fun.

Listen to what your body tells you and watch what goes into it

It is an anatomical fact that your brain maintains an intimate, two-way communication with the rest of you via a nervous system of staggering complexity. It has taken about 1.5 billion years to achieve this level of sophistication. You can therefore be quite sure that the methods it has developed for telling you that something is going wrong are reliable. Most of the signs that we are overdoing it usually arrive via the sympathetic nervous system. We spend much of our day routinely enquiring of others about such symptoms as headache, palpitations, dryness of the mouth, butterflies in the stomach, loss of appetite, nausea, neck ache, dizzy feelings, tiredness, sleep disturbance, loss of interest in sex and recent changes in body weight. Every now and then, it is a very good idea to run this checklist against ourselves. Every car needs an annual MOT, and we would suggest at least this frequency of check-up, however you do it or whoever you do it with.

Often, the earliest signs that we are working too hard, or not coping too well with the work in hand, are far subtler than those we look for in our patients. Funny twinges, little niggly aches, woozy spells, twitching eyelids or lips and especially tiredness towards the end of the day are several of the symptoms that we most easily overlook or take for granted as a natural consequence of a day's work. Most of us tend to have a musculoskeletal 'weak spot' in our bodies, which, through years of misuse, tends to get tense or achey when we are in need of a break; the commonest spots are the temples, forehead, upper neck or anywhere along the spinal column, although some may find that it occurs elsewhere. Often, such people may have a particular history of injury or strain to that area.

The dividing line between an acceptable and unacceptable degree of tiredness is also exquisitely sensitive to our beliefs about our ability to cope and is thus easily dismissed as a warning sign that we need to alter our working style. Feeling a little tired at work is perfectly normal, and grabbing the odd snooze or rest is sworn by some to be a perfect way of maintaining peak efficiency; however, it is easy to over-sell this. Many individuals sustain themselves with the false belief that it is normal to go to bed as soon as one reaches home and that having any energy left over for anything else in one's life is an impossibility except during the holidays. If work is reaching the point at which you have little time or energy to do anything else other than rest, you are in serious need of a rethink. If the act of going to work is a struggle in itself, again you need a rethink.

Your sleep pattern is one of the clearest ways in which your body will let you know if things are getting out of hand, particularly in those crucial moments after you switch out the light. Do you go to sleep straight away or within a few minutes? Most of us should do. If you are a natural insomniac, then ask yourself if you are more so than usual? The important thing to look out for is a *change* in your sleep pattern compared with normal. Are you dreaming more than usual? Is there a recurring theme to the dream? What is it? If you do find that you are losing sleep worrying about your work, or waking early or in the middle of the night, don't automatically diagnose a depressive episode or begin to panic. Instead, try to be totally honest with yourself and ask what it is that is keeping you awake. Often it comes down to a particular thought or matter. As we shall see, identifying this is the essential precursor to remedial action.

Another useful indicator is your appetite. Do you still feel hungry and enjoy food? Has your weight changed much, up or down, since you started work? Has your diet changed over time, from decent meals to junk and hasty snacks? Given that most of us tend to gain a pound or two for every year that we live over the age of thirty-five, and that few of us are naturally programmed to look like film stars, be honest and ask yourself whether you are really happy with your weight and what you look like.

It is also a very good idea to pay the occasional thought to what goes into your body recreationally as well as nutritionally. Although younger people commonly display an enviable ability to turn up for a full day's work after many nights of full-on cruising and boozing, most mortals start to lose this ability once they turn thirty. Many of us also use food and drugs as a way of fending off any warning signs that we are overdoing it. It is advisable to keep an eye on one's intake of alcohol and other substances. You should automatically know what the sensible limits are for the legal drugs. Be very wary of illegal drugs; random workplace urine screens may become routine. As members of a profession that is heavily invested with respect by society, don't expect to be treated leniently if you are caught in possession of any drug, whether it is class A, B or C. If you ever feel even the *teeni-est* bit of guilt about your intake of anything, the odds are that you are overdoing it. It makes good sense to have at least one or two alcohol-free days per week.

Another warning sign of not coping well involves not the quantity of food and drugs being consumed or the frequency of consumption, but the context in which they are consumed. Doing so in the company of like-minded others is usually safer than doing so by oneself. People who drink in isolation stand a much greater than average chance of developing substance misuse problems in later life. Don't be fooled into thinking that tea and coffee are innocuous beverages, either. Three heaps of instant coffee daily contain enough caffeine to give quite a few people a pounding headache by mid-afternoon.

Keeping up a reasonable degree of physical fitness can help a lot, although the word 'fitness' is subject to a very wide range of definitions. Because one man's gymnasium is another man's torture chamber, we recommend that a sensible care worker tries to maintain, at the very minimum, a lower level of baseline physical fitness. If you can walk briskly up two flights of stairs while maintaining a conversation, you will have passed our test. It is actually a lot easier to achieve this than it seems. Refraining from using lifts when out on visits is one way, whereas avoiding use of the car for home visits close to base is another. Getting into the habit of doing these things automatically is just as important. It is great if you happen to enjoy cycling or running to work, but you don't need to be an athlete to be a happy healthy care worker. However, it is worth remembering that regular exercise for 20 minutes, three times a week, is all that is needed to stay aerobically fit.

How to watch what goes on in your head

All of us have different ways of making sense of our world but, fortunately, most of us use the same language, internal and external, to describe it. Although there is no straightforward correspondence between the thoughts and images in our heads and what comes out of our mouths, it is helpful to try to remain aware of the general themes of our language, both private and public. This may actually involve a degree of honesty that some might find uncomfortable, but what is there to lose? No one is ever going to have access to what we find out unless we tell them.

If you had to use a single adjective to describe the essence of your day-to-day thoughts and feelings in the workplace, what would it be? Happy? Content? Tired? Fed up? Undervalued? Notice how here inside our head, our thoughts and feelings don't seem to be quite so separate from each other as they do when described in externally expressed language. It is a fact that, at any one instant in our lives, our emotional state constantly influences the sorts of things that we choose to think about and colours the ways that we think about them. And because our moods can change for all sorts of reasons and in all sorts of ways, so can our ways of interpreting, understanding and thinking about things. Cultivating the habit of observing this process from time to time can help us to act more consistently and so deal more effectively with the job that confronts us.

Another method of watching what goes on in your head is to cast an occasional eye over your fantasies – the things that you would dearly love to do if you had the nerve, the time and the money. Are these things eating you up or cropping up in your head more often than you would like. What sort of feelings do they engender? Laughter? Sexiness? Anger? Guilt? Alternatively, try to identify the themes that your thinking takes on when you have to react to something disappointing in the workplace. Is it all doom and gloom? Could have been worse? Do you use humour to deal with things at work? What makes you laugh? Gallows humour or *Schadenfreude* perhaps?

Another technique for monitoring yourself is to use the cinema trick, variously employed by psychoanalysts and actors. Imagine that your current life is not happening to you at all but is, instead, being enacted up on the silver screen. You are seated in the cinema watching, a few rows from the back. What sort of film is it: a comedy, a tragedy, a soap? What are the motives and emotional states of the main characters? Who are the good guys? What do you think is going to happen?

It is important not to ascribe values to any particular thought, mood, impulse, image or fantasy that these methods may dredge up from your unconsciousness. An urge to torture your supervisor or salacious thoughts about an attractive patient on your books are not necessarily unhealthy or abnormal. There is no 'correct' way

195

to feel about any of these things. To consider it in such terms is to miss the point. Rather, all that these tricks aim to do is to cultivate the invaluable skill of emotional honesty – a tried and tested method of holding on to your sanity in the workplace. The alternative, namely to sail along blithely, ignoring what you think and feel about your work, carries a far greater risk of difficulties as a result of exhaustion, gloom and burnout.

Similarly, there is no 'correct' action to take in response to your mental discoveries. Of course, there are better and worse ways of remedying any problem but, usually, the worst thing to do is absolutely nothing. If what you uncover is little more than peace and contentment, skip the rest of this section and count yourself among the lucky 1% of care workers who are totally at ease with themselves and their work. If, however, you find yourself staring into the oncoming headlights of tiredness, desperation, resignation or worse, do something. It doesn't matter what you do, as long as you do it. Freezing and hoping that it will go away doesn't work for ostriches or road-bound hedgehogs. It doesn't work for care workers either.

Watching your behaviour – what your brain tells your body to do

Your behaviour is that part of your emotional, intellectual and physical activity which is on permanent display to the world. If your behaviour is like a coat, then emotion is its inner lining. It is the thing by which you will be judged by both patients and colleagues alike. No matter how vain you are, other people have to look at you and listen to you much more than you do yourself. Others, therefore, are often in a better position to notice subtle changes in your mood and behaviour. Keeping an occasional eye on 'how you come across' is thus a very useful habit to cultivate. Concerned glances, solicitous comments or people avoiding you or reacting differently to you are all significant.

Indecisiveness and procrastination are two of the commonest signs that it is time for a holiday or a change of scene, especially if your degree of indecision is greater than usual. A good place to observe this directly is on your desk. Is paper accumulating at a greater rate than usual? How often are you picking something up only to put it down again a few minutes later, unaddressed? Are you going to great lengths to reduce your contact with patients or confining your work with them to the absolute bare minimum that is necessary? If any of these questions strike an uneasy chord, do something about it.

In addition, watch your emotional behaviour. Do you often moan and complain to anyone who seems willing to listen? It is important to try not to. We have already considered the importance of humour as a defence against the difficulties of the job, but how often do you laugh during your average working day? In a similar way to keeping fit, it varies greatly from person to person, but there is still a basic definable minimum. Even the worst curmudgeon should smile, or preferably laugh, at least once in any 24-hour period, even if it is only in private. The opposite goes for irritability. Irritability in the work place is almost always abnormal and is usefully defined as disagreeing with more than one colleague in any 24-hour period. If you find yourself breaching any of these clear-cut definitions, the solution is easy. Smile more. Try to make a positive effort to be nicer, even if you don't mean it. Most people don't think about whether you mean it or not, and returned smiles might even make you feel better.

The Friday afternoon test

Because of the nature of the work, sooner or later all of us are going to run into difficulty with a particularly challenging case, take on too great a workload or make a mistake. We would not be human if we didn't. After a while, all of our cases and decisions can begin to take on a stale, unprofitable quality. No one seems to get better. Try to stay aware of the way that you think, feel and react to these things. If we can identify the subtle point at which new cases change from being challenges into stresses, we can avoid the tiredness, despondency and burnout that we so often see around us. We have already suggested several ways to remain vigilant to this eventuality, but here we propose one more simple method of psychological self-help. On a Friday afternoon, think of any time in your life when you were *really* happy. Try to focus on the memory of the emotion itself. If all that you can summon up is a blank, it's time for a holiday.

How to develop as a professional while having fun

Every day that you come to work (with the odd exception) should, in one way or another, lead to your becoming better at what you do, being promoted or generally improving in whichever way that you want. The secret is to work at it, even if you are not quite sure what it is that you want. Doing your best all the time will usually suffice until you have an idea. To this end, always make sure that there is regular, dedicated time in your working week for personal study, reading, writing or attending courses. It is *essential* that these activities are a core element of your work, rather than being a luxurious addition.

It is important to keep up with what is happening not only in your field but also in the world of mental health care in general. Our understanding of the causes, patterns and treatments of mental illness never stands still, and keeping abreast of the broader picture is not only a fascinating and rewarding topic of study in its own right but also something that will make you a much better care worker. It will help your patients gain access to information and treatment much faster, involve you in all sorts of useful conversations with other people, and result in your emanating that knowledgeable, confident glow that makes colleagues and patients feel that they can trust you.

However, this is not to say that you should immediately go and take out a subscription to the *Journal of Clinical and Experimental Neuropsychology*. By strategically focusing on the more general journals and confining one's attention to the abstracts, reviews and general news sections, one can rapidly gain a thorough grounding in events and progress without having to complete a thesis. Good journals start up all the time (and some close down); Table 7.2 lists a few of the texts that contain the right blend of news, editorial content and clinical research and which will repay perusal by the thoughtful care worker. Just spending an hour or two a week in a postgraduate library reading what you fancy can be most interesting.

Most articles have carefully worded titles. Therefore, scanning the contents pages of the journals need take only – literally – a few minutes of your working week. Keep an eye out for key words and make a quick note of the ones that seem interesting. In-depth reviews usually need reading in full, but original research articles often provide a handy way around this in the form of an itemised abstract. This is a helpful innovation that is becoming increasingly accepted as the norm in many journals. At the beginning of each article there is a short summary detailing

Table 7.2 ● Journals worth reading

Professional	
Regularly	*Community Care*
	Psychiatric Bulletin
	Evidence-based Mental Health
For editorials (mainly)	*British Medical Journal*
	The Lancet
	British Journal of Psychiatry
For heavy (but occasionally great) articles	*American Journal of Psychiatry*
	Behaviour Research and Therapy
	Social Psychiatry and Psychiatric Epidemiology
	British Journal of Criminology
	Health Service Journal
	Hospital Medicine
General	
Regularly	A Saturday or Sunday broadsheet newspaper (whichever you fancy)
	Private Eye or *Viz*, or whatever makes you laugh
	A weekly journal, e.g. *Economist, Spectator, New Statesman,* etc.

what the paper is about (including aims, methods, results and conclusions). Very often, all that you need to know is contained in this section. Alternatively, there may be useful boxes somewhere within the text of the article labelled 'Conclusions' or 'What this paper adds to our knowledge'. Try this out for a few weeks and you will be surprised how effectively this method substitutes for a detailed reading of the entire article.

Having praised the precis, however, there are several reasons why it is worthwhile building up a consolidated knowledge in one or two areas. The first is the epicurean pleasure of being an expert in something. The second is that it can lead to all sorts of interesting opportunities. It is a good idea, therefore, to try to corner the market in one or two subjects in which you take a particular interest. This is exactly what successful architects, violinists, bond traders, brain surgeons and nuclear physicists do, for example, and there is no reason why you shouldn't. Within the field of community care itself, there are many areas in which it profits to become widely read: the ethics and practicalities of compulsory treatment, comparative mental health law in different countries and cultures, the role of family education in the management of chronic schizophrenia . . . the list is endless. Become an expert in any one of these and, sooner or later, you'll find yourself at a conference in some exotic location.

Don't just confine your reading to the professional literature – keep an eye on what your patients and their families are reading too. Try to keep up with what is happening in the news. At any one moment, a mental health story is breaking somewhere. As you read this, virtually every newspaper, film or television company is considering some idea or other to do with mental health. Madness, sadness, badness and struggles therewith are the very stuff that boosts ratings and sells newspapers. More often than not, the images of mental illness that we see through the strange looking-glass world of the media are grotesque (and sometimes downright harmful) distortions of the truth. It is worth remembering that the media is probably the main source from which people draw their ideas about mental illness and those who experience it, as well as those who attempt to treat it.

Consider the career of the actor Jack Nicholson. He has effectively become a multi-millionaire through his cinematic depictions of misfits, psycho-killers, manic depressives, addicts and obsessive compulsives. As mental health professionals, we ignore what the television and newspapers say at our peril. If a new film, play or book about any aspect of mental health is released, read it or go and see it. In recent years, *A Beautiful Mind* (schizophrenia), *Girl, Interrupted* (borderline personality disorder) and *As Good As It Gets* (obsessive compulsive disorder) have been outstanding and are available on DVD. If a story breaks in the news, read about it in both a tabloid and a broadsheet and keep the cuttings. Similarly, if something remarkable in the field of mental health or illness crops up on the television, record it if possible. Today's bulletin is tomorrow's audiovisual aid for teaching, giving a presentation or for enlightening a long away-day.

Going to the movies or reading books and newspapers is not enough if done in isolation. Discuss them with others, especially like-minded colleagues or those who you respect but who appear to have different opinions on or approaches to these matters. Make an effort to get away from clinical work to attend courses. Most departments nowadays have a budget allocated to employees' ongoing professional development. Find out who the budget holder is and what you are entitled to and claim it. Don't be afraid to go on courses that may not seem to be directly related to your day job. As we saw when we considered the content of the humdrum week, courses on time management, speaking with confidence, the psychology of football and the role of dog dreams in Dutch lesbian cinema, for example, are all legal, as long as you can justify it to a senior.

Get involved in journal clubs or go along to debates, discussions and conferences. This will help you to form your own opinions more clearly and help you to grasp the details of a complex issue to the extent that they will trickle over into your own clinical work. If you can, don't confine your deliberations to verbal discussions but also write about them. Very few of us in front-line posts can find the time or energy to participate in proper research, but don't underestimate the extent to which your own experience is a valuable source of data. Even if you only write a letter to *The Sun* about one of their more egregious depictions of mental illness, it is time well spent. If you can manage to keep it up over time, the publications section of your CV will grow as surely as your chances at the next job interview. Remember, the *British Medical Journal* posts all its letters on its website, so just by writing you can claim some cyberprint at least.

Is there life after work?

Sustaining an interest in matters mental is important, but don't overdo it. Watch that your familiarity with human interactions doesn't creep too far into your personal life. There are few things more annoying than a chum in the mental health trade cheerfully dispensing psychodynamic explanations of your choice of breakfast cereal or why you keep getting dumped. Bringing fun to work with you is one thing. Taking work home is another. If you aren't on call, switch your pager off when you head for home, and guard your home phone number like weapons-grade plutonium. Make sure that you are ex-directory and never take clinical work home with you. Similarly, never leave clinical notes unattended in a car or anywhere else, home included. People who conduct CPA meetings and attend ward rounds over the telephone whilst on holiday need help. They all too often have gaping holes in their private lives into which they pack work as a sort of addictive, pain-relieving stuffing. With a few exceptions, anoraks, trainspotters and social misfits do not make particularly good care workers.

Do your best to keep as varied an existence as possible. For example, play games, travel or read more, or take up macramé or bullfighting. Make sure that you take all of your entitled holidays, study days, days in lieu, bank holidays and any other days that you can think of – many don't. Cherish those mates who don't have a clue what you do all day. Try to avoid eating lunch with the same crew in the canteen, week in, week out. Bunk off for your idea of a treat every now and then. The people who get the most out of life are those who love many things, of which their work is but one.

Become a political animal

Mental health work overlaps with philosophy, politics and current affairs more than any other branch of the caring profession. Only in the field of mental health does one find legislation that allows us to treat someone without their consent or even against their expressed wishes. No other group of illnesses is so heavily weighed down by stigma, prejudice and misunderstanding. In spite of all the assurances by politicians over the past 50 years, mental health seems set to remain the Cinderella of the services for the foreseeable future. Even the idea of what constitutes 'mentally ill' is constantly changing.

A shrewd care worker appreciates the importance of analysing this kaleidoscope of fact, opinion and reaction. Given that, in some respects, your job requires the definition of abnormal thoughts and behaviour, you cannot afford to be unfamiliar with the more fundamental arguments surrounding such ideas. This will come naturally if you heed our advice to follow what is happening in the literature, in newspapers and on television. However, what we are advocating here is a little more substantial. Have an opinion. Get involved. Just what you decide and how you choose to express it are entirely up to you, but doing more than simply staying aware of the complex moral and ethical issues that surround your job will make you much better at it. It will also make you appear much more confident and knowledgeable at job interviews.

Perhaps another way to consider this is in terms of language, the medium by which we communicate our opinions about everything in life. Observing how language is used or misused to affect the lives of those on your caseload can provide all sorts of insights. For example, consider the pronunciations of several senior politicians in the late 1990s when, stirred by rising public anxiety over the apparently large number of homicides committed by people with mental illness, they stated that 'community care had failed'. The 95% of individuals who had gained from the move out of the asylums over the past 50 years were, in a few short speeches, turned into a political football. Or consider the way that euphemistic management-speak is increasingly being used by those who seek to tell us how we should be thinking about our work. Unless you can spot a cash-releasing efficiency saving (CRES) for what it is, it is difficult to take a stand against it. In fact, spotting managerial gobbledegook, apart from being a necessary skill in halting the downward slide into mediocrity, is a satisfying hobby in its own right. An entire dictionary could be devoted to this fascinating and fast-growing dialect.

One short, final word on care worker survival needs to be added here. Throughout this chapter, we have described ways in which we can protect ourselves from the stresses and strains of a demanding but rewarding job. Most of what we can do to take care of ourselves we can also do for our workmates; they too have to deal with the same knocks and pressures. Every now and then, you will spot a comrade who is showing some quiet, early sign of buckling under the weight of it all. A hint of irritation, bags under the eyes, a sustained loss of sparkle or the faint whiff of booze on a Monday morning. No matter how tired you are, strive to be good to them. Listen to them and help them if you can. You never know, one day it might be you that fails the Friday afternoon test.

Danger zones – risk management – what, why and how

8

Introduction

As we have noted, there are many paradoxes at the heart of community care that pose a challenge to the care worker. The process of caring for someone involves an intervention of some sort. Implementing a care plan means doing something with someone. This will always involve the care worker taking at least some control of, or responsibility for, an aspect of the patient's life that involves their illness. When the disturbance of behaviour, judgement or insight is marked, this intervention can be quite extensive. Yet the central philosophy of community care is exactly the opposite of this interventionist approach; the aim is to do everything possible to foster patients' autonomy and independence, helping them to make their own decisions about their lives, their symptoms and their treatment.

In the old days of the asylum, it was quite feasible for carers to exert a very large amount of control over a patient's environment. Indeed, the concern that this control had gone too far – as immortalised by the infamous Nurse Ratched in the 1975 film *One Flew over the Cuckoo's Nest* – was one of the things that led to the closure of the asylums. Nowadays, in the community, most of our patients are out of our sight and therefore our control for most of the time. 'Care' stands for involvement, whereas 'community' stands for the normality of freedom from involvement. Herein lies the first paradox of community care: we are providing community care properly when we are not providing it. At first glance, this may seem like a pointless play on words. In fact, it reveals the art of community care for what it truly is: an endless – and in some ways impossible – balancing act between freedom and influence. Or, to put it another way, a balance between your patient's rights and your responsibilities as a care worker. This balance is not confined to patient and carer alone. In the business of community care, it seems that everyone holds a stake. Ask yourself what the public expects from community mental health services. The answer can be given in one word: *safety*. Therefore, here is another paradox: we think that it is our job to care for sick people, whereas the rest of the world thinks that it is our job to control them. We expect to manage patients. Others expect us to manage risks.

If we are seen as failing in this regard then, rightly or wrongly, many people believe that we should be held to account. Because of the very strong feelings that mental illness provokes, this judgemental tendency can often reach extremes. It is almost as if the care workers themselves are somehow responsible for the thoughts and deeds of their patients. On the occasions that someone with a mental illness harms themselves or, far more rarely, harms someone else, the media can be unforgiving in their accusations of failure and neglect, or their exhortations to 'lock up the psychos'. With the possible exception of recent efforts, successive governments have done little to challenge these inaccuracies, their pronouncements on community care often driven more by vote-winning assurances to a nervous public than by the real needs of people with serious mental illnesses.

Left- and right-wing governments alike have broadly agreed that 'community care has failed' (e.g. Frank Dobson, House of Commons, 1998), even though the evidence points to the opposite conclusion. In 1999, a government White Paper endorsed 'safe, sound and supportive' services. It is perhaps no coincidence that the only word in this phrase with any connotation of care comes last. Considered in the light of the history of community care, outlined in Chapter 1, some unpalatable conclusions become clear (see Box 8.1). These lessons are so important that the rest of this chapter is devoted to the ways in which we can learn from them.

Box 8.1 Eleven key lessons for the care worker

1. The public think that it is our job to protect them, quietly and efficiently but preferably invisibly, from the behaviours of people with mental illness

2. The public is nevertheless quite fascinated by our patients harming other people and they like to read about this provided they or their families aren't the victims

3. Whether we like it or not, it is a central part of our job to assuage the public's sense of anxiety as best we can, by any means available

4. Anticipating, identifying and knowing exactly what to do in a risky situation is an essential part of this job

5. Writing something down on a piece of paper or holding an inquiry into something that has gone wrong is a very good way of creating the impression that something is being done; however, it does not necessarily mean that anything has been done, is being done or will be done

6. The government will willingly pay the *real* cost of modern, sophisticated community mental health facilities when hell freezes over

7. Community care workers will experience the discomfort of working between a rock and a hard place for the foreseeable future

8. Murphy was right: no matter how good your treatment plan, things will always have the potential to go wrong

9. Sharon Campbell, Christopher Clunis, Ben Silcock and Michael Stone (patients all) have done more to alter community care in 15 years than any politician or clinician has managed to do in half a century

10. The media are powerful players in the game. We ignore them at our peril

11. Successful prevention is invisible. Most people only think about, or agree to support, mental health services when something goes wrong, so the better we get at our job, the harder it becomes to justify our funding

The inexorable rise of risk

As we have noted, the last 50 years have seen a major shift in our thinking, away from the idea of social responsibilities towards a much more individualistic, rights-oriented view of our world. Indeed, so high is the price now placed on an individual's entitlement to comfort that we have almost come to see discomfort as undesirable, even unnatural, rather than as an essential accompaniment to the brighter side of life. Take death, for example. Only 70 years ago, the sight of a corpse was commonplace. Yet today, apart from in a few deeply personal moments of our lives, the closest that we will come to death – especially through violence or infectious disease – is via the television or the newspapers. It is almost as though we have convinced ourselves that we can somehow keep death at bay. In a similar way, the concept of depression as a widespread illness simply did not exist 70 years ago. Instead, sadness was regarded as being a natural part of life. It was taken for granted that life was not always a bed of roses. This obsession with the control of all things uncomfortable is one of the reasons why risk has become such an issue.

Over the last 25 years, risk has become big business. Risk seems to be everywhere: in asteroids heading for earth; in crossing the road; in contaminants in our food and even in the air that we breathe. We talk of identifying risk, assessing risk and eliminating risk. We pay good money to 'risk management experts' so that they can tell us what to do about it. It is almost as though we have begun to think of risk as a real thing, like some sort of ghastly toxic fungus.

All of this obscures some points about risk that are important to the care worker. The fact is that, unlike fungus, risk is not a 'thing' in the concrete, objective sense. We like to think of it as real because it makes the uncertainty that it stands for seem more manageable. We noted this falsely comforting tendency to reify an abstract idea when we considered the non-existent place called 'the community' in which we are supposed to be working. This tendency to reify, or treat something abstract as if it existed as a real object, can have potentially disastrous consequences.

In spite of the apparent complexity of risk, it is, in fact, a very simple concept: risk is simply the chance that an event will or will not happen. That event may be good or bad, but risk is nothing more than a probability or a chance. Seen as an abstract, mathematical notion of probability, it becomes clear that risk should never be thought of in isolation. For it to exist, it must always be concerned with *something* that might or might not happen. Usually, it relates to a decision. Any meaningful attempt to address risk, therefore, must involve thinking about all of the things to which that risk relates. By talking up the idea of 'risk!' as an entity in its own right, we are completely missing the point. It is as if we are in a stadium cheering on 22 men running around a football pitch without a ball.

Such a magnified view of risk can also exert a subtle but profound effect on the way that we think and work. The dramas and attendant bad publicity that community care has attracted since the 1988 Spokes inquiry have led people, erroneously, to conclude that mental illness is a highly risky business. In such a climate of worry and uncertainty, it is very easy for us to stop seeing our work with patients as a collaborative effort to get people better. Instead, we start to see our patients as living bundles of frightening possibilities that must be contained at all costs. Might he commit suicide? Will she neglect herself? Will he become violent if he relapses? Risk can transform us from carers into obsessional custodians.

Virtually all of the inquiries that have been carried out from Clunis (1994) onwards have reached the totally obvious conclusion that 'not enough was done' to identify, communicate, assess or manage risk. As a result, risk management has come to occupy centre stage in our work with patients. Increasingly, we find ourselves obliged to undergo 'risk training' or to abide by risk guidelines and risk protocols. Risk assessment forms, usually separate sheets of alarm-coloured paper, now decorate the inside front covers of case files. If one of these forms is not filled in, or is completed incorrectly, the reasoning is that risk has not been adequately assessed. If something subsequently goes wrong – and Murphy warns us that sooner or later it always will – the form creates a convenient sticking point for the apportionment of suspicion in the aftermath. If the form has been correctly filled in and filed and something subsequently goes wrong, it seems to exert a mysteriously protective effect upon the signatory. Thinking of risk as a thing to be measured and recorded in this way not only increases our preoccupation with pieces of paper but also breathes life into the comforting illusion that something useful has been done. In the uncomfortable climate in which we work, such comfort seems welcome. But it is a false comfort because, by placing this 'thing' at the very forefront of our thinking about and recording of our work, we also start to see it as something separate. We see it as a uniquely important facet of our work with a patient, located to a specific point in time and space, rather than as an abstract sense of chance that is inexorably woven into every aspect of a case, at all times and in all places.

Risk assessment forms, or 'tools' as they are even more unhelpfully known, are really only useful at the time they are completed. Once completed, they may cause us to lower our guard. A 'tool' may tell us that a deluded, crack-addicted, ex-marine with a machete is dangerous at the moment, or has been at some point in the past, but it tells us very little about the risk that he is likely to pose five Thursdays from now. The only way to do this would be to fill out a risk assessment tool every time that we see him. Or, far more sensibly, take all of our knowledge about his history and mental state into account every time that we see him, think about him, write about him or discuss him with others. This is otherwise known as 'doing one's job properly'. It should not routinely need an extra piece of paper. Rather, risk assessment should be placed exactly where it belongs, as part of the much larger story of a patient's life and clinical history.

This is not to say, however, that there is nothing useful about the method of posting specific, pertinent risk factors in a prominent place in a patient's record. The government's unsuccessful attempt to introduce supervision registers in the mid-1990s was, in effect, an attempt to do this. What we wish to emphasise here is that no specific risk-monitoring device should ever be relied upon unduly or in isolation. 'Homicidal when relapsed' is all very well emblazoned inside the front cover of the case notes but, if our treatment plan does nothing more than acknowledge it, this warning is likely to be a complete waste of time. Instead, risk assessment must always be an ongoing thing, constantly following the ebb and flow of hazards that attend the lives of all our patients.

The problems of risk assessment

Placing undue emphasis on risk at the expense of less sensational aspects of a patient's history, mental state and care plan can have other less visible but far-reaching consequences. One of these is to de-skill and demoralise front-line staff.

The more that we come to think of risk as a special aspect of a patient's care, the easier it is to conclude that it is a matter best left to a specialist to handle. Faced with the disconcerting possibility of someone being hurt, this urge to defer to expert opinion 'because I'm not good enough' can be very powerful. In the late 1980s and early 1990s, as forensic psychiatric care was establishing itself as a distinct speciality, many experts in what was then known as 'dangerousness' were perfectly happy to go along with this illusory shift of responsibility for what might happen. Only when our forensic colleagues began to grasp the sheer quantity of risk 'out there' did they quietly retire from this position. In some areas today, our forensic colleagues will only emerge into the community if the risk is so obvious as to be detectable by a sensible 12-year-old. As any truly candid forensic psychiatrist, social worker or nurse will admit, they are little better at gauging the risk posed by any given patient than the rest of us.

Much of the evidence in this area points to the same conclusion, and even the government itself has openly admitted that the assessment of risk is 'at best an inexact science'. The one tool that forensic staff do have on their side, which front-line care workers simply do not have, is more time. A forensic worker will rarely complete an interview in under an hour (often longer) and will expect every file from every involved agency to be neatly stacked and ready for his or her perusal. How else, they ask with enviable ingenuousness, can we possibly be expected to do the job properly? How else indeed. But the idea that being anything less than obsessively thorough (a luxury that front-liners will simply never be able to afford) is somehow synonymous with doing the job less than properly is a destructive form of self-doubt. It is a doubt that we must work hard to resist, especially in the current climate in which so much seems to be at stake.

Another problem with risk is that it leads to an irreversible change in the way that we view a situation. Once the 'risky' label has adhered to a patient, it can prove very difficult, if not impossible, to remove. This can have all sorts of negative effects and illustrates the way in which risk can involve a *good* thing *not* happening just as easily as a bad thing actually happening. Consider the following, not uncommon, situation. A young man with a remote history of violent assault against care staff during his first psychotic episode now presents 4 years later with an early relapse. Even though he may have moved on from everything that led to the original behaviour, such as illicit drug use, a chaotic personal life, etc., the admitting team is still more likely to place him on a locked ward at the earliest sign of unrest or give him higher doses of tranquillising medication than another patient who is identical in all respects other than the risk history. Because of the way that his behaviour is now viewed through the 'halo' of his past, his progress through admission is significantly changed. Even discharge to aftercare may be compromised by the increasing unwillingness of many (often privately run) community facilities to accept someone with such a history, no matter how remote. Why should they, when they can take any of dozens of clients with a comparatively clean record?

Although such judgements may appear to be highly irrational, even unfair, they underline the fact that, when confronted by emotive issues of risk, dangerousness and harm, rational argument stands little chance of success. Nowhere is this clearer than in respect to judgements made about probability. Risk, as we have noted, is essentially about a decision made in the face of a probability that an outcome may or may not happen. As any experienced poker player or estate agent will tell you, the human brain is simply not very good at calculating odds when feelings are running high. For example, the odds of being killed at random by a psychotic stranger are around 13 million to one, far lower than the chances of being killed by a fire in one's own home or even being struck by lightning. This also happens to be, roughly, the odds of winning the national lottery. Therefore, any rationally minded person would have little fear of a community psychiatric unit being opened in their neighbourhood and would never dream of wasting hard-earned money on a lottery ticket. But because of the high emotions that accompany sensationalist reporting of the latest community care scandal, or the enticing fantasy of being a millionaire, we deceive ourselves into thinking that these events are far more likely to happen than they truly are. Few of us do the sensible thing, which is to stop worrying about psychotic axe murderers and spend our lottery ticket money on a smoke alarm instead.

The powerful emotions aroused by risk can disrupt far more than our ability to make rational decisions about individual cases. It can affect the way that we spend our money and design our services. Numerous inquiries into serious incidents, and the government policies that have arisen from them, have repeatedly stressed the need to identify those most at risk. Given that community mental health services seem set to remain under-resourced for the foreseeable future, this means that any available funds will be targeted to these risky individuals. Again, we see how the idea of risk is pointless unless we ask what the risk is about and to whom it pertains. The patient? His family? The public? The story of the last 30 years has made it clear that the resources provided for the 'safe, sound and supportive' services of the 21st century are to be directed at the risk to the public rather than anyone else. At face value, this might sound sensible, but when we take a closer look at the tools that we must currently rely on to decide just who is and who is not risky, things start to look a lot less certain.

Risk assessment tools are based on a variety of factors (e.g. previous assaults) that history has shown are associated with a higher probability of an undesirable event occurring. In keeping with our argument that risk should only ever be considered within the context of a particular clinical situation, we will not dwell upon these specific factors here. For now, we need only accept that certain factors do appear to increase the chance of a person with a mental illness becoming violent. Ostensibly, our risk assessment test should provide us with a way of distinguishing between those who are potentially violent (i.e. few false negatives) and those who are not. This is what statisticians call the sensitivity and specificity of a test. Sensitivity is an indication of the ease with which a test will correctly identify someone as being potentially violent, whereas specificity is an indicator of the ease with which a test will reject those who have a low potential for violence. This may seem sound in principle, but transferring neat mathematical principles into the real and sometimes nasty world of mental illness is a completely different matter.

For example, suppose that there are 10 truly violent patients in a group of 100 and that we look for them using a risk assessment tool that has a 90% sensitivity and a 95% specificity – figures that are very high by anyone's standards. This level of sensitivity means that, out of the 10 truly violent patients, 9 will be identified correctly. For a specificity of 95%, 85 out of the remaining 90 people will be correctly identified as being non-violent. Therefore, the probability of positively predicting a truly violent person using our test is $9/(9 + 5)$, which is approximately 64%. Similarly, the probability of predicting a truly non-violent person is approximately 99%. If we were to use this test alone as the basis for deciding whether or not to release our 100 patients from hospital, we would end up detaining 36 people who were not truly violent. Conversely, of the 86 individuals whom we saw fit to release on the basis of a negative test, only one would be truly violent.

These figures might seem acceptable if we were to apply them to the inmates of a maximum security prison, but suppose we use the same test amongst a community sample of, for example, 1000 patients, of whom 10 are truly violent. The probability of predicting a non-violent person is still high, with only one truly violent person released out of 1000; however, the cost of identifying the remaining nine violent individuals is now very high. The probability of a positive prediction has now fallen to $9/(9 + 59)$, or 13%. Of the 68 individuals who remain incarcerated by our tool because they are potentially violent, 59 are quite safe. Leaving aside the obvious problem that human beings do not fall into neat categories of violent versus non-violent, this simple arithmetical demonstration shows that, when it comes to risk assessment, the circumstances under which one makes the assessment are crucial.

In spite of this very wide margin of error, risk has such a grip upon contemporary thinking that risk assessment tools are still being used as a way to allocate resources across general populations. A far more sensible approach would be to offer the basic minimum of best available service to everyone evenly across the board. This way, everyone would stand a better chance of receiving decent care whilst, at the same time, providing a statistically good chance of containing the riskier patients.

The current fashion for trying to target services towards those individuals perceived as high risk leads to another paradox: high risk is low risk. Compared with the total number of people who suffer a serious mental illness, the number who pose a high risk is actually quite small. In their lifetime, probably less than 1% of patients with a psychotic diagnosis will pose a significant threat to others. Assume for a moment that we were successfully able to not only identify but also successfully contain the risk posed by these individuals. Thus contained, these individuals would now pose a much smaller risk but would be consuming a significant proportion of our effort in the process. In a system with a finite capacity to cope, this energy would, of course, need to be diverted from elsewhere, namely from the far greater number of individuals who appeared to pose a smaller risk at the time of assessment. Because risk is a complex, changing thing, which cannot be divided into convenient categories of high or low at the filling in of a questionnaire, sooner or later, some of the individuals outside the scope of our intensive management are likely to pose a significant risk. But, as we noted, it is very difficult to let go of a risk once identified and contained. Instead, we divert more of our energy from elsewhere to contain each fresh source of risk as it arises, drawing ourselves into an ever-shrinking circle of reward. Those of our patients who remain outside this forensic noose receive an ever-poorer service and our own practice becomes increasingly defensive, driven more by custodial than compassionate principles.

This critique of risk as it applies to community care should not be taken to mean that we regard risk as an unhelpful concept. The crucial point that we are seeking to make is that risk is nothing more than one important aspect of our work. It must always be considered in the context of *everything else* that we are trying to do, not only with our patients but also with their families and the public. The dangers of risk that we have outlined here occur only when we make the mistake of considering risk in isolation. As we will see when we look at specific risky situations, effective risk assessment must go far beyond the simple application of a checklist of risk criteria. To be really useful, risk assessment requires a far more subtle and complex approach.

An empirical knowledge of risk factors in general always needs to be combined with detailed knowledge of a particular case, acquired over time. Time is the second most helpful aid to risk assessment, because nothing predicts the future like the past. To this must be added the most important factor of all – the dilated nostril of experience. Over time you just learn to smell risk. This ability has its roots in whatever it is that can be learnt but not taught. Nothing can replace time spent in the field cultivating this indefinable sixth sense. As Murphy says, you can't get it right all the time. You just have to learn from those times when you don't. This brings us to the most unsettling paradox of all: in order to save some, you have to lose some. This is a truth that, at present, very few people seem willing to contemplate.

Handling suicidal patients

Few aspects of mental illness hold more grim fascination than suicide. The 'suicide rate' is one of the few mental health statistics that has made its way into common folklore. Almost everyone seems to think that it is common in Sweden, or that in Japan it is seen as honourable. People think that lemmings do it en masse, even though no one can find a zoologist who agrees.

Suicide interests us in a way that other mental health problems do not. For example, one study of the press coverage of mental health crises over several years found that, whereas reporting of homicidal people with mental illness almost invariably portrayed them as evil unpredictable maniacs, coverage of suicide was far more balanced. Moreover, sympathy was often expressed for the victims and – perhaps most importantly – some attempts were made to understand their behaviour. There are many good reasons for this. For a start, suicide rings some very private bells for a lot of us. Many people, if not most, have toyed with the idea of killing themselves at some point in their lives, usually, but not always, when depressed. But our fascination with the subject goes beyond mere commonality. The idea of taking our own life touches on some of our most sacred beliefs: that we are free to choose our own actions and that life itself is the most precious thing that we possess. This reflects what we sometimes call 'the will to live', the idea that no matter how bad things get, where there is life there is hope. Suicide, with all its irrevocable, awful certainty, offers us the confusing possibility that these precious truths may be wrong. For some, the issue of 'to be or not to be' amounts to the most important philosophical question of all: what is the point of life? Or, to put it another way: 'Why not kill myself?'

The world around us reveals that these questions amount to more than philosophical dabbling. It was only in 1964 that we ceased to punish people for attempting to kill themselves. We still talk of 'committing' suicide as if it were an offence. In some civilised Christian countries, successful suicide victims are still forbidden a Christian burial inside a churchyard. Coroners in the UK are still shy of passing a verdict of suicide unless the evidence is incontrovertible, because of the shame and guilt that often accompanies the grief in such settings.

The fact that suicide questions some of our most cherished beliefs can also have an effect upon the relationship between the care worker and the patient. Many nurses and doctors, especially those with relatively little experience of mental health issues, find themselves confused when a patient's utterances seem to reject the very things that the caring professions stand for: the promotion of life.

CARE WORKER: 'So, how can I help you?'
PATIENT: 'By getting lost. I want to die.'

Confronted by this scenario, which is basically a rewrite of the philosophical conundrum we saw above, many people respond with a bewildered mixture of irritability, rejection, sympathy and uncertainty.

This scenario is not exactly a rare one, either. In accident and emergency units all over the world, presentations following self-harm are commonplace, from hasty overdoses and lacerated wrists to comatose people dragged from fume-filled cars. Amongst the younger age groups, both successful suicide and what has variously been called parasuicide or deliberate self-harm (DSH) have increased at an alarming rate. Indeed, the stark fact that, in many Western countries, suicide now outstrips road accidents as the commonest form of death among people aged from 15 to 25 raises poignant questions about our supposedly successful civilisation. Attempts at self-harm are common and seem set to become more so over time. Therefore, knowing how to talk to a suicidal person, convince them that you can understand them and engage their interest in a plan that successfully contains their risk are core skills for a competent care worker.

Understanding the suicidal patient

Given the powerful emotions that the issue of suicide can evoke in us all, the first lesson in the management of the suicidal patient is to be aware of these feelings and not allow them to obstruct one's efforts to devise and apply a clear plan of action. This is not always as easy as it sounds. The second lesson can help with the first. Of all the patients who tell you that they want to die, very few of them really mean it, even the ones who end up killing themselves. As we shall see, there are many reasons for telling someone you'd rather be dead, and truly wanting to die is only one of them. Most of those who really mean it are to be found in mortuaries rather than talking to you. Nine times out of ten, the fact that they are talking to you at all implies that they are willing to consider other options. The one out of ten, on the other hand, is a little trickier, and all the more so when you see several hundred such cases over the course of a few years.

Understanding why anyone should want to think and talk of killing themselves is probably the single most important aspect of managing the suicidal patient. Unless you can establish why they are talking – or behaving – in this way, it will be very hard to achieve your main aim: helping the patient to accept alternative ways of thinking and acting. Before we consider how to manage the challenge posed by such a patient, it is helpful to look at some of the reasons that can make a person act in a suicidal manner in the first place.

The causes of suicide/reasons not to be cheerful

The most important reason is, of course, because a person sincerely and genuinely wishes to end their life. Surprisingly, these cases are often the most straightforward. The person's history and mental state usually yields enough detail to make the need for prompt intervention quite clear. Far more commonly, however, suicidal behaviour is not a purposeful step through death's door, but a way of trying to cope with life's difficulties amidst a fluctuating mental state.

Suicide as a coping strategy

All of us have a personal threshold for how much hardship we can take. This threshold varies with time and a good many other factors, but it is clear that some, for example those who survived Auschwitz, have a higher threshold than others. Although it is by no means a hard and fast rule, those who are in possession of a reasonably stable, robust and confident personality formed out of good breeding stock and an emotionally and materially stable upbringing, usually cope better with life's vicissitudes than the rest of us. When confronted with seemingly insurmountable problems, many people often find themselves indulging in various fantasies of escape: wishing they were more confident, even superheroes; wishing they were somewhere else or dead. In our darker moments, the absolute certainty of death can exert an alluring comfort that some find hard to resist. Harming oneself is propelled not so much by a wish to die but by a misguided search for a better way of dealing with one's problems. Only later, when confronted with the consequences of their near-misses, do people admit that a sincere wish to die was not their actual intent but rather that hurting themselves seemed like a good idea at the time. Often, it transpires that what someone wanted at the time was not so much a way out of life but a way out of responsibility for their situation.

Others may seek the temporary oblivion of drugs and alcohol as a way of buying time. To the outsider, a handful of swallowed pills and a bottle of vodka may look like a pretty serious suicide attempt, but once the patient has recovered enough to talk straight, they will tell you that their carefully premeditated goal was simply 'to get completely out of it for a bit'. The occasional patient who may come to your attention after having ingested paralysing quantities of booze and drugs may not have had death or oblivion on their mind but instead have simply been an over-enthusiastic partygoer who ended up in the suicidal basket by mistake. For others, this pursuit of oblivion may be an attempt to place their future in the hands of a higher authority, be it you, the gods, fate, chance, providence or whatever. For this spiritually minded subset of survivors, the typical refrain is 'I wanted to see how it would all work out'. Again, the wish here is to get out of control rather than out of living.

Of course, suicidal behaviour is a very powerful language in its own right. Some people will resort to it as an exclusive form of communication, so effective is it at signalling distress. These people often tend to lack the emotional and/or verbal ability to communicate their feelings by other means or feel that all attempts to communicate via more civil methods have come to naught. Others with a leaning towards the more impulsive, flamboyant corner of the human colour chart may simply revel in the drama of it all. Among these often fascinating characters, we may find some for whom the attention of a kindly nurse, offering a mouthful of activated charcoal, is about as close as they have come to being cared for in a long time.

For a small, but clinically significant, group of patients, the powerful responses generated by suicidal behaviour can be a strong reinforcing factor for further suicidal behaviour. It is as if, in the face of recurrent distress, suicidal behaviour becomes the most favoured way of coping. Often, the 'stress' that people respond to in this way is not so much taking place in their environment but inside their heads.

People with high levels of anxious or angry overarousal, who may have very strong negative views of themselves and who often have an early history of neglect, isolation, abuse or worse, seem to find a strong release of tension in the process of harming themselves. The actual wish to die seems to have only very little relevance to a small group of recidivist self-harmers who present with great frequency to the emergency mental health services. Instead, it is as though, over time, they have developed the firm belief that they are bad, that they deserve to be punished and that a 'good' thing to do is to punish the bad. The anticipation of the act of self-harm through to its enactment by whatever means – cutting, bingeing, purging, exercising, head banging, hair pulling, suffocating – takes on a powerfully satisfying quality. It is surprising how many unhappy young patients – often female – describe a characteristic pattern of thinking, feeling and doing. The urge to harm steadily builds up to a self-harming act, which is accompanied by a strong sense of bittersweet satisfaction and relief. This is swiftly followed by an urgent sense of regret, helplessness and self-reproach at the useless, repetitive nature of the behaviour.

Who is at increased risk of suicide?

Over the last century it has emerged that some people, by virtue of history, circumstance or mental state, are at greater risk of harming themselves than others. A substantial body of research now allows us to identify certain subgroups of individuals on the basis of certain factors that are associated with a higher risk of self-harm. This can provide a useful net with which to sift the endless stream of potentially suicidal people passing through your care. However, because this research is essentially epidemiological, it carries the usual drawbacks of statistical methodology: it will tell you that 20% of such and such a group is at a high risk of suicide but it won't tell you *which* 20%. Once again we meet the problems of sensitivity and specificity. We need to be careful, therefore, not to rely on this list of factors as though it was a handy tool (see Table 8.1). Instead, the items on the list should be embedded into our practice with all our patients in such a way that they come into use almost automatically. Attention paid to age, disease, drug misuse and so on should only ever form the skeleton of our suicide risk assessment. On to this we must always add the uniquely individual flesh of every case.

Table 8.1 ● Suicide: associated social and diagnostic factors

Diagnostic factors	Depression
	Schizophrenia
	Alcohol/drug dependence
	Personality disorder
Social factors	Male gender
	Increasing age/retired
	Single/alone/unemployed
	Physical illness (especially if painful)
	Family history of depression/suicide/alcoholism
	History of childhood losses/previous self-harm
	Impulsive/aggressive/labile personality traits

Social factors associated with suicide

Gender is an important social factor that is associated with suicide. Although men complete suicide more often than women, women attempt it more often than men. Suicide also becomes more common with age, especially for men. However, this should not divert attention away from the fact that large numbers of young people are attempting and completing suicide with increasing frequency. Social status and social network are equally important factors. More single, widowed or divorced people, or those who are isolated for other reasons, attempt suicide than those who are married or have a more established network of social contact and support. Recent changes in social network because of a change in lifestyle, a bereavement, an illness, unemployment or some other stressful event also carry an increased risk of suicide. Conversely, having someone to care for, such as a child or an elderly relative (or even a pet), seems to exert a protective effect, as does religion or a sense of belonging to some other social institution.

Beyond the patient's immediate network, wider environmental factors also seem to exert an influence. Suicide is more common in the spring and on Mondays, whether in the northern or the southern hemisphere. Some studies have found this seasonal variation to be more pronounced in rural than in urban areas but, generally, life in more urban environments carries a higher risk. Whether this is because of the pace of city life itself or because cities can act as traps for unemployed, isolated and impoverished people remains unclear. Broader social events also have an effect on suicide. The suicide rate drops in wartime and at other times of enhanced social cohesion.

There is also a curious relationship between suicide and its portrayal in the media of the age. This was noted after publication of the novel *The Sorrows of Young Werther* in 1774 by the German writer Johann Goethe (1749–1832). The book told a romantic tale of self-destruction through unrequited love. In the years that followed its release, numerous young men killed themselves in a similar fashion, many going so far as to dress in the style of the book's hero before they shot themselves. This has since been dubbed 'the Werther effect' and has been reported in response to news stories, films and even television soap operas. Perhaps more than any other issue, suicide shows us that we are more sensitive to our environment than we realise.

Psychiatric and general medical features associated with suicide

Suicide, it is nice to know, appears to be much less common among those in good mental health. One much-quoted study of 100 successful suicides found that 95 of the victims had suffered from a recognisable mental illness around the time of their death and that a substantial minority of them had been in contact with psychiatric services up to the time of their death. Three psychiatric disorders in particular have been repeatedly shown to have a strong link with suicide: depression, alcoholism and schizophrenia. We should always keep the possibility of suicide at the back of our minds in all our dealings with patients given these diagnoses, no matter how remote the possibility of self-harm may actually seem, especially in those with a dual diagnosis (e.g. depression *and* alcoholism).

Of all the factors associated with suicide, major depression has the strongest association of all. People with this condition are 30 times more likely to take their own lives than similar but non-depressed members of the general population. Within the cluster of features that comprises the depressive syndrome itself, insomnia and poor concentration are particularly important factors associated with suicide, as are a history of alcohol misuse and self-neglect. Apart from frank suicidal ideas and plans, recurring themes of hopelessness and intense pessimism are important features of the patient's mental state. Many authorities warn of the need to be vigilant for a sudden, unexplained lift in the patient's mood, which may be the only outward sign of the relief that accompanies the final decision to act. Sadly, it is often only those who are close to or in frequent contact with the patients who detect this sign, and an immediate and appropriate response to it is difficult to provide in the uncontrolled setting of the community.

Approximately 10% of patients who receive a diagnosis of schizophrenia die by suicide. Such patients often tend to have a more severe, relapsing pattern of symptoms and to be young and male, with a relatively good insight into their impairment. High risk also surrounds discharge from hospital, particularly when this is associated with discontinuity of care, which may foster feelings of isolation. Stigmatised attitudes towards mental illness, including active denial or intense fear of the diagnosis, also seem to be relevant. The complicating factor of alcohol abuse, on its own or in association with schizophrenia or depression, enhances all these risks. Limited impulse control, often associated with alcohol dependence and traits of a formal personality disorder, seems to be a key factor in promoting suicidal completion.

People suffering with chronic or malignant illnesses are also at a greater risk of killing themselves. It is tempting to assume that some illnesses create a suicidal state of mind in their own right, almost as if this is part of the disease itself. This is a diversion from the fact that all chronic disease, depending on severity, can affect a patient's life. Suicide risk is much more strongly associated with those physical illnesses that carry connotations of irrevocable loss of autonomy or function. In this sense, insightful schizophrenia is understandable as a 'physical' illness. Movement disorders and neurodegenerative conditions, chronic pain syndromes, disfiguring injuries and any other illnesses that carry the prospect of a decline in the quality of life without hope of recovery all carry a significant risk of suicide. Add to this the isolation of increasing age and the loss of friendships or family, and the risk multiplies even further, especially in older men.

Talking with suicidal patients

There are two ways in which you will come into contact with a suicidal person. Either someone will come to you because of concerns that they might be suicidal, or a person will come to you after a suicide attempt. Although the basic goal is the same in both situations, namely to engage the person in a way that safely contains the risk of their killing themselves, the inevitable difference between the two cases requires a different approach. Talking with a survivor of a recent attempt is usually easier than talking with someone who has yet to display their intentions via their behaviour. The event itself provides an important starting point for the interview. In the absence of an event, however, we need to start our work one step back, as our patient resembles an unopened book, one that may or may not tell a story ending in self-harm.

Regardless of the situation that you are faced with, the way in which you conduct the interview should be the same. Pay careful attention to your own emotions from the outset. A sense of urgency may cause you to forget your surroundings, and many patients may not feel able to discuss the futility of life in a busy, public area. Try to be serious and empathic from the outset and avoid the use of any humour until you are certain that you have established firm trust. The style and wording of one's approach must always be flexible enough to suit the patient's age, culture and mental state. Be prepared to give the patient more time than usual when forming replies. A marked disruption of mood, concentration or both may make it very difficult for the patient to gather thoughts and form replies to what are, after all, likely to be the most important questions of his or her life.

It is impossible to plant ideas into a patient's head. The idea that enquiry into suicidal ideas encourages suicidal action is untrue and may be a rationalisation of the unease that many of us feel when talking to suicidal people. Descriptive statements and open-ended general questions about mood, for example 'You seem very low at the moment ...' or 'How long have you been feeling like this ... ?', provide a useful way into the issue of suicide. Encourage the patient to speak about the events and circumstances that led to their current distress before moving on to more specific questions about suicide itself. As a rule, it is better to build up a rapport by exploring the edges of an issue before popping the big question. In the process, try to show that you understand how the patient feels: 'When it gets this bad, do you ever think of killing yourself?' Little will be gained from asking more specific questions when the patient is still making ambivalent comments. Only narrow things down when you feel that the patient is likely to give an honest answer. Then, be confident and explicit: 'What do you think you might do exactly?' Even if the reply to this question generates cause for concern, do not jump to the conclusion that suicide is imminent. Rather than leaping into action and organising respite care or hospitalisation, take the interview further by following through the implications of the affirmative reply. Find out what death really means to the patient, not only in terms of the reasons for dying but also in more practical terms. It is a safe bet that anyone who has given serious consideration to the idea of taking their life will not have struck upon the idea shortly before the interview. If you find yourself forming this suspicion, it is almost certain that the patient is using suicidal talk as a way of communicating distress rather than signing off from life.

True suicidal intent is almost always accompanied by some degree of reflection over ways and means. This can range from the vaguest of notions, such as 'maybe take some tablets', to loosely formed plans, such as 'take some of the sleeping pills Mum keeps in the bathroom', to the thoughtfully worked out, for example 'I shall visit four different pharmacies and collect 32 paracetamol from each ...'. Try to find out just how far down the line of preparation the patient has gone. Explore the method (especially if it is a bit unusual), remembering that men usually use more violent methods than women but that, when women choose such methods, they usually mean it. Does the patient have personal or occupational access to potent tools, such as firearms, poisons or powerful drugs? Most farmers own guns. Does the patient have a debilitating illness, such as diabetes, that might provide the wherewithal (insulin) for self-dispatch? If patients talk of hanging, jumping or drowning, explore the geography of their ideas. Where will they hang the noose? Which high building? Which river? Recall that cultural factors can often influence the choice of method and site. Beachy Head in southern England, for example, exerts a magnetic effect on suicidal Britons. A cherry grove outside Osaka draws people from all over Japan. Knowledge of the local variants of these sad places can prove invaluable not only in gauging the seriousness of the intent but also in convincing the desperate person that you know exactly how they feel. By convincing the patient of your near-telepathic ability to understand just how they feel, you begin to erode that terrifying loneliness that accompanies the hopelessness and despair of the truly suicidal mind.

Apart from choice of site and method, explore the extent to which preparations have already been put in place. Have bank accounts been closed or has money been spent on air tickets, firearms or other material aids to self-elimination? Has the patient instructed a solicitor recently or even given the matter some thought? Have final letters or notes been written or even posted? Has there been a change in the patient's usual routine?

Begin to explore the way in which the suicidal ideas involve other people. Has the patient had any recent, unusual communication with significant others in his or her social network? Any odd comments or sad farewells in recent days and weeks? If the patient has thought of leaving a note or actually gone so far as to write one, was it thoughtfully worded or hastily scribbled? What was the theme of the letter? Anger? Blame? Regret? Apology?

Broaden this questioning about others into the possible consequences of the suicidal plan, particularly the way in which the death will affect others. The discovery of 'the body' is a useful way in to this area of the conversation: talking through the event as though it has already happened sometimes encourages the patient to think more coherently and calmly about the fuller implications of their ideas. Would you conceal yourself? Would you do it at a time when no one else was around? Who would be likely to find your body? Try to keep it personal – 'your' body, not 'the' body. Also, explore what the patient thinks will be the impact of the discovery upon significant others. How do you think your mum/husband/brother/mates will take the news? If this fails to yield valuable information about the seriousness of the intent, explore the aftermath. Who will come to your funeral? What sort of music do you want played at the memorial? Burial or cremation? This line of questioning is not just voyeurism – it is a means of getting the patient to think again about their suicidal intentions.

The other important issue to address is the 'why now' question. Often, this will reveal a story of steadily accumulating grief, culminating in a 'final straw' moment. Of course, this will then beg the question of just why the patient is now talking to you rather than acting on his or her ideas. It is also helpful to approach this why now issue from the opposite angle. What has stopped you from acting on your ideas so far? Is there anything that might make it easier for you to cope with the way that you feel at the moment?

At times throughout the conversation, try to draw the talk away from the central theme of death and destruction and explore for hints of future orientation. If, for example, themes of redundancy or exam failure appear to be relevant, gently try to tease out any evidence of a willingness to consider signing on for unemployment benefit or re-sitting an exam. Try hard not to sound as though you are deliberately looking for inconsistencies or contradictions in the patient's story. This will only undermine the trust that you are trying to build and, in cases in which the patient's primary motivation is to elicit care rather than signal a wish to die, it may lead to more vociferous protestations of imminent self-destruction, as if the patient has taken themself hostage. The slightest hint of a future orientation is extremely important and touches on something that comes close to being a hard and fast rule in the uncertain world of suicide: if you can think of the future, you don't really mean it.

Talking to a survivor of a recent suicide attempt

When an attempt at suicide has already been made, it can provide a useful way in which to organise the interview. Think of the interview as a target with three concentric rings and a bullseye. The inner ring represents the attempt itself, the middle ring, the background to the attempt, and the outer ring, the patient's personal and family history. First, go through the attempt chronologically, exploring it in the sort of detail that Hercule Poirot would be proud of. Where did you get the tablets? Where did you take them, in the bedroom or the bathroom? With water or alcohol? Did you lock the door? Was anyone else in the bathroom? In the house? Were you expecting anyone to arrive? Did you leave a note? What did it say? When did you write it? Where did you leave it? After you swallowed the tablets, what did you do? Did you expect to be found? How were you found and by whom? Often, the most revealing question is simply: 'Who called the ambulance?' Going into such obsessive detail reveals not just your concerns and the full seriousness of the attempt; it also almost always reveals the true reasons behind it. It also helps the patient to face up to the full consequences of their intentions.

Before moving on to the big question, move out to explore the middle ring. This does not usually need to be as detailed as the inquiry into the attempt itself, but try to identify not only the key events but also some idea of how the patient felt about them. Try to ascertain why the patient has chosen *now* to react in the way that he or she has. Then, move on to the outer ring and try to form a picture of the person's background and broader history. This will very often reveal details that resonate with the motivation behind the recent attempt and throw valuable light on what needs to be done to resolve the situation. By the time that you have completed this inquiry, you will not only know a lot about the person but will also have created a fairly clear impression that you understand and wish to help. This is by far the best climate in which to pop the 'to be or not to be' question. When you finally do, try to avoid a closed style that closes down on the patient's need to keep thinking. Tying the question to actions is useful, for example: 'If you were to leave here now, what would you do?'

What to do next: admit or not admit, call on the home care team, phone a friend?

Having won the trust of your patient, you will hopefully have a clear idea of the way that they intend to act upon their thoughts and feelings of suicide. From this, the answer to the next most important question may seem obvious: whether or not to call on special resources or even to admit the patient. In the relatively uncommon situation in which your assessment indicates that life is imminently endangered, this decision is straightforward. Getting the patient to a safe place, compulsorily if necessary, is the only sensible thing to do. However, whether or not that place should be an acute psychiatric unit is another matter. This is another example of the way in which a risk decision always has two sides. Bringing a truly suicidal patient into an acute unit staffed by people who know just what to do will definitely reduce the risk of self-harm. But it may also carry some less predictable disadvantages as well.

Many psychiatric units, especially in the inner cities, are so overcrowded, cash-strapped and geared towards the treatment of other forms of mental illness that admission of the suicidal patient may ultimately do more to disrupt their engagement with help than encourage it. For many, psychiatric hospitalisation may reinforce the false belief that all is lost. More realistically, the stigma of psychiatric hospitalisation as a 'suicide case' [especially if under a Mental Health Act (MHA) section] may have serious implications for a person's future prospects of finding work, education, a mortgage or life insurance. These may seem like comparatively trivial issues when matters of life and death are at stake, but they return us to that important point: most people who threaten suicide don't always have the wish to die at the top of their motivational agenda. In fact, for some of these individuals, the attention and support that comes with hospitalisation may even reinforce further suicidal behaviour in the future. This is particularly so in cases in which a past history of repeated threats of suicide is quite clear, either from the case notes, the computerised record in A&E or the patient's wrists.

Such cases often crop up at clinical meetings as being 'difficult to manage'. The ensuing discussion often carries recurring themes. The care worker who actually saw the patient in crisis – more often than not out of hours – is usually a less experienced, younger worker. During the assessment, they rightly concluded that the risk of suicide seemed high from the patient's words and deeds but that the long history of similar words and deeds in the past suggested a different conclusion. Furthermore, the junior doctor, nurse or social worker may often feel under pressure not to admit the patient and so take up one of the precious few remaining beds in a service where 120% bed occupancy is the norm. They may even be wary of being seen as a soft touch in the eyes of colleagues, among whom the idea of appearing firm in the face of apparently manipulative behaviour is desirable. Even contacting a senior colleague for advice may feel difficult, especially if it is 2 AM and the senior is known to be a bit tetchy on the phone.

On hearing the case presented several days later, long after the sense of urgency has passed, more senior staff may airily suggest that, when confronted by such uncertainty, 'it's always best to admit and sort it all out in the morning.' Anyone who has ever been on the phone at 3 AM to a more experienced (and less conscious) senior member of staff will at once recognise that the play-it-safe decision is a common one. Such a view, be it expressed from a warm bed or a comfortable chair in a conference room, fails to get to the heart of the problem that the front-line staff find so taxing. By playing safe and admitting the patient, we are often treating our own anxieties about what might otherwise happen as much as we are treating the patient. Senior staff often fail to take the fears of the assessing worker into account when giving advice on the matter.

It is all the more difficult to strike the right balance in this dilemma when one considers how the atmosphere in which we work has become so litigious in recent decades. It does, after all, take a lot of experience – and not a little courage – to be able to stand up in a coroner's court and explain that the connection between the patient's last recorded utterance of 'Goodbye, cruel world' and their subsequent demise isn't quite as clear as it might appear. To the sad, angry relatives in the front row or the happy journalist busily scribbling away at the rear, such a connection may seem like an open-and-shut case of death through negligence. It is this real-world knowledge that gives the more experienced worker the reason for his or her quiet, seen-it-all-before smile and justification to 'always admit'. Seeing the admission of the patient within the whole picture helps the care worker to stand by the decision to admit in the face of moans of 'Oh, no, not him again' from ward staff, to whom the patient's life or death may seem to pose much less of a dilemma. Even if admission is, possibly, an inefficient use of ward time and space, at least it should secure the certainty of life; in any case, the long-term process of encouraging patients to make more appropriate claims for help can only begin if they are in touch with care rather than out of it.

If the decision to admit to hospital requires thought, the decision to keep the suicide-threatening patient in the community is just as challenging. Several rules can help here. The first is always to draw the patient into some form of agreement about what is to be done. Some people even go so far as to draw up some form of non-suicide contract on paper. Before you can let the patient out of your sight, this agreement must fulfil at least two central points. The patient has to agree to remain in contact with the caring services and a precise time, place and date must be agreed for a follow-up meeting. It is usually better to stick to these two easy-to-agree points rather than getting caught up in the issue of whether or not the patient still wishes to die. Some less experienced workers cannot let the matter rest until they have wrestled an outright rejection of suicidal intent from their charge, turning the interview from an empathic exchange into a gruelling interrogation in the process. Many a patient confronted thus may well respond with increasing obtuseness, outright threats of self-destruction or, more commonly, a 'maybe I will' form of ambivalence. This can prolong the interview unnecessarily and make it feel more like the Cuban missile crisis than an attempt to help someone. A patient who can commit to the future doesn't really mean to die; an agreement to keep in touch and come back at another time is a good enough indication of this. Even better, an available phone number and a willingness to have someone visit soon or to stay with relatives or friends can seal the deal.

Apart from an unhealthy obsession with recantation it is important not to get too caught up in the trap of second-guessing the suicide-threatening patient. The moment that you begin to question whether the patient can really be trusted when they agree not to harm themselves, you enter an uncertain world of bluff and double bluff, in which nothing spoken is of reliable value. Worse still, it detracts from the important idea that the patient is a responsible person whose utterances can be relied upon. When moving the interview towards the final agreement, it is always a good idea to make this trust explicit: 'If you give me your word that you are not going to harm yourself and agree to come back and see me in the morning, that's good enough for me'. This may seem risky if the patient has a history of lying, but if you can't reach some form of agreement then you probably shouldn't be letting the patient go in the first place. If you are unhappy about taking their words at face value, sooner or later your local inpatient unit will be full to overflowing with sorry, but very alive, individuals who may or may not intend to harm themselves. And, sooner or later, they will have to go home.

Having decided against admission, the next step is to find somewhere equally safe in which to manage the patient until the agreed time and date of review. This must always involve other people. Preferably, these should be members of the patient's own family or social network rather than professionals, although in situations in which loneliness and social isolation are significant, finding such individuals may not always be easy. Nevertheless, a potentially suicidal patient must never be left alone for any length of time, especially if the case is not familiar to you. If no one can be found to monitor the patient, reconsider hospitalisation. The time between your first contact with the patient and your follow-up, as well as the intensity with which the patient should be monitored, will be proportional to your concern at the risk of an attempt: the riskier the patient, the quicker you should review them. A crisis intervention team, if available, now becomes a first port of call – this is just the kind of job they are designed to do.

Deciding just who will look after the patient until review – for example at home – requires some consideration. Be very careful when assigning this responsibility to young people, no matter how worldly wise they may appear. In fact, identifying who will be involved is something that should begin early on in your assessment. Patients who present in a suicidal state rarely do so alone and it is essential to include the opinions and accounts of accompanying friends and relatives whenever possible. The information that they can offer about all three rings of the target is often invaluable in formulating the management plan. As you listen to each one, weigh them up and ask yourself whether they would make a reliable member of the support network you intend to construct. Pay attention to their feelings as well. From your detached clinical point of view, the case may be just another attempted suicide. To the person who found the patient semi-conscious in a bathroom and called the ambulance, your arrival may be the first source of hope in an unpleasant drama that has already lasted many hours. The individuals who are charged with the responsibility of monitoring the patient until review must never be allowed to feel out of their depth. Try to explain the management plan as explicitly as possible, and make sure that they have a very clear idea of what to do if they feel that their ability to contain the situation is breaking down. Ensure that they have prompt 24-hour access to some form of specialised support, be it the local acute ward, casualty department, crisis team, GP, telephone helpline or whatever else is available locally.

The environment in which the patient will spend the time before review also requires some thought. Ideally, the patient should be monitored somewhere familiar, preferably their own home or that of a friend or relative. It is important to remember that suicidal patients, who have settled with careful reassurance and planning during your assessment, may often feel further impulses to self-harm that can overwhelm them with frightening speed. As far as possible, try to minimise the easy availability of physical methods for further attempts at self-harm. Visibly removing sharp knives, razors, ropes, car keys, domestic chemicals and other potential hazards from the patient's vicinity not only reduces exposure to further dangers but also sends a very clear signal that you mean business. Patients who are taking medication should be given access to only very small quantities. If patients self-destructive behaviour continues in the face of these efforts, it is advisable to reconsider admission, even if the risk of them killing themselves is more by accident than true suicidal intent.

If there is one overarching aim of your work with a patient in a suicidal crisis, it is to always try to give the impression that things are going to be different as a result of your assessment. Often, the assessment will have identified a specific problem that led to the suicidal ideas in the first place. Always try to encourage the view that for every problem, no matter how insurmountable it may seem, there exists a solution. Sometimes this will involve a quick bit of on-the-spot negotiation with a significant other who has accompanied the patient at your assessment. Extracting an agreement from a frustrated partner to put a temporary hold on a threatened separation, for example, may buy precious time in which to persuade the patient to take a fresh look at the meaning of his or her life. A systematic approach to problem solving can prove to be very helpful in securing such agreements.

Suicidal patients who pose particular problems

As if the management of the suicidal patient was not enough, occasionally a patient will pose a particular challenge by virtue of drunkenness or by choosing to remain largely silent throughout the entire interview.

Alcohol intoxication (i.e. being drunk) is very commonly associated with suicidal attempts for a number of reasons. Alcoholism not only carries a greater risk of suicide, especially later in life, but also many people use alcohol to find the chemical courage to carry out an attempt at self-harm. Others might act out suicidal behaviour whilst disinhibited by drink without any true underlying attempt to harm themselves. At some point, most care workers will confront an intoxicated patient who has swallowed a potentially life-threatening quantity of medication and who is acting in an angry, help-rejecting manner. Negotiation with a drunk person can be difficult at the best of times; doing so with a patient on the verge of an incipient coma is even more disconcerting. The central problem here is not how to treat the patient as much as how to persuade the patient to accept any treatment at all.

A principal rule of law is that the patient has the right to autonomy. That is, they have the right to determine what is and what is not done to their body. A worker who decides to initiate care of a patient – even life-saving care – without the patient's expressed consent may leave themself open to charges of battery or even assault. This is a perplexing area in which the cold letter of the law is at odds with the warmer aims of the caring profession. An essential component of a patient's autonomy in the legal sense rests on whether or not they have the capacity to understand the nature of their condition, its implications for their health and what treatment will involve and might achieve. In a situation in which a patient clearly lacks this capacity, it is reasonable – and safe – practice to intervene on a patient's behalf. Unfortunately, where suicidality, drunkenness or mutism are concerned, the issue of whether or not a patient has capacity is not always clear cut. In law, drunkenness itself is not usually regarded as sufficient evidence of incapacity. Workers in this situation, therefore, may find themselves confronted by a dilemma: either accept the apparent wishes of the patient and leave them to die or detain them, save their life and run the risk of a lawsuit.

Of course, such a curmudgeonly outcome is very rare. In such a situation, most people wake up gratefully hung-over, but this scenario does show how important it is to understand the law in regard to suicidal patients. It is essential to know where you stand not only in cases of life and death but also when ethical and legal matters are at stake. If you are unsure how to handle a help-rejecting patient, it is always better to act in favour of saving the patient's life rather than in favour of legal niceties. This way, your patient gets another chance at life, and any reasonable judge called upon to rule on the matter is more likely to take a sympathetic view of the case if you can demonstrate that your actions were at all times driven by the best interests of your patient. In fact, provided that you have used an accepted form of treatment and have made it clear (*good notes are vital*) that the patient's health and safety are your primary concern, you are essentially untouchable under the law.

Sometimes, the possibility of detention under a section of the MHA may help the patient to engage with treatment. There is, of course, a large difference between indicating your intention to use mental health law and actually doing so but, for many patients, the very suggestion of compulsory hospitalisation is enough to make them reconsider their intentions. Mental health law is quite specific about what can and cannot be done here. The current MHA applies only to people who are suffering from a mental disorder. Being drunk and talking of suicide is not by itself sufficient evidence of mental disorder. Mental health law gives no powers to treat a patient for a purely physical disorder such as paracetamol poisoning. This may seem to rule out the use of the MHA in such a situation, but a little imaginative thinking, talking and writing can provide a very useful degree of flexibility in the use of legal sanctions for suicidal individuals. First, a drunken refusal of treatment probably does not constitute sufficient evidence of an intention to decline treatment. As the guidance on the current MHA puts it, there must be 'unequivocal and reliable evidence that the patient did not want the treatment.' Drunken shouts of 'piss off and leave me to die' do not exactly meet this criterion.

Second, mental disorder is defined as 'any disorder or disability of mind'. Although the act explicitly excludes those in whom the presentation is entirely due to alcohol or drug misuse, we can take advantage of the fact that, in real life, as opposed to law, this distinction is often far from clear. Very few patients who present drunk and in a suicidal state do so suddenly out of the blue and in the absence of any antecedents. Interviewing others who have accompanied the patient, paying careful attention to the patient's recent history or going through any medical records that may be available can often uncover evidence of some form of mental disorder. Sleep disturbance, low mood, social withdrawal or vague suicidal ideation expressed before the patient started drinking may all justify an attempt to detain a patient legally on the grounds of a depressive disorder when all else looks like failing. It some senses, it is almost immaterial whether the suspicions of underlying mental illness turn out to be true. By the time that the patient has been admitted and exerted his or her right of appeal against the detention, the crisis will have passed, enabling the matter to be dealt with in a more sober and, hopefully, informal manner. Care workers may feel uneasy about the idea of detaining patients in this manner and clinical decisions should, whenever possible, always respect the patient's rights; however, these include the right to expect that care workers will exercise their duty to protect life wherever possible.

It is worth repeating that, whenever confronted by this or similar ethical dilemmas, careful and clearly written (timed, dated and signed) case notes are crucial. It is helpful to remember that case notes are legal documents. Before you write anything down, always think about how it would sound if read out in a court. With any decision that involves a degree of risk – for example allowing a harm-threatening patient to go home – it is always a good idea to err on the side of inclusiveness when putting your reasoning down on paper. As far as a court or an inquiry is concerned, if it is not written down then it did not happen.

Before putting your thoughts down in ink, it is often a good idea to jot down the key issues in rough or make a mental sketch of the major issues or problems as you see them. Be careful of your own emotions at this point, especially if your pulse is still high from a near miss with an angry patient. Take a breather before you write up your thoughts. Once you start writing, try not to be too telegraphic. Adopt a style that you might use when explaining your actions to an intelligent layperson or journalist. Try to make it clear that your concern lies not only with your anxieties over the current event but also with the bigger picture. Stock phrases and sentences can often come in handy here, especially when you are tired. Box 8.2 provides an example that can often be adapted into a useful entry.

223

Box 8.2 Example of a written assessment of a suicidal patient

Suicide risk formally assessed: although patient presented expressing ideas of self-harm, in my opinion, this behaviour is motivated primarily by a need to elicit caring responses from others rather than indicating a true wish to end her life.

At interview, the patient displayed clear future orientation and has a history of previous attempts in a similar manner that have not resulted in serious self-harm.

In my opinion, it is advisable to decline admission to this patient as it would do little to further minimise the risks of self-harm in the short term. It would not address the issues that underlie the present behaviour. Indeed, hospitalisation at present could reinforce further self-harming behaviour in the future.

I acknowledge that there is a small risk that the patient may come to harm as a result of the decision not to admit to hospital but this risk needs to be balanced against the overall care required for this patient to succeed in the longer term. In my opinion, were this patient to come to harm, it would be more likely to occur accidentally than by a premeditated intention to end her life.

Most care workers will encounter this situation at some point and, when they do, it is essential never to make important decisions in isolation. Always discuss the management plan with a senior and record the fact that the discussion has taken place. Decisions in risky cases should only ever be taken on the basis of a measured evaluation of the evidence and should not, as far as possible, be influenced by worry about adverse public opinion. Difficult judgements should never be made 'on the go' and a phone call to a senior, even at 3 AM, is a good way to avoid this happening.

Handling aggressive patients

An interview with an angry, threatening or violent patient is probably the most challenging situation that a care worker is likely to face in the course of his or her work. Most assaults against care workers happen early on in their careers. The relative inexperience of junior staff is probably only a partial explanation for this. Violence against public servants in general appears to be on the increase. Junior staff also spend more of their time in contact with a range of different kinds of patients compared with their more senior counterparts. Fortunately, violence against care staff, be it verbal or physical, is a relatively rare event, but not so rare as to justify being unprepared for the possibility.

The resources and abilities needed to anticipate and deal with the aggressive patient comprise another essential aspect of the core skills of the care worker. Some of these skills cannot be taught via the written word. Training in breakaway techniques, calming and restraint should be given to all workers who are likely to encounter aggressive patients in the course of their duties.

This underlines the fact that resources are the most important issue in the management of the potentially aggressive patient. As we saw above, mental health services have long been accustomed to working at the limits of their capability, all too often with inadequate resources. A care worker who is expected to interview a potentially violent person in an ill-equipped environment without adequate training, supervision and practical support has every right not to go ahead with the interview. The manager of every mental health team has a responsibility to provide not only adequate facilities but also absolute clarity regarding the safest way to deal with aggressive patients. Unless there is a clear, unequivocal policy in place for dealing with such cases, and it is used rather than merely referred to after an event, staff will feel increasingly pressurised and demoralised. Undue anxiety and underconfidence can drastically affect the way in which we manage this important group of patients. They are, as we have seen, one of the standards by which the public judges our service.

Effective management of the aggressive patient, therefore, begins long before the interview. This should not only be reflected in departmental policy but also in the physical structure of the workplace. It is important to give careful thought to the layout and design of the room where the potentially aggressive patient is to be interviewed. The service should have a room designated for this purpose. Its size and shape are important. It should be neither too small to allow for a safe, comfortable distance at interview nor so large that it allows the patient to get up and run around. The room should also be free of cul-de-sacs or other features that might allow the erection of a hasty barricade. The door to the room should never have an inside lock and should open outwards to prevent blockade from within. It should have a clear window of unbreakable glass so that others can monitor the progress of the interview. Decor and lighting should be unobtrusive and conducive to a relaxed atmosphere.

It should not be possible to convert furniture and fittings into blunt objects or missiles; a fresh cup of coffee can be a frightening weapon in angry hands. The positioning of furniture is also important. A table or desk placed between the two chairs may create a more formal atmosphere, but it also provides a convenient barrier if the interview becomes difficult. Chairs should not face each other, as this encourages a head-on pattern of eye contact that can upset an angry or suspicious patient. Chairs placed at 45 degrees to each other allow eye contact to be made and broken at will without either party appearing to be shifty or evasive. The structure and style of the chairs is also important. The interviewer's chair should be firmer, higher and armless, to allow for a swift exit, whereas the interviewee's chair should be lower and softer. It is much harder to move quickly out of such a chair and may make a frightened patient feel more secure. The lower eyeline also makes it much harder to adopt a dominant posture whilst seated. Any service that ever anticipates aggressive behaviour should always be equipped with some sort of alarm system. At its most basic, this should involve a second person remaining within earshot throughout the interview. If it employs more sophisticated technology, such as a personal alarm or a panic button, it is essential that staff at both ends know how it works. An untrained receptionist may overlook a flashing light that is the only indication that you are taking a pasting in an adjoining room.

Working with police officers when assessing aggressive patients

Occasionally, you will be called upon to assess a potentially dangerous patient away from the relative security of your base. Often this will occur at the patient's home, where he or she will have a strategic advantage in the event of violence. Such an assessment should never be undertaken alone, no matter how well you know the patient. If you ever anticipate the possibility of violence on a home visit, always notify your base of your intentions, your whereabouts and your company, and always involve the police.

Working alongside the police is not always as straightforward or as easy as one might hope. Police officers are very busy people and do not always view mental illness as a priority. Furthermore, the culture in which they work is emotionally much harder than that of the care worker. Appearing too sensitive and compassionate can lead to some officers being thought of as 'soft' by their colleagues. This is hardly surprising: it is hard to display caring sensitivity towards a frightened, psychotic and aggressive person when many of the people you encounter during your work are unpleasant, aggressive and totally sane.

A welcome by-product of the publicity given in recent years to the small but significant link between mental illness and violence is that police forces are starting to incorporate mental health issues into routine training. Unfortunately, much of this theory has yet to trickle down into actual police practice. As a result, assessments of potentially dangerous patients often tend to start off on the wrong foot, with the police and care staff communicating poorly, ignoring important information and rushing to 'get the nutter in the van a.s.a.p.' There is much that a thoughtful care worker can to do avoid this outcome.

The first thing is that if you anticipate the possibility of violence, inform the police as early as possible, preferably more than 24 hours in advance. This often allows the police to do their own risk assessment (i.e. to check previous behaviour/lawbreaking) and to allocate those with training in such problems to the case. Such preparedness should also be carried over to the site of the operation, which should be addressed with a seriousness and clarity of military precision. Never rush into a patient's dwelling without first having clarified the precise reasons for the visit with all professionals gathered. Spending 5 minutes in a windswept car park identifying who is who to the police assigned to the job – no matter how disinterested or impatient they may appear – is always time well spent. Identify which officer is of senior rank and address them foremost. Give them as much information as you can, not only about the patient but also about the layout of the dwelling. Draw a map if necessary, particularly noting ideal ambush points, lockable doors and the whereabouts of the kitchen – the likeliest repository for domestic weapons. Also, if you can, try to give them some idea of the sad human story on the other side of the door. If there is one, try to target the WPC in the team, especially if the patient is female.

In addition, pay close attention to the manner and verbal style of the police officers and form an opinion of which are likely to be the most sensible if things get verbally colourful during the assessment. Police are often unable to distinguish between angry thought disorder and imminent assault and are often unaccustomed to the long silences that may occur during an interview with a psychotic person. Mistaking this for a waste of time, they may occasionally decide to take over the interview, to get it over and done with. Often, this can lead to fisticuffs and wrestling, which might otherwise be avoided. Having an idea of the tolerance threshold of any of the officers, no matter how hastily formed, can often tell you which ones to interrupt and which to leave alone when the interview becomes colourful. If you can, try to keep control of the interview.

Preparing for the interview

Assuming that you are satisfied with the support and safety of the setting in which you are working, further preparations are essential before you begin any interview. Try to find out as much about the patient as you can beforehand. This involves far more than a thorough reading of the case notes or simply compiling all of the 'known facts' about a case. Emotional information should be compiled as well.

In many cases, the reputation of a patient with a history of violence will reach you well before the patient does. Because of the strong emotions that violence provokes in all of us – even the most experienced – it is often very hard to reach an unbiased opinion about a difficult patient. As far as you can, try to be honest with yourself about your own possible fears and prejudices, particularly in the light of any unpleasant experiences of your own. In the last chapter, we described ways of monitoring your own emotional state. It is important to use these methods here. Does the patient fulfil any of the stereotypes that you associate with higher risk? Although it is impossible to ever fully eliminate the distortions of perception and expectation that can arise from our own fears, bearing this in mind can help to keep it to a minimum and possibly prevent the interview from slipping into a self-fulfilling prophecy of anger and suspicion.

It is important to pay close attention to the way that other people think, talk and feel about the patient, especially those who have actually met him or her. Be especially wary of those who appear to exaggerate or play down a patient's reputation for aggression. Compare such views with the objective record and ask yourself if this view of the patient is justifiable. Also, be wary of those who claim to have developed a special 'knack' for engaging a particular patient. Such people are often trying to bolster their own nervousness and their claims can help to create the false idea that there is some mysterious, proper way to deal with an aggressive patient that somehow evades you. Such a view will result in your going into an interview feeling less, rather than more, confident. In truth, all interviews 'go wrong' in one way or another. As with the breaking of bad news, there is never a right way to interview an aggressive person, but some approaches can prove to be a lot less disastrous than others.

Having gathered all of the information that you can from others, study the case notes carefully. Never delay reading them until after you have seen the patient. Pay particular attention to the known markers for violence (see Box 8.3). Particular risk factors are a young or male patient, or impulsive, unstable or aggressive traits in the pre-morbid personality. Do alcohol or drugs feature much in the history? If so, then for how long? Is there any evidence that the patient has turned over a new leaf? If so, what is the evidence that this new-found peace will reign during your interview? The most important factor to be gleaned from the notes is, of course, a previous history of violence.

Box 8.3 Risk factors when assessing violent patients

- Socially deprived upbringing including abuse (sexual and/or physical)
- Pattern of broken relationships, unstable living situation (e.g. temporary accommodation)
- Young male living on his own
- History of previous assaults/fights
- Weapon carrying or using, e.g. knife
- Use of drugs, especially alcohol, cocaine or amphetamines
- Paranoid ideation, believing oneself to be under threat or physically interfered with
- Inarticulate, semi-mute or confused

Given the inexactness of risk assessment in general and the prediction of violence in particular, the old adage is still the best: nothing predicts the future like the past. How often has the patient been violent before and in what sort of situations? How do these situations differ from the present, if at all? What was the nature of the violence? Did the violence occur with or without weapons? Were there any signs or evidence of premeditation? In the past, has the clinical picture been influenced by substance misuse or some particular aspect of the mental state, such as delusions or command hallucinations? If you have not considered these questions, you should not go ahead with the interview. Even if you have, there are still one or two other preparatory questions left to answer, i.e. what has been happening to the patient in the last hour and who will be with you during the interview.

Setting eyes on the patient before they set eyes on you can often hint at what lies ahead. If possible, watch patients whilst they are in the waiting area and scan for signs of possible trouble. Are they sitting or standing? Can they keep still? Are they sweating, clenching their jaws or flexing their muscles? Do they look fit and fast, slow, sluggish or tired? Look closely at their posture for signs of intoxication or disinhibition. Often, the receptionist who has greeted them will provide useful information on their mental state. Find out whether the patient has been waiting long or has arrived early or late. A patient who mistakenly arrives at 10 AM for a 2 PM appointment may feel, and act, as though they have been kept waiting for 4 hours (which in their mind they have been!).

Give careful thought to your company during the interview. If you anticipate even the slightest chance of any physically aggressive behaviour, ask yourself if you should be going ahead with the interview without adequate backup. An interview conducted whilst sandwiched between two burly male colleagues may not send the most disarming of signals to the patient, but one's physical integrity is far more important than any interview and a bodyguard at least sends the unequivocal message that the patient is being taken very seriously. Also, be wary of interviewing the patient in the presence of others from the patient's own social network. It is safer and wiser to subject such people to the same degree of caution as that reserved for the patients themselves; however, a sensible mum or dad can be a very useful and calming presence.

How to talk to a very angry person

Although it is virtually impossible to describe good interviewing skills in writing, this hasn't stopped hundreds of people writing books on the subject, present authors included. When it comes to handling interviews with an aggressive or violent person, the how-to-do-it sort of manuals are often full of hilarious stock phrases, for example 'I can see from the way you have your hands around my throat that you are angry with me', or useful suggestions, such as 'run away'. Because any interview with another human being – let alone a potentially explosive one – is such a complex, unpredictable thing, we can do little more here than identify several essential principles. The rest comes down to practice, discipline, confidence and a little luck.

The first essential point is always to keep control of the interview. The best way to start the interview is by initiating some form of physical contact, ideally a handshake or a gentle touch of the elbow as you guide the patient to the softest seat. Note the firmness of the grip and the warmth of the glance that comes with it. Try to remain impassive at the refusal of a proffered hand or the swift recoil from touch, but lower your threshold for an early ending of the interview. Always maintain a polite and formal style from the very outset and respond promptly and clearly to any deviation from this by your subject. It is useful to think of the interview as a ritual in which both parties act according to certain rules. Unlike casual conversation, in which both sides usually have equal status and access to information, the patient/professional ritual entails a set of assumptions that confer privileges and restrictions on both sides. Information flows in a more unidirectional manner compared with informal conversation, and the professional is usually unable to use personal details of his or her own to reach an understanding or gain sympathy.

The way that you start the interview can also be vital in carrying it through and making it successful. Tell the patient that you want to talk, to hear their point of view, to hear their version of what the matter is. Also tell the patient that you are here to try to help, that you are a nurse or doctor or social worker – provide identification (always have this on you) to validate your role. All of this may seem blindingly obvious, but getting these little details right often makes the difference between success and failure when situations are on the edge. Emphasise that you are a health worker and not a police officer or agent of the state/housing/customs authorities, which can be especially important when dealing with immigrants or asylum seekers. In addition, tell the patient that you will need to ask some questions, directly or after he or she has had their say, and that you will be taking notes. Paranoid people quite easily become suspicious about notes, so write them openly on a desk or table in front of you and always let patients see what you are writing, especially if they ask. (Keep a hand on the notes, though, because there is nothing more frustrating than having someone run off with them, usually the action of a patient who is angry but not, as a rule, psychotic.)

If a patient asks you not to write something down, for example a particular phrase or a comment about somebody that is rude, agree not to and openly cross out the offending remark. Of course, if that remark reflects a vital aspect of the patient's psychopathology, keep it in mind and add a note later (assuming that you still have the notes!). If the patient insists that no notes are kept, try to point out the advantages of note keeping – the right details documented, a copy for the patient if he or she wishes and a clear record that the patient has been listened to. It is very rare for absolute refusal, but think about closing out soon if this does happen. A non-committal remark should be taken as agreement unless obvious dissent ensues. Remember also to think about time – suggest at the start of the interview that you will need to talk for about 20–30 minutes, a reasonable enough commitment to make someone feel that they are being taken seriously. However, don't be too precise about this. If you do need to finish in that time frame – because the problem is sorted out or because you have other duties – the patient usually won't feel short-changed. If you do go on for a bit longer, or even for an hour or so, the patient will feel rewarded, even special, because you will have given something extra. Don't think of such approaches as being 'tricks' of the trade; they are also standard practice in the duller worlds of banking, business, commerce and sales – straight out of the 'how to make friends and influence people' tradition.

Within the confidential framework provided by the interview, the patient can express deeply personal information without fear of being judged or exploited in a way that might arise during a more informal conversation. The instant that any of these rules are broken, for example by insult, shouting or overfamiliarity, try at once to re-establish authority by politely pointing out the nature of the transgression and proceeding with the interview. This may involve telling the patient that the interview cannot proceed and that it may possibly end unless the patient makes an effort to calm down. Occasionally, it may be helpful to allow the patient some breathing space or 'time out' of the interview to regain control of their temper. If you have even the slightest concern that this is unlikely to succeed, halt the interview.

Defusing aggression

Often, a patient's anger is not driven by a wish to subvert or gain control of the interview but from a sense of inadequacy or fear of being seen to lose face. Directly acknowledging the patient's strengths can often defuse a potential conflict. By being

229

upfront with the patient, and even admitting that, if it came to a fight, the patient would very swiftly gain the upper hand, one can often neutralise the inferiority that feeds the patient's hostility at interview. Other features can act as a warning that one is losing control of the interview. Invasion of personal space, which means any degree of physical proximity that makes you feel uncomfortable, the refusal to reply to any questions at all, unusual movements or facial expressions and shouting or the use of dehumanising language, such as 'you are nothing but a pill-pushing parasite', are clear signs that loss of control is irretrievable. If these lines are crossed, do not attempt to regain control. Instead, end the interview at once. The question of what to do next is one that should be asked and answered elsewhere.

Another important point is to pay as much attention to what is communicated non-verbally as to what is spoken. All live interactions between human beings are rich in non-verbal information. Much of this is read and responded to without us being fully aware of it. Given the similarity of this non-verbal behaviour to the communication patterns used by most other higher mammals, it is likely that these patterns of posture, gesture, facial expression and movement are largely innate. Many anthropologists believe that they evolved during the pre-verbal era of human history, when 'body language' was the most significant way of denoting status within a group.

Cultivating an awareness of such subtle signs is largely a matter of practice. There is a lot of 'man-watching' mumbo jumbo that ascribes meaningless significance to specific gestures, but some general observations about non-verbal language do seem to hold true. For example, the total amount of movement shown by both parties is significant. When two people of reasonably equal status are involved in free, relaxed conversation, both sides make pretty much the same amount of movement, be it nodding, leaning or gesturing. Next time that you are alone in a busy cafe, take a look and you'll see what we mean. Any interview that becomes heated is, by definition, an attempt by one party to gain a form of dominance over the other. This is reflected in a visible change in the way that movement is shared. The more we become aroused, the greater and swifter our total amount of movement. Eye-to-eye glances increase in frequency and length, and truncal and limb movements become more pronounced. Always watch closely for any early signs of increased general movement, as well as more focal features such as jaw clenching, rapid breathing, sweating or tremor. All but the most explosive of psychopaths will inadvertently use their bodies to signal an assault. If you fear this, try to keep the patient talking. People very rarely punch and talk at the same time.

Conversely, one's own body language can play just as large a role in shaping the progress of the interview. As we grow more anxious or become intimidated by an aggressive patient, we send out non-verbal replies that show how we feel about the patient's attempts to gain dominance. It is precisely for this reason that one should never begin an interview without having at least a reasonable degree of confidence. As the interview proceeds, those who lack confidence will display a gradual decline in overall movement, keeping the arms closer to the trunk, and will resort less to expression and gesture. Even smiling will look like a rictus of disgust or even a sneer to the paranoid patient. Shoulders will hunch up, bowing the head into a submissive gesture, which greatly reduces the opportunity for eye contact. We acknowledge this when we use the phrase: 'I couldn't look him in the eye'. The best way of looking at someone, so that they feel as if you are paying attention to them but not staring them down, is to look mostly at their mouth. This means that, every now and then, you can look at their eyes while monitoring their facial expression overall. Nods, frowns and smiles – appropriate to the tone of the conversation – should also be used regularly to show that you are alert to what the patient is saying. This may all seem a bit actorish, but you are playing a role, that of the professional therapist who has to know how to listen. In this regard, don't be averse to a spot of video interview training – we all get better with a little ironing out of our interpersonal habits, such as the semi-voluntary 'okay' after every reply, which reeks of inattention.

Apart from actually hitting someone, standing over someone is the loudest non-verbal shout of all. Never continue an interview with an aggressive person who is standing over you unless you are extremely sure of, or very close to, fully trained backup personnel. Instead, try to regain control by calmly explaining that the interview will end unless they return to their seat. If this is unsuccessful, halt the interview. Becoming aware of the way that people use their bodies in an interview can help to reduce the chances of things going pear-shaped.

Skilful self-monitoring of motion and emotion is also one of the best indicators of how an interview is progressing. It is a physiological fact that our emotional reactions to events begin some 300 precious milliseconds before they reach our awareness. In cases in which a patient's angry arousal leads to sudden aggressive impulses, particularly in psychotic or stimulant-intoxicated states, a sudden sense of fear may be the first and only warning that you will receive of imminent assault. Therefore, it is essential to learn to monitor your own emotional state during an interview just as closely as you watch that of your patients. With time and prac-tice, it becomes possible to 'read' the subtle ebbs and flows of your own arousal to track the progress of an interview.

It is important also to watch yourself for anger. As we grow irritated or frus-trated with someone, the theme of the interview can move subtly from obtaining information towards creating an effect in the listener. Occasionally, this may be put to good use, for example using a mildly exasperated tone to ask 'How can I possibly help if you keep shouting at me?' but, as a rule, it is unwise to allow such exchanges to become the main theme of the interview. If they do, end it immediately.

Tiredness is the other emotional state that can act as an important indicator of how an interview is progressing. Talking with a potentially violent person is a draining process. Those of you who may not notice, or acknowledge, a subjective sense of fear or anger may instead find yourselves growing intensely tired or men-tally muddled as the interview progresses. If this begins to coincide with a sense that your thoughts are somehow 'frozen' or confused, or perhaps that the patient's utterances are becoming increasingly incomprehensible, do not waste precious time puzzling over phenomenology. The problem is far more likely to reside in your own brain. If you find your mental flexibility becoming replaced by a frozen fearfulness, end the interview at once.

Ending the interview properly

The ending of an interview with an aggressive person is easy to overlook. If feelings have run high, you may feel a strong urge to finish up and leave as soon as possible. Always resist this urge if you can and try, instead, to leave the patient with some-thing useful at the end. Try to summarise all that you have heard and show that, as a direct result, you are going to do something that may be of specific use to the patient. Choose your words carefully, adjusting them to a level of complexity that you feel stands the best chance of being understood, given what you now know of the patient's mental state. Beware of euphemisms such as 'I know how you feel', which may at best sound patronising and at worst enrage the 'empathised', feeling as they often do, *un*-understood. Remember that the worst thing that you can do for a patient who has struggled to keep in control of angry impulses throughout an interview is to let the patient think that their efforts have been a total waste of time. This has the drawback of leaving yet more problems in store for the next interview. Writing something down, for example a list of problems/tasks, etc., can be helpful. Offering to write to the patient outlining what has been agreed, with a copy of the letter sent to the patient's GP or the housing department, can leave a perplexed smile on the even most cantankerous patient's face. Table 8.2 summarises how to deal with aggression.

Table 8.2 ● Handling aggression

Before assessment	Obtain training in breakaway techniques, control and restraint (C&R), and mental state assessment and at-risk symptoms/behaviours
	Ensure appropriate environment: room design, furniture
	Check that the alarm system is working and monitored
	Carry out a pre-interview risk assessment and history review
	Ensure adequate staffing numbers and support; involve the police?
During assessment	Monitor patient's posture and movement
	Remain polite, concerned, formal
	Explain the reasons for questions, notes, etc.; emphasise that you are here to help
	Keep the patient in sight and seated but not too near or between you and a door
	If frightened/uncomfortable, leave as quickly as possible
	Never reject, oppose or downplay the patient's concerns
After assessment	Write up a care plan, with good clean notes of what was said *and* how you felt
	Contact all relevant individuals, e.g. family, GP, colleagues, regarding your experience/concerns
	If violence occurring/imminent, *call the police*. Consider use of the Mental Health Act
	Discuss with colleagues your next steps and future contacts

When it all goes wrong: coping with a serious incident

'No battle plan survives contact with the enemy'
(*The Art of War, c.* 500 BC, attributed to the Chinese general Sun Tzu)

No matter how hard you work or how well thought out your treatment plan, sooner or later, something will go wrong. And because we work with disorganised,

unpredictable and occasionally suicidal people in a cash-strapped service, surrounded by a public who expect the impossible, sooner or later, someone will die.
Most, if not all, care workers can expect to lose one or two patients to suicide
within the first decade of their career. An unlucky few will have to endure the
rigours of a homicide committed by a patient on their caseload. Either way, such
events go with the territory – if you never lose anyone, you're not working with the
people and problems who most need your help. There are many difficult, 'malig-
nantly unwell' people out there. Remember that the best surgeons don't spend their
time doing day-case cosmetic operations on fit, fussy, young actresses; they are
in at all hours seeing anyone who needs them – old or young, chronically ill with
loads of complications or fit as a fiddle but needing an emergency intervention.

Coping with these awful events is always difficult, but facing up to their inevitability is one of the first and most important steps towards this. Acknowledging the
inevitable can help to sustain our rationality in a situation in which our emotions
put us at a high risk of irrational thought and action. Handling our own feelings
during a serious incident can be difficult; without a doubt, one of the most uncomfortable questions that one must ask is: 'Was it my fault?' There is a more realistic,
rational and useful way to pose this question, however. Could I have done anything
differently that might have changed things and, if so, why didn't I do it? Whereas
the former question employs the 'glass half empty' approach, which has its roots
in blame, guilt and anticipation of punishment, the latter is a 'glass half full'
approach, with its roots instead in ideas of recovery and growth.

In the days after the bad news has come through, it is almost impossible to avoid
the agonising soul-searching that comes with the event. However, it does highlight
one of the few useful things that can be said about what to do at this stage: monitor
your own mental state closely and try to keep themes of blame, anger, apology and
regret out of your head or at least in proportion. Above all, don't make any important decisions at this stage. Do not offer to resign, telephone the family, commit
hara-kiri or arrange the funeral, or yield to any of the other odd but powerful urges
that will come into your mind. All of these can, and must, wait and will need to be
addressed in due course by a proper process. And in that due course, they should be
weighed against a backdrop of history, mental state, diagnosis, caseloads, resources,
exhaustion and countless other factors that one simply cannot grasp at the outset.

Apart from one's own personal angst and self-doubt, the next hardest thing to
handle is the response of others. It helps to be able to spot the sometimes extraordinary hypocrisy that emerges when a suicide or a homicide occurs. Consider the
following two case histories:

A 34-year-old mother of three is readmitted to hospital in the advanced stages
of disseminated breast cancer after 8 years of intensive surgery, radiotherapy and
chemotherapy. She is suffering excruciating pain from secondary growths in her
bones. Finally, she dies in a state of reasonable comfort, provided by palliative care
specialists. Her family were at her bedside.

A 34-year-old mother of three is readmitted to hospital with a severe depressive
psychotic disorder. Numerous treatments, including cognitive behavioural therapy
(CBT), antidepressants, neuroleptics, mood stabilisers, electroconvulsive therapy
(ECT) and a close relationship with a care worker have only partly helped. Finally,
she kills herself by jumping from her apartment balcony in a 17-storey council
block. Her ex-husband keeps her children away from the funeral.

Were both of these deaths equally inevitable? Do we feel that, in both cases,
the carers did all that they could? Because we have a much clearer grasp of physical than mental events, we tend to be much more accepting of the inevitability

of death when there is a clear physical antecedent. After all, dying is about as physical as it gets. Because of this, we are much more forgiving, even grateful, towards those who battled to save the woman with breast cancer. Unfortunately, this attitude of 'thanks, we know that you did your best' is far less often extended towards those working in the mental health field. The reasons for this are important. Certainly, these double standards have not been helped by decades of under-resourcing or the intense publicity that has surrounded a handful of tragedies, but because mental illness still has a capacity to frighten and confuse, these emotions still obstruct the process of acceptance and forgiveness.

Thus, often well before all the facts are known, the immediate conclusion that many reach about death related to serious mental illness is that there was a mis-judgement or that something more should have been done. It is as though, where mental health care is concerned, all conditions are essentially curable. If only the nurse or doctor or therapist or social worker had somehow sussed the problem, exorcised the psychic wound or got the medication right, all would have been well. Furthermore, we have to be seen to have gone the extra mile before the public will acknowledge that we too have tried our best. For now, at least, our culture is reluctant to accept that we also have our 'malignant' cases. This certainly helps to propel the powerful sense of shame, guilt and self-reproach that we all feel when we lose a patient, which is why discussing difficult 'cases' with others and being aware of their potentially 'poor prognosis' should be part of regular reviews.

Self-doubt after an incident is not just propelled by our uncertainty over mental illness. Ironically, it can also be caused by the reactions of one's colleagues, sympathetic or otherwise. This is particularly so when the event is in some way poignant or spectacular, and homicide is always spectacular. Because of the real world in which we work, each of us constantly has to deal with the possibility that the next serious incident, rather like the doodlebugs of World War II, might be 'the one landing on me'. When an incident is close, but mercifully not a direct hit, the event unleashes a powerful feeling of 'there but for the grace of God go I'. This will manifest itself in the form of phone calls, cards, letters and open expressions of sympathy from colleagues. Even worse, some will stop to offer you the benefit of their own handy formulations of your mental state. Beware particularly of those smug colleagues who tell you that you are worrying too much or that you are becoming paranoid. It is not just you, though. People *really are* out to judge you.

This sudden display of support and emotion is – in most cases – well intentioned, but what it can easily do is nourish that growing sense of isolation that many of us feel when we suddenly find ourselves under the spotlight of a serious incident inquiry. No matter how experienced you are, it can make you feel very alone and very incompetent. So, listen closely to your colleagues words of support and sympathy, and home in on the ones who spontaneously say 'It could have been me' or 'I'm surprised it wasn't me'. These are the ones with whom to discuss your thoughts and feelings about the forthcoming inquiry. For inquiry there must be. But before that happens, there are a number of other important steps that must be taken not only to limit your own psychological damage but also to help others and smooth out the sad ritual that inevitably arises from an untoward incident.

What to do after a serious incident

Apart from one's own responsibility to oneself there are a number of obligations to others that must be carried out in the immediate aftermath of a serious incident. Some are demanded by law, others are driven by simple decency and common sense.

In the UK, there is a legal obligation to inform the authority charged with the investigation of all unusual deaths. In England and Wales, this is the coroner, whereas, in Scotland, it is the procurator fiscal. It is also sensible to inform the police as early on as possible, especially if the event carries even the faintest hint of possible homicide. All community mental health teams have a robust protocol that details just what to do in the case of such difficult events. It is your professional duty to know about this document and to follow it. In return, the management of your trust should take responsibility for ensuring that this document is up to date and that statutory communication takes place. As the care worker involved, these tasks should never fall to you directly, especially if you were the first on the scene. Instead, they should always be carried out by a senior clinician or manager; however, it is always wise for you to check that the correct procedure has been followed from the outset. The clarity and transparency that arises from firm adherence to an agreed protocol can be very helpful in the event of someone trying to invoke 'poor communication' as a reason for shovelling blame back down the line. Informing the police is also very helpful in dealing with one of the most unpleasant jobs of all: telling the next of kin.

Just who should inform the family of the deceased is a matter of judgement. As a rule it should always fall to more senior staff members, although a care worker will often have a much better personal relationship with the family, which may make the care worker's involvement more appropriate. Having two or three people (never one person alone) meet with the family as soon as possible, to sympathise, support, explain and offer further help, is an absolute must. The best way to do this is as for the breaking of any other piece of bad news, but it is a pretty safe bet that you will have to deal with unusually strong feelings of anger, despair and accusation in the process. When confronted by such issues, it is very important not to be drawn into a defensive debate about neglect and responsibility. Apportionment of blame should always be left for a more clear-headed moment. Whatever your involvement with the family in the early days after the event, do not allow this to become your only contact with them. It is easy to avoid those whom you feel that you have upset but, by keeping at least some contact with the family during their grief, you may well help them to cope better with the initial shock as well as form a clearer judgement of your efforts to help as the inquiry gets under way.

Of course, it is impossible to define the correct procedure for dealing with a family bereaved by suicide. When considering whether to send a card or flowers and, particularly, whether to attend the funeral, it is always best to play it by ear. However, a good general rule with regard to the funeral is 'if in doubt, go'. Attendance at formal ceremonies is much appreciated by the bereaved; if they truly don't want you there (which is very rare), they will say so. Close attention paid to the words and deeds of the family, other carers and the patient's broader network should allow you to gauge the degree of hostility to or acceptance of your condolences. In all cases, though, a personal touch is most important; however, responsibility for this should never be yours alone. A formal expression of regret and condolence, however worded, is the responsibility of the head of your team.

Keep your eyes on other people

In the days and weeks after a serious incident, it is easy to become absorbed in your own experience of and reaction to the event, especially if you were the worker closest to the patient or perhaps even the one to discover the corpse. Suicides and homicides never affect one person in isolation and can often exert unpredictable effects on the morale and behaviour of teams as a whole, especially once an inquiry gets under way. Pay the closest attention to those who are most involved, particularly the corpse-finder assuming this was not you. Make sure that these people have someone to talk to, should they feel a wish to do so. Watch out particularly for the less qualified or less experienced staff members. Doctors and nurses encounter extremes of suffering and death as a routine part of their training, but not all front-line workers will necessarily have the toughness born of this experience.

Make sure that affected staff are offered a few days off work along with adequate cover for their caseload while they are away. Don't assume that they will have got over it by their return, either. Keep a quiet eye on their spirits. It is best not to make too much of a show of this, as any inquiry can easily be misinterpreted as being patronising, accusatory or worse; however, a quiet word when the time feels right is always preferable to a pregnant silence. Keep a similarly sympathetic eye on your seniors too. Although it is the job of a consultant or senior manager to take such events on the chin, because of their status, they often do not have quite the same degree of support and supervision as that of the front-line care worker. 'You okay, boss?', tactfully expressed at the right moment, can go a long way to helping your seniors cope with the inquiry, which is, after all, what they are paid to do.

The other group of people for whom a completed suicide has a very powerful effect is, of course, other patients, particularly those who knew the deceased or identified with him or her in some way. News of a suicide spreads faster than fire and can lead to distressed acting out or even 'copy cat' suicidal behaviour in some cases. Pay close attention to patients for whom suicide has recently been a pertinent issue and do not be afraid to mention the issue in the course of work with them. If a patient attended a day centre or was recently on a ward, it is only fair to make sure that everyone knows about the death. The relevant ward or day centre team can help with this by organising a meeting or individual contacts as they see best. It is also very easy to forget to inform the patient's GP (or other staff, e.g. occupational therapist), especially if they were not involved in the details of the patient's mental health care.

Some teams use a routine 'debriefing meeting' after every major incident, believing it to be a helpful way to enable the team to accept, understand and learn from what has happened, as well as to prepare for the forthcoming investigation. Some organisations even go so far as to provide guidelines for a 'psychological autopsy' (see Box 8.4). We hold the view that such a mandatory approach detracts from the flexibility that is always necessary in difficult situations. Formal meetings can all too easily turn ugly and become inappropriate forums for the ventilation of anger, blame and recrimination, directed at people either inside or outside the meeting. If such a debriefing is to be held, it is very important to decide what such a meeting can and cannot achieve before people sit down together. Answers to the questions of how and why the death occurred, let alone the apportionment of blame, should never be on the agenda. Instead, these issues should remain the remit of other institutions: formal inquiry panels and courts. Trusts now conduct internal reviews, and a regular suicide audit, collating findings over time, should be part of good practice and clinical governance. The point of all of this is to improve constantly on how things are done and to learn from every incident.

Box 8.4 Guidelines for a 'psychological autopsy'

1. Identifiers: name, address, age, etc.

2. Suicidal act: time, place and method, who discovered it

3. Psychiatric and medical history, including previous suicide attempts, diagnosis and treatment

4. Family psychiatric history: illnesses and suicides/parasuicides

5. Personality and lifestyle

6. Typical pattern of reactions to stressors

7. Recent stressors or major life events

8. Role of alcohol and drugs, previously and in relation to suicide

9. Interpersonal relationships: sources of support

10. Suicidal ideation: when and how often expressed

11. Deterioration or improvement prior to death: mood, vegetative signs

12. Strengths: reasons to live, plans for the future

13. Assessment of intention

14. Lethality of method

15. Effect on others, e.g. staff, family, other patients

16. Additional information

Modified from Bartels SJ (1987) The aftermath of suicide on the psychiatric inpatient unit. *Gen Hosp Psychiatry* 9, 189–197.

How to handle an inquiry

With the exception of being beaten up by a patient, finding yourself in front of an inquiry panel or a coroner's court is likely to be one of the most unpleasant moments of your career. It is also likely to be one of the most interesting. As a care worker, you are far more likely to have to face an internal inquiry than a coroner, but there are numerous ways to reduce the horror of both. The first is to accept that, no matter what happens, it may well be an unpleasant experience. At least you can console yourself with the fact that it hardly ever gets any worse than this. The second is to remember that, no matter how unpleasant it may seem, you are a witness and not the accused. This distinction may not always seem to be so clear once you find yourself climbing into a box and taking an oath or sitting before a stern-looking panel of strangers while a tape recorder or stenographer listens to your every word. Work hard to keep up this distinction between blaming and informing, as it is the best way to come out of the entire event feeling sane, alive and wiser.

The next thing to do is to make sure that you are prepared well in advance of the hearing. In some ways, preparation for an inquiry should begin before the event has even taken place. Every department has its own serious incident protocol, which clearly spells out who should do what in the event of an untoward incident. It is part of your job to know what this document says and to follow it. Familiarity with local procedure also helps to make the chilling unfamiliarity of the inquiry procedure feel a little less uncomfortable at a time when you may feel that you are being subject to an unpleasant degree of scrutiny for simply having come to work in the morning.

However indignant one may feel about an individual case, and whatever the rights and wrongs of the inquiry process (and, as we have seen, there are quite a few of these), it is important to cooperate with the inquiry. As a front-line care worker, you are not in a strategic position to identify and challenge the shortcomings of the process, no matter how much it may feel like an unfair witch hunt. Fighting at this stage almost always ends up doing more harm than good – if you do feel as though you need to rail against the corrupt iniquities of the system, remember that the one-eyed monster of the inquiry is much bigger than you are. Hold your fire, think long term and use your experience to improve and update matters as required.

The first stage in cooperating with the inquiry process lies in providing it with clear reliable information. This is done in two ways: in writing and by oral submission. Thankfully, your contribution to most inquiries will rarely go beyond the written stage, but it is important to realise that written information is the raw material upon which the giant of the inquiry actually feeds. There are two brands of written inquiry fodder: case notes and formal written reports. If you have paid heed to the discussion on keeping proper written records in Chapter 7, you will find that conjuring the latter out of the former is a simple process. You stick them together in a continuous narrative that clearly describes what you did and said, what the patient did and said, and what happened overall. Therefore, the best way to cope with a serious incident is by keeping case notes that read as though a serious incident is imminent in all of your cases at all times. Of course, in the real world, such a goal is almost impossible to achieve and, even if it was, it would probably cause just as many problems as it solved, but this does illustrate the point that our case notes are not ours alone. They are legal documents which, in the event of an incident, show the public that their public servants have been coming up with the goods.

If you undergo this strange process of public scrutiny, you will inevitably begin to notice a fundamental truth about inquiries that we have already considered. No matter how objective the inquiry process may appear, it is, in fact, a highly irrational process, subject to all sorts of biases, illusions and distortions (see also Chapter 1). Of these, none is quite so powerful as the distorting effect of retrospect. The human brain is hardwired to detect patterns. Once we have found a means of putting information together in a way that makes coherent sense, it is almost impossible to ignore it, even if that 'sense' subsequently turns out to be nonsense. Inquiries have a tendency to create a feeling of sense, and even pattern, when none in fact ever existed. Because none of us ever keep perfect case notes on all of our cases all of the time, sooner or later, when something happens with one of our patients, a less than perfect record of the event will help to muddy the picture of what actually happened. *You* may know that when you noted verbatim the patient's utterance 'I have had enough' he was referring to extra strong lager rather than life but, unless it was recorded as such, it simply didn't happen like that. And, as if these distortions were not enough, one must inevitably handle the inaccuracy of the entire process whilst simultaneously attempting to manage all one's other personal worries and thoughts about the event, not to mention the other 19 patients still on one's caseload and the forthcoming memorial service.

It won't be surprising, therefore, if, in the middle of all this, you find your mind turning to the idea of tampering with the notes. After all, if the entire inquiry is just a farrago of distortion, bias and misinterpretation, why not feed the monster with a few well-chosen extra pieces of non-information that might make the beast look elsewhere for a victim? Under the spotlight of an inquiry, it can feel very tempting to rewrite history. Just take out that leaf of A4 and modify that page of history, in all its different hands and inks, to recast yourself as the prescient, blameless, non-stick Teflon clinical superhero. The response to this urge is simple – *don't* – and there are several good reasons for this.

First, the inquiry has enough of a job on its hands trying to make at least some sense out of an overwhelming amount of information without you muddling the matter. As we saw above, serious incident inquiries, with especially formed external inquiry panels, can all too easily turn into meaningless paper juggernauts that incur enormous personal and financial costs. Second, when you are caught in the headlights of an oncoming inquiry, it is very easy to forget that the event is unpleasantly distorting for pretty much everyone, panel members included. Third, over the weeks of an inquiry, the case notes take on an almost mythical quality. Remote and hitherto unseen files on the patient that you never dreamt existed, for example a school report showing that your patient used to own a hunting knife, may suddenly become viewed as the document 'that could have changed everything if only we had seen it'. When previously mundane case records are subject to this degree of scrutiny, it becomes horribly easy to spot a tampered script, artificially enlightened by *post hoc* wisdom.

Therefore, if you do want to clarify something that you did, to add something to the record, it is far better provided in the form of a written report. If it must be inserted into the case file, make sure that it is clearly timed and dated and that it obeys the rules of report writing. Everyone likes crisp, typed summaries much more than page after page of scrawled notes, so the mere presence of such a beacon of clarity will advance your cause significantly.

How to write a report for an inquiry

The basic and most important rule when writing a report for an inquiry is simple: stick to the facts. Very often, people end up going far beyond this uncomplicated remit and instead provide reams of adjective-laden analysis and explanation that can all too easily read like a traumatised confession. Instead, don't complain and don't explain. If the inquiry wants explanations, it will seek the clarification that you may regard as essential. In fact, the panel probably won't be all that interested in focusing upon your personal contribution to the greater scheme of things. They are far more likely to direct this sort of attention to your manager than to you, therefore, let him or her do the work.

Apart from trying to make your report as objective as possible, the other rule is to keep the language as clear as possible. Adjectives and adverbs should be kept to an absolute minimum. Stick to short, sharp sentences that calmly say what was done, by whom and when, rather than saying how it happened and why. It is easier to stick to this if you follow a familiar format. Use plenty of headings and lay the document out in the same way that you might when writing up an assessment or a detailed referral. Before you submit your document to its intended destination, which should be spelt out in your local protocol, sleep on it for a few days and revise it for clarity, conciseness and lack of emotionality before you post it. If you can, show it to someone who you feel understands your situation and get their opinion on the revision before the final dispatch. This time, the law of the letter is the other way around. If it hasn't got your name and signature on it, you haven't said it.

Another paper-based practice that some people find useful during inquiries is to keep a diary. This can prove particularly helpful if the event is in some way unusual, as homicides always are. If you find your incident turning into a political football, as can easily happen in these cash-strapped cynical times, a private record of who said what can come in very handy when dealing with outside authorities, such as the local health authority, police or even the press. But remember, don't talk to the press, even 'off the record'. There is no such thing when it comes to ordinary folk like you – news hounds just want a nice, meaty story that will sell papers and they want it now, hot and fresh. Therefore, if you demur, don't ring back and say 'no comment' enough times they will soon go elsewhere for titbits. Your health trust will have a media policy and a communications manager to go with it whose prime task is to deal with this. They will be putting out statements, possibly setting up a news conference and getting the chief executive or communications director to make the right noises and take the lead in trying to control the story. Refer any media approach to this person and keep out of the headlights. You might fancy being seen on the 10 o'clock news but people can be made to look awfully foolish and the interest soon fades, leaving you looking very naive.

Giving oral evidence to an inquiry

Giving oral evidence to an inquiry will not happen very often in one's career. The rules here are broadly similar to those governing written evidence: keep to the facts and don't scare yourself into thinking that you are the accused going before a court. It is meant to be an informal process and you are attending voluntarily. You can refuse to go if you want, and some people do, but we would not advise this in general. After all, the point is to clarify the facts, with you as an expert, helpful witness. Bring along a friend and any notes that you need, turn up on time, look smart and friendly and try to be cooperative. However, beware of answering 'When did you stop beating your wife?' types of question. If you find the line of questioning moving towards the realms of guilt and blame, say so and make sure that what you say is recorded.

An incident inquiry panel has no legal authority to apportion blame or reach any meaningful conclusions about liability. That is what courts are for. In an inquiry, you are not allowed to cross-examine, submit your own evidence, answer a question with a question or enjoy the rights to representation that you would automatically expect in a court. However, you are entitled to courtesy, respect for your professional experience and opinion, an acknowledgement of the stress associated with your involvement, and a full record of what was asked and what answers you gave. Likewise, the chairperson of the inquiry panel should always explain to you their terms of reference (i.e. the purposes of the inquiry), showing you a written copy if you prefer, should introduce you to the panel members, and should make you welcome as a participant rather than as an interviewee. If you need a break for a drink, a cigarette or to go to the toilet, do say so. No one will mind, and others might well need the same. Note any problems or concerns and remember that, before finishing, the chairperson will always ask you if there is anything that you want to ask or if there is any other comment that you want to make. Don't feel that you have to say anything but, if something is bothering you, now is the time to speak. A long whinge or a prepared speech full of obsessional details won't go down well, but an apposite comment or inquiry can nicely make your point. In our view, this is why it is almost always best to attend an inquiry.

However unfair it may seem, the person who doesn't show up is by inference seen as being stroppy, lazy or even guilty. There may be a right to silence in British courts – which is increasingly being eroded with inferences being allowed to be drawn from so doing – but if you don't give your version of what happened, you create a vacuum into which all sorts of negative notions may creep. Put bluntly, you can easily become the one who gets dumped on.

Inquiries usually use methods of deliberation and set thresholds for reaching conclusions and recommendations that are usually far lower in intellectual quality than those that might be reached by an average judge. If the event is not a court, don't turn it into one. Taking along a lawyer rather than an intelligent, supportive colleague might help you feel better in some ways but it will feed into a creeping sense of legalism in the longer term. By all means take the legal advice of a respected professional defence organisation at any point during the process but, in our opinion, it is usually wiser to keep this separate from the inquiry as far as you possibly can. Discuss the case with other colleagues who will also be attending. Be quite frank about this and do give your views on what might have helped (if anything) achieve a better outcome. This is not just an investigation; think of it as an opportunity to make some improvements in terms of resources or arrangements.

Appearing in court

It is possible that you may have to appear in court during a trial for homicide or some other offence committed by one of your patients. A suicide may mean you having to attend a coroner's court. Whichever of these it is, the likelihood is that you will be there as a non-controversial witness of facts, for example to describe your level and range of contact with an accused or your knowledge of their illness or treatment. Nevertheless, it can be daunting. Remember that your duty is to the court: you are there as a professional witness to assist the judge and jury in sorting out the facts of the case. As with an inquiry, bring any notes/records that you need – if you wish to consult them, this is perfectly all right – dress quite formally and soberly (weird ties or scruffy jeans undermine you at once) and keep your answers simple, factual and to the point.

When you enter the witness box you will be asked to swear an oath, either on the Bible or another religious text or just as a general 'affirmation'. Both forms are equally binding in law, and you may choose what fits with your beliefs (the affirmation is for agnostics/atheists). These formalities reinforce the rule that you must tell 'the truth, the whole truth, and nothing but the truth'. You will then be addressed by 'your' barrister (i.e. from the side, defence or prosecution, that has called you as a witness) and asked to give your name and professional details. You may also be asked about your experience so have a couple of lines prepared, for example: 'I have worked as a community psychiatric nurse for 8 years in an inner-city mental health team and have been qualified for over 15 years. I have special experience in caring for those with severe mental illnesses, such as schizophrenia, a caseload of about 20 patients whom I see regularly and I also work on the crisis/duty roster as required.' You may be asked additional details that are relevant to the case in hand, for example 'How long have you known Mr B?', which should be easy to answer from your routine clinical work.

Be careful of jargon as the jury may become confused and the judge annoyed. If you use shorthand terms, for example 'a CPA meeting', explain what actually happened: 'As part of the regular care programme approach, we met every 2–3 months to assess how Mr B was doing, what further help he needed and to keep everyone up to date with things.' Only explain things that you know about and if a question is outside your experience be prepared to say so. Don't respond to snide remarks from barristers – if in doubt, stay silent – and only speak when asked questions. You can also ask for a question to be rephrased if you don't understand it, and remember that your barrister will quickly leap in if he or she feels that you are being unfairly questioned or harassed by the other side.

If you are feeling bullied, you do not need to hide your feelings – the jury may well sympathise with you and see you as one of them (i.e. not a bewigged member of an elite profession). They will respond positively to you if you use plain English and show honest emotions. Think before you speak, showing that you are trying to get things right and to be as helpful as possible. Never try to engage in point scoring with the barrister; lawyers are trained for this and will easily outwit you and get the last word. Finally, remember to address the judge as 'your Honour' and be prepared to answer questions from him or her (it's usually a him) as well. Don't be put off by this – he'll probably want to clarify some aspect of your evidence, much of which he will have taken notes on.

Conclusions

We have gone into considerable detail in this chapter to try to get under the skin of what is meant by risk assessment. We have concentrated very much on our personal experiences of difficult situations, whether of at-risk patients, stressful inquisitions or the feelings engendered by both. Some may feel that we are a touch cynical, others that we have been patronising or overdetailed in our advice. Much of it is plain common sense, but we hope that it reflects our combined experience of 50 years of working in psychiatry and that a number of technical, practical and psychological issues have been dealt with.

These situations are part and parcel of modern community mental health work and being able to deal with them, and even enjoy them because you are confident that you are good at your job, is one of the most rewarding aspects of the profession. You and your team will be enhanced by your ability to cope with them. However, if dealing with risky crises leaves you drained and feeling bad, you should think seriously about a career move. You won't be letting anyone down because you must enjoy your work if you are going to be an effective care worker. There is plenty of work to be done elsewhere in mental health that might suit your temperament better. Either way, think of crises as a way of gaining wisdom – of finding out about yourself, knowing what you can do and knowing what not to do.

The rules of the game
(Or the Mental Health Act and all that)

9

Introduction

Hearts pump, kidneys filter and lungs breathe but the brain is the only organ in the body that can vote, choose or argue. Because of this, there is a considerable overlap between mental health work and philosophy, politics and the law. Among the peculiarities of working in the mental health field, therefore, is a need to understand the law relevant to issues of mental health. Many Acts of Parliament touch upon mental health, for example the new Incapacity Act, the Police and Criminal Evidence Act and the National Assistance Act; however, the most important Act in this field is the 1983 Mental Health Act (MHA), supplemented by the 1995 Patients in the Community Act. These two statutes outline the definitions and procedures that concern 'the reception, care and treatment of mentally disordered patients, the management of their property and other related matters'. In other words, they legally enshrine the process of 'being sectioned'.

As legal documents go they are reasonably accessible and there should be one of each to hand in any well-equipped community mental health team office. It is not necessary to know them word for word but you should be familiar with them. When you are involved in dealing with patients who, because they often cannot think clearly, may be unable to recognise what's real and what's not real, there has to be an agreed and recognised means of ensuring their health and safety and the safety of other people. Most other branches of medicine act under what is called 'common law', although the importance of obtaining 'informed consent' for an operation or the need to define capacity relating to all sorts of issues are very much legally driven and increasingly so in today's litigious world.

The essence of the MHA is very simple. If someone is considered to have a mental disorder 'of a nature or degree' (i.e. serious enough) that it may put themself or others at risk, they can be taken to hospital against their will. Many, of course, will voluntarily seek help and accept treatment. However, some don't see themselves as being ill – usually because lack of insight is part and parcel of the illness process – and so have to be 'compulsorily detained'. To achieve this, the patient is examined by a doctor (or two doctors) who will write out his or her recommendations on a standard form, stating the reasons for detention. Then, an approved social worker (ASW; see below) or nearest relative (also see below) signs another standard form making an application for admission to hospital. Once all the forms are signed, the patient can be taken to hospital and kept there until their illness risks have resolved. If necessary, force can be used (i.e. the police) although, in practice, many patients, once told they have to, come grudgingly and without needing to be restrained. The details of the commonly used sections of the MHA are outlined in Table 9.1.

Table 9.1 ● Commonly used Mental Health Act sections

Section	Potential length	Name	Signatories
2	4 weeks	Assessment and treatment	Two doctors (one approved) + ASW or NR
3	6 months	Treatment	Two doctors (one approved) + ASW or NR
4	72 hours	Emergency treatment	One doctor + ASW or NR
5(2)	72 hours	Inpatient treatment	One doctor
5(4)	6 hours	Nursing detention	One RMN
136	72 hours	Police detention	Police officer
37	6 months	Hospital order	Two approved doctors + court
41	No limit	Restriction order	Two approved doctors + Crown Court

ASW, approved social worker; NR, nearest relative; RMN, registered mental nurse.

Like most legal documents, the British MHA is not an easy read. Because the law has to establish black and white definitions of the culpability of people's actions, it has to rely on test cases that are constantly being argued in the courts to refine its basic principles. Interpretation of this accumulated 'case law' is a demanding intellectual discipline. However, because all of the possible circumstances that one might meet in mental health and illness cannot be dealt with in detail, the Secretary of State (for Health), under Section 118 of the MHA, has been empowered to prepare and produce a *Code of Practice*, which should also be available in every community mental health team office. The most recent *Code of Practice* was published in 1993 (HMSO, London) and is designed to fill in the often significant gaps between the principles of the MHA and what actually happens to you and your patients in the field. For example, the MHA does not attempt a precise definition of mental illness. It uses terms such as 'mental disorder' or 'severe mental impairment', the former meaning 'mental illness, arrested or incomplete development of mind, psychopathic disorder and any other disorder or disability of mind'. Cut away the jargon and this is very non-specific, echoing that Shakespearean joke, 'to define true madness, what is it but to be nothing else but mad?'

In a sense, every MHA is a heroic yet flawed document that is always a little out of date. Consider, by analogy, the rules of football, for example. People argue all the time, referees are abused and interpretations are seen as 'harsh' or 'lenient'. If the ball hits a defender's hand in the penalty area, should that be a penalty kick? The referee has to decide whether the action was 'intentional' without the benefit of telepathy, detailed interviews, witness statements or video evidence. Likewise, there will always be times when it may be hard to decide whether someone has a mental illness, whether they could form 'an intent', what the risks are and whom to believe. But remember, almost every country in the world has an MHA or a version thereof. Deciding how to help those who cannot help themselves is part and parcel of living in a civilised society. Some countries merely empower the police, and many use the courts or magistrates much more regularly than we do in the UK. But, wherever you go, there are agreed and special procedures to protect those who are deemed to be mentally ill.

A bit of history

Entire libraries have been written about the relationship between crime and mental illness. Certain famous cases have profoundly affected public attitudes. These include the cases of James Hadfield, who shot at George III in Drury Lane Theatre on 15 May 1800, and Daniel McNaughton, who shot the then Prime Minister's Secretary, Drummond, on 20 January 1843. Being obviously deranged both were jailed (rather than hanged), and they elicited public sympathy and various legal changes as a result of their actions. By and large, in the UK, the principle of habeas corpus ('you may have the body') has also meant that depriving a citizen of their liberty requires an order from the local judiciary (magistrate's court, Crown Court, etc.). Until 1959, families had to apply to the magistrate's court for a certificate (hence the notion of 'certifying' someone) to have a mentally ill person taken into care against their will. This still pertains in many countries and some argue that we should return to such a system. After all, considerable stigma is attached to psychiatrists and approved social workers because of their powers to haul people off to hospital. Perhaps mental health professionals should be involved only in giving advice and treatment rather than in the messy, time-consuming and occasionally risky business of going out and detaining people.

Compared with many statutes, mental health law is relatively recent. If one looks at the various acts that have accrued over the last 400 years, until the early 19th century, only the Poor Law of 1601 and the Vagrancy Act of 1744 could be used to confine people in hospital. Of course, this didn't stop 'lunatics' being locked in the attic, chained in the cellar, quietly disposed of or driven out of towns and villages. No one wanted the cost or bother of having to deal with such troublesome folk. Wandering vagrants were accepted as part of the landscape. Criminal behaviour led to fairly arbitrary arrests and punishments (until the Criminal Lunatics Act – passed in 1800 – mental illness was no defence), and 'mad doctors' were deeply distrusted. Not a lot has changed.

During the 19th century there was a constant legal debate over whether the responsibility for criminal behaviour could be attributed to mental disease, exemplified by the Hadfield and McNaughton cases. The 1812 murder of the Prime Minister, Spencer Perceval, by his deranged Secretary, and seven attempts on the life of Queen Victoria, mainly by individuals who were obviously mentally unwell, created a climate in which the 'insanity defence' became quite controversial. A critical step was the decision to base any judgements on the 'McNaughton' rules whereby if the perpetrator did not know 'the nature and quality of the act' being committed because of a 'defect of reason, from disease of the mind' or, if he did know it, 'that he did not know what he was doing was wrong', then he could be excused on the grounds of insanity. Until the abolition of capital punishment in 1965, this defence became central to many murder trials. The responsibilities and definitions that were generated regarding mental illness also became embedded in the various acts that were passed, and have strongly influenced current practice.

As has already been noted, the major mental health acts in the UK were passed in 1890 (Lunacy Act), 1930 (Mental Treatment Act), 1959 (Mental Health Act) and 1983 (Mental Health Act). This pattern of decreasing intervals between fresh legislation predicts a new act sometime in the first decade of the 21st century. It is a moot point whether this will be more or less restrictive, depending on the climate of opinion at the time (see below). What has been established, however, is that someone suffering from a mental illness, however defined, who is *also* at risk to their own or other people's health or safety because of that mental illness can have their civil liberties taken away. To put it another way, all those who suffer from a severe, incapacitating mental illness *should have the right* to be treated against their wishes. It is as if one is viewing a patient with a mental illness in the same light as a patient who is unconscious and in urgent need of an operation. This right to treatment also embodies the humane acceptance that behaviour deemed to be immoral and antisocial may be due to an illness rather than simply being 'bad'. Such an approach is surely an advance on the medieval beliefs in the supernatural or witchcraft whereby 'mad folk' were often blamed for their behaviour, with their madness being regarded as a punishment visited on them by divine intervention. Part of the stigma of mental illness that still persists today reflects just these kinds of attitudes.

The nature of the current MHA

The 1983 MHA consists of 149 paragraphs, or sections as they are usually called, which are divided into 10 separate 'parts' covering all areas of practice under the MHA. The parts that apply most to regular community work are Part II (compulsory admission to hospital or guardianship) and Part III (patients concerned in criminal proceedings or under sentence). Part IV deals with consent to treatment, Part V with mental health review tribunals, Part VI with the removal and return of patients from and to the UK etc., and Parts VII–X with various practical aspects, such as the 'management of property' and the 'miscellaneous functions' of local authorities and the Secretary of State. The MHA also contains a special section (Section 141) that is entirely devoted to the process of dealing with a Member of Parliament who might be suffering from mental illness. As far as we know this section has never been used, but we should all be ready and waiting!

Throughout the MHA there is a tacit assumption that mental illness is a disability requiring special assistance. Those suffering from mental illness are deemed to have a form of diminished responsibility, and the whole purpose of the MHA is to protect them and the public from the consequences of their illnesses. It is not surprising, therefore, that the MHA has its critics, especially those concerned with notions of social control, and that there is a considerable potential for abuse when dealing with those considered to be social deviants. The notorious use of suspect mental illness categories (i.e. 'sluggish' or 'latent' schizophrenia) to put away political dissidents in communist Russia has heightened awareness of just what can happen to human rights if they are not carefully protected. Built in to the MHA, therefore, are a series of safety nets, including the requirement for specialist training and approval for those signing the forms, the right to a tribunal as well as a managers' hearing, and the right to a second opinion in matters of consent to treatment. There are also certain key personnel in the MHA, whose roles and responsibilities are carefully defined.

Key personnel in the Mental Health Act

The patient

This is the term that is used in the MHA and this is the person whose interests, illness and treatment must never be forgotten. In the subtitles to the 149 sections of the MHA, the words 'patient' or 'patients' are used 36 times. By contrast, the word 'persons', usually in the form of 'mentally disordered persons', is used 10 times, whereas 'prisoners' and 'nearest relative' are used four times each. This emphasizes the point that the MHA is about helping people who are suffering and that this suffering requires treatment of a medical nature. It also recognises implicitly, and by the fact that most of the sections are to do with the practical aspects of care and where people should be looked after, that the social and environmental situation of patients is just as important as anything to do with treatment. Although the term 'patient' is not defined, the MHA is meant to apply to anyone who is suffering from a 'mental disorder'; apart from 'mental illness' (which is not further defined) this includes 'severe mental impairment', 'mental impairment' and 'psychopathic disorder', all of which are defined! However, people who are suffering 'by reason only of promiscuity or other immoral conduct, sexual deviancy or dependence on alcohol or drugs' are very carefully *excluded*. Getting involved in the compulsory treatment of those who retain control over what they are doing (sex- and drug-wise) is like taking a picnic in a minefield. You can't put someone away because they keep getting drunk. Of course, explaining the consequences to the patient may be rather tricky.

As can be seen from some of these terms, the MHA appears to be somewhat out of date in terms of its language. This is enhanced by the constant use of the male pronoun ('he' or 'him'), making it seem (to those who are more gender conscious today) as if there is no provision in the MHA for the detention of women. However, because the forms that are used to write out section orders do include the phrase 'him/her', it is probably unlikely that a legal challenge to the MHA on gender grounds would be successful. Despite this rather stiff language, however, most of the MHA is reasonably clear and not difficult to follow. It is also comforting to know that carrying out one's proper duties under the terms of the MHA renders you *not* liable to prosecution yourself.

Because no other diagnoses are mentioned, anyone with a mental illness can be considered 'liable to be detained' under the MHA. Again, this notion of mental (as opposed to physical) illness is a little out of date, because the psychoses such as schizophrenia or manic depressive disorder are seen by most psychiatrists today as being largely due to brain malfunction. Even the neuroses, such as obsessional compulsive disorder, panic syndrome and the anxieties and depressions, are often treated by medication as well as psychotherapy, indicating an acceptance that they too involve a physical disorder. Putting aside these vexed questions, it is clear that patients can be detained for the problems of learning disability ('mental impairment') and personality disorder ('psychopathic disorder'). By contrast, people who expose themselves or have sex with sheep, as well as those who are drug addicts and alcoholics (most frustratingly for many relatives), are excluded. Of course, if a drug addict or alcoholic *also* has a mental disorder, for example severe depression, the fact that they are dependent on drugs or alcohol does not exclude them from getting treatment. Likewise, if someone has a physical illness (e.g. a brain tumour)

247

that causes them to have what are termed mental symptoms, such as hallucinations, they can be detained for the treatment of their mental symptoms but not (oddly enough) to have their tumour removed (see below).

Families

Families, or rather 'nearest relatives', have a central role to play in the practice of the MHA. The nearest relative can not only sign an application order to have a family member detained but can also refuse to agree to a Section 3 (treatment order) and discharge a relative under certain circumstances. Sections 26–30 of the MHA outline the 'functions of relatives of patients' and are quite revealing. For example, in case of arguments, there is a kind of batting order as to who is deemed to be the nearest relative, starting with the partner (husband or wife) and moving on to any children, parents, siblings, grandparents, grandchildren, uncles or aunts and nephews or nieces. It is important to note that 'relatives of the whole blood' are preferred to 'relatives of the half blood' (i.e. full sisters take precedence over half-sisters) and that the elder of two equal relatives takes precedence. However, if the patient *lives* with a particular relative, that relative wins out over anyone else. Likewise, there are certain exclusions if, for example, the patient and their spouse are separated or the spouse has deserted the patient or the nearest relative is under 18.

Without going into all the details (and working out just who is the nearest relative may be quite interesting in itself) it is clear that the MHA sees the family as having a considerable influence, as well as rights, with regard to a patient's mental health. It goes without saying, therefore, that the family should always be consulted when the MHA is being used and that they need to be aware of their rights. A particular problem can arise when the nearest relative is unwell or even shares the delusion of the patient that you wish to detain. Such problems can usually be circumvented but you need to know the MHA. The nearest relative can actually be displaced (Section 29) but this has to be done through the court and a delay is always thereby incurred. It is especially important to clarify what is called the 'availability' of the nearest relative and to assess how practicable it would be to consult him or her given the urgency of the situation.

In our experience most families are very happy to cooperate with something that they see as being in their relative's best interests. In fact, families will often complain that patients are not taken in early enough, particularly when someone is good at covering up or masking their symptoms. Thus, the family member who has overheard the shouting at night or endured the hostile remarks of a demanding, psychotic relative may give an entirely different story from the patient. Listening carefully to the family's perceptions and needs is good practice, an integral part of the MHA and in the spirit of the MHA.

The approved social worker

In terms of the MHA, the ASW is the equivalent of the nearest relative when it comes to *applying* to have someone detained for treatment. In fact, ASWs only came into official being in the 1983 MHA. They are social workers who 'have to be specially designated and trained in the care of mental disorder', and their particular duties in applying for admission are outlined in Section 13 of the MHA. They can also apply for guardianship orders and can 'displace' a nearest relative (see above) if that person is 'incapable' because of mental disorder or other illness or is unreasonably objecting. Of course, they cannot make an application to have a patient detained for treatment until they have received the medical recommendations, and so they are always required to take the medical evidence into account alongside their own assessment of the patient and the patient's situation. There have been some interesting arguments between doctors and social workers regarding 'diagnosis' – for example should an experienced social worker accept the diagnosis of a doctor if it doesn't seem right – but social workers' training should equip them to make reasonable judgements. In many countries there is no such position as an ASW, with the relative, the police or magistrates – for better or worse – taking on the role instead.

The crucial role of the ASW is defined under Section 145(1) of the MHA, which states that an ASW is 'an officer of a local social services authority appointed to act as an Approved Social Worker for the purposes of this Act'. In addition, Section 114 states that local social service authorities should appoint 'a sufficient number of Approved Social Workers for the purposes of discharging the functions conferred on them by this Act'. However, although one can't be appointed as an ASW unless 'approved by the authority as having appropriate competence in dealing with persons who are suffering from mental disorder', there is no indication of how one is meant to obtain this appropriate competence. If in doubt it appears that one has to consult the Secretary of State, as the MHA goes on to say that the approval process should 'have regard to such matters as the Secretary of State may direct'. Oddly enough, ASWs (Section 115) can actually 'enter and inspect any premises' in which 'a mentally disordered patient is living'; they have to produce a 'duly authenticated document' and have a reasonable cause to believe 'that the patient is not under proper care'. Usually, ASWs seek a Section 135 (court order) to enter a person's house and one wonders why Section 115 is not more widely used. Perhaps the inability of anyone else to enter with them makes this a rather risky procedure.

In terms of the individual professional responsibility of an ASW, the *Code of Practice* gives further details in Chapters 2.10–2.17. The ASW is seen as having overall responsibility for 'coordinating the process of assessment' and for 'implementing that decision'. In other words, the ASW does all the dirty work: contacting people, ensuring that the timing is right, sorting out the signatures, checking out the family and getting the patient into hospital. Apart from identifying yourself (if you are the ASW), you should interview the patient in a 'suitable manner' and alone if that seems safe, consult with other professionals (as well as the family; see above) and explain to everyone what is going to happen or whether an admission has been arranged. Such procedures can be a major hassle or can be very simple.

A good training programme should be undertaken, usually lasting 8–12 weeks; this will mean accompanying experienced ASWs on a number of MHA assessments in the community. The programme should include practical training on the meaning of the MHA (often not a particularly exciting form of education but vital) and provide continuing updates as the law progresses. Remember, there are always new case law decisions coming down from the courts and it makes sense to regularly audit your use of the MHA. The ASW who always seems to be making Section 4 applications (emergency orders) may be seen to be 'too quick on the draw'. Yet, refusing to make an application (when everyone else wants one) needs to be carefully thought through. Keeping well-written, clear and dated notes (and ASW decisions must be formally documented), discussing any situation that arises with all relevant people and knowing the MHA are the keys to good practice.

The doctors

Oddly enough there are no doctors in the MHA; instead, they are termed 'medical practitioners' or even 'consultants'. They are responsible [and the term 'responsible medical officer' (RMO) is particularly used when it comes to the granting of leave] for deciding if someone is suffering from a mental disorder. This means, of course, examining the patient, obtaining information about the patient's history and background (from the relatives, old notes, the GP), and trying to make a diagnosis. However, an exact diagnosis is *not* necessary for a recommendation to be made. The MHA has intentionally been framed to provide a broad remit for the term 'mental illness'; however, it does ask the doctor to describe the symptoms that the patient has (on the official forms used for writing out section orders). It is also important to understand that doctors can only *recommend*, and not apply for, admission for treatment. Many doctors talk about 'sectioning' patients but it is the patient's nearest relative or the ASW who actually signs the part of the order that results in a patient being detained.

One of the medical practitioners who assesses a patient has to be 'approved' by the Secretary of State as having 'special experience in the diagnosis and treatment of mental disorder'. Such doctors will, by definition, be experienced psychiatrists, and a list of approved doctors is kept for each region. They have to apply every 5 years for re-approval, but there is no formal training course or exam (as yet) under the MHA. However, some training forms part of the membership exam of the Royal College of Psychiatrists, and more and more departments are adding on specific MHA training courses, for old and young alike. Nowadays, approval is unlikely to be given unless the doctor has attended a recent (in the last 3–5 years) approved MHA training course.

Although any registered practitioner (i.e. doctor) can sign an emergency order, which lasts for only 72 hours (under Section 4; see Table 9.1), the rest of the orders usually require two doctors to sign. This is a kind of safety measure, deriving from concerns that doctors might detain people unnecessarily or for their own nefarious reasons. Ideally, an order should be signed by someone who is approved, i.e. a specialist psychiatrist, and the patient's GP, i.e. someone who has a 'previous acquaintance with the patient'. If you can't get hold of the GP, the second doctor should also be approved, if possible. However, two doctors from the same hospital are not meant to sign an order, again because of concerns about collusion. If a patient is going to be admitted to a private hospital, a doctor on the staff of that hospital *cannot* sign an order. Similarly, if a doctor is likely to get any specific fee for looking after a patient (again in private practice), that doctor is not allowed to put that patient under a MHA order. There is also a general duty for the doctor who is actually treating a patient to be consulted.

Overall, the role of the medical practitioner under the terms of the MHA is to act as a specialist giving professional advice. It should not be forgotten that doctors only 'recommend' and, therefore, they have to be part of a multidisciplinary team to work under the terms of the MHA. There is no doubt, however, that some doctors mistakenly seem to think that their decisions should be accepted without demur or discussion; this may not be altogether surprising because, as they are often the 'responsible' individual, they are liable to be panned if things go wrong. The best community mental health teams make sure that everyone understands their role under the MHA, that all team members work as equals and that all specialist skills are respected.

Other people in the MHA

Because the MHA deals with those who have been sentenced by the courts, it follows that prisoners, judges and members of tribunals all pass through its pages.

Also included in the MHA are the Lord Chancellor's visitors and, if a member of the House of Commons is involved, the Speaker of the House (Section 141). For practical purposes, it is the hospital managers and members of tribunals that are most important in understanding the MHA. The former are actually defined under Section 145 but this is merely to point out what it is that they manage in terms of the phrase 'in relation to'. Oddly enough, these managers are not the same NHS managers that run trusts and health authorities. According to the *Code of Practice*, the health authority has to appoint a committee or subcommittee to 'undertake the duties of the managers'. This is supposed to be made up of informed members of the health authority and/or informed persons from outside. This loose definition has created considerable problems, and although most trusts carefully vet people taken on as managers, give them training and support, and try to ensure that they are sensible and informed people, their role is really quite anomalous in the modern NHS. The managers are meant to check that all of the admissions procedures are valid, check any documents and ensure that information is given to detained patients and their nearest relatives (Sections 132 and 133). In particular, they are meant to ensure that a patient's detention is regularly reviewed as required and they have the power to discharge certain patients. In other words, a patient can attend a manager's hearing and be discharged, and the multidisciplinary team has no means of blocking this apart from signing another section.

Perhaps more important are the people who work on mental health review tribunals, whose role is outlined in Part V of the MHA, Sections 65–79. In essence, tribunals are the watchdog of the system. Any patient can appeal to a mental health review tribunal, although there are certain limits on how often they can do so. Tribunals presently consist of three people, namely a lawyer, an experienced consultant psychiatrist and a layperson, usually someone who has some interest in mental health and who is aware of the issues involved. They are able to discharge a patient if they feel either that the patient is no longer suffering from a mental illness (or whatever) or that the illness that the patient is suffering from isn't severe enough ('of a nature or degree') to require continued treatment in hospital. Tribunals act as a civil rights safeguard for all patients and a patient can be represented by a lawyer; however, apart from having the power to discharge patients, directly or on a deferred date, tribunals have no other powers whatsoever. Thus, they cannot change the terms of treatment or advise on continued management. Their proceedings tend to be rather formal, although they strive for informality, and presenting a case to a tribunal requires considerable clarity of thinking (as well as knowledge of the MHA). In this sense they are very good for everyone, because they make one think afresh about why a patient is being detained.

Principles of the Mental Health Act

In Table 9.1 we have summarised the main sections of the MHA that community mental health workers are liable to be involved with. There are, of course, a number of other sections to do with court orders, in particular Section 37 (whereby the court, upon the recommendation of two doctors, orders treatment for a patient, the court taking over the role of the ASW). A Crown Court can also impose a Section 41 restriction order alongside a Section 37; this can impose any condition on a patient and requires the specific remit of the Home Secretary to change any aspect of it. However, most patients will be under the routine sections, namely Section 2 (assessment and treatment), Section 3 (treatment) and Section 4 (emergency treatment).

Section 136 empowers a police officer who comes across someone who is 'mentally disordered in a public place' to take that person to a place of safety for assessment by a doctor and an ASW. This order can last for up to 72 hours. Although controversial, research shows that Section 136 has been used very effectively by the police in that they are able to correctly identify mental illness and it circumvents the tedious business of going to court, prison and so forth. The legal/custodial process is slow and counter-therapeutic, can take months before the patient actually gets to hospital for treatment and is wastefully expensive. Prisoners cannot, by definition, be treated against their will under the MHA when in custody.

The basic theme of the MHA (as already stressed) is that some people need help even though they don't think that they do. On the other hand, as any reading of history tells us, giving one person power over another is known to be extremely dangerous. Thus, the law demands, if possible, at least three official signatures on any documents and insists that those signing such documents are trained, have experience in the nature of psychiatry and/or know the patient very well. There is also a general principle that the shorter the period of detention, the better, and that the mentally ill are extremely ripe for exploitation. Thus, there is an instant appeal system (i.e. for anyone detained for longer than 72 hours) and it is the duty of the managers to ensure that all patients have their rights read to them and that detailed written outlines of the detention rules are given to them.

The process of being 'sectioned' is also a very intrusive event for the patient. Being sectioned under the MHA involves a loss of rights, a loss of freedom and being taken away from your home. If patients reach the stage of a Section 3 (treatment order) they cannot marry, vote, leave the UK, apply for a passport or driving licence or write a will. In other words, it's a fairly serious impairment in terms of doing important things. The only parallel form of deprivation (excluding of course being charged and detained because of a criminal act) resides in one aspect of the National Assistance Act, whereby it is possible for someone to be removed from their home because they are a risk to public health. In other words, the MHA is one of the most powerful statutes on the books in terms of personal liberty. A patient can, of course, be given leave under the MHA (Section 17), usually with conditions attached (i.e. to take any medication); this allows the patient out of hospital although still 'liable to be detained'. It is up to the RMO to decide how and when this occurs.

The MHA also includes the notion of guardianship, whereby it is assumed that a patient can no longer look after his or her own affairs. This again is humane, but being a guardian to someone who is resistant to help and without insight is rather different from helping someone who is dementing or mentally impaired. In the former case, it has a very limited impact, whereas in the latter case, it can ensure that people live a decent life, as these individuals want help rather than resist help. Nevertheless, the role of guardianship has been subjected to both doubt and criticism, with some people feeling that it is not used enough and others suggesting that it is rather a limited power for dealing with the mentally ill. (The same concerns apply to the supervised discharge order of the 1995 Patients in the Community Act; see below.)

Another key feature of the MHA is that there is a duty to provide aftercare (Section 117), an order that is, in a sense, the father of the current Care Programme Approach (CPA) arrangements. Under this section, it is the duty of the health authority and the local social services to provide 'in cooperation with relevant voluntary agencies, aftercare services for any persons to whom this Section applies'. It does not, of course, define 'aftercare', but the *Code of Practice* suggests that the purpose of aftercare is to enable a patient to return to their 'home or accommodation other than a hospital or nursing home'. It requires proper record keeping, a care plan, the involvement of the multidisciplinary team (including the RMO, a hospital nurse, a social worker, the GP, a community psychiatric nurse and so forth) and that account should be taken of the patient's own wishes/needs as well as the views of relevant relatives. It also stresses the importance of identifying any 'unmet need', which may lead to considerable controversy because identifying unmet need is not the same thing as being able to deal with such a need. Nevertheless, this type of aftercare planning is largely sensible because it focuses the community team on what they need to do to try and keep patients stable after leaving hospital, prioritises the more severely unwell (that's why they get sectioned) and forces the hand of reluctant local authorities to stump up the housing/social support required.

Supervised discharge orders (Section 25)

A recent addition to the range of powers available under the MHA has been the supervised discharge order as part of the Patients in the Community Act 1995. This order makes it possible for the RMO to insist that a sectioned (Section 3) patient lives in a particular place on discharge, to insist on visiting the patient at that home or hostel and to be able to 'convey' the patient from place to place. Oddly enough, it does not give the RMO any powers to treat patients. Quite how one is supposed to break into someone's house, toss them in the back of a car or van, drive them to an outpatient department and then somehow think that they will accept treatment is difficult to imagine. However, this is now the law and it has been used since its introduction, although to a very limited extent (the exact numbers are not known). Many people feel that it has less to do with therapy and more to do with giving powers that seem to be more relevant to the police and social control. On the other hand, if a patient is on a supervised discharge order and this discharge is not supervised (i.e. an untoward incident occurs), clearly blame will fall very heavily on the supervising team and/or consultant. It seems to have been introduced as a panic measure to provide a sop to public (and political) concerns, despite considerable opposition from professional and patient groups. The fact that it got passed into law shows how ignorant our political masters often are about how community care works.

Problems of the 1983 Mental Health Act

In general, the MHA provides a reasonable framework for trying to insist that people who need treatment get treatment but that people who are just socially deviant don't get bullied into unnecessary limitations on their lifestyle. The difficulty is that it is becoming increasingly out of date. This is because of the changing nature of treatment, societal attitudes and the law (e.g. human rights legislation). Specific problems include the following, some of which are being addressed in current proposals for a new MHA (see below):

1. The MHA gives no consideration to the idea of compulsory treatment in the community. It assumes that 'treatment in hospital' must be a natural concomitant of any kind of compulsory treatment. Therefore, no account is taken of modern drug treatments, such as depot injections, or of the importance of such medication in maintaining stability in psychotic patients. You have to deprive someone

of their social liberty, in other words incarcerate them, in order to treat them. You cannot simply treat them at home under some form of community treatment order, which might be much nicer for everyone if given the choice.

2. The important legal case of *Hallstrom* v. *Regina* (1985) put an end to the custom of bringing patients (e.g. on leave from a Section 3) back into hospital the day before a Section 3 expired, signing another order and then sending them back out. This was merely a practical way of getting around the fact that you wanted to keep someone under permanent treatment, although on leave from hospital, because you knew quite well that as soon as they were discharged they would stop taking their treatment. In Scotland (which has a separate legal system), however, there has been no such court case and so the process remains legal. Although there is no doubt that bringing someone to hospital for just one night and signing a treatment order on them was against the spirit of the MHA, this custom nevertheless showed the need for continuing treatment and the extent to which these things can become a kind of game, of which you have to know the rules to ensure that patients stay well. For example, recently, another court case, *Gardner* v. *Regina*, readjusted the Hallstrom ruling. The judge pointed out that the term 'treatment in hospital' could include any use of the hospital as part of a patient's continuing treatment programme. It did not necessarily mean full-time inpatient care; if a patient had to come in regularly for medication, occupational therapy, nursing or medical review, for example, then that could be deemed hospital treatment. He thus considered that it was legal to detain a patient on a continuing Section 3 order, even if he or she was only attending as a day patient several times a week, for example.

3. Although patients have the right of access to a tribunal, this is not automatic. It is voluntary and patients have to apply for it, even though they may be frightened, thought-disordered and, perhaps, mute. This seems intrinsically unfair, because those who are most unwell and confused and unable to make judgements are those who are most in need of close review by a neutral body. Furthermore, tribunals can be a frightening experience, which puts patients off applying and/or attending. Making tribunals automatic could promote a change in procedure making them more informal yet just as efficient.

4. In all of this, the care worker in the community mental health team remains central. To opt out of this role is to deny the role. However, if the care worker is also the individual who signs a section order, there may be a breakdown of the therapeutic relationship. Should it therefore be part of the care worker's role, if they are an ASW, to sign section orders? It has been suggested that we should revert to the courts and have a specific court officer (as used to happen) organise the section under recommendations from both the doctors and the community worker.

5. Many members of the public feel that there *is* such a thing as a community treatment order and they are often surprised at some of the complexities of the MHA. They do not understand that people cannot be treated against their will in the community. They do not understand why crowds of social workers, nurses, police and doctors gather outside people's houses at odd times. Furthermore, the recent supervised discharge order has created the myth that somehow a community treatment order has now been introduced. To the average citizen, the notion of community care without a community treatment order is something of a paradox.

6. Perhaps the most interesting part of the MHA remains Section 141, concerning the detention of MPs. This complex procedure, requiring that the Speaker of the House of Commons be informed if an MP is sectioned and that a special tribunal be organised by the President of the Royal College of Psychiatrists to review the process, seems to suggest that MPs are rather paranoid. Maybe this is true, maybe not, but one wonders why this procedure has to be followed for MPs and why everyone else does not receive an automatic tribunal.

Possible future updates of the MHA

In our view it is quite clear that community care requires some form of community treatment order. This order, which would need to be reviewed every 6 months or every year, would mean that tribunals were automatic. Such review requirements would be a positive reform, resulting in the law and high-quality legal minds being much more involved in MHA proceedings. It is also quite clear that the care worker's role needs to be redefined. Why shouldn't anyone be able to sign a MHA application? In New Zealand, this is already possible, with the local policeman, a neighbour or any good friend able to do so, provided that they can explain to the judge why they did it. Such a sensible approach fits the spirit of practical English case law.

Regular reviews of mentally disordered offenders, i.e. under Section 37 and/or 41, should be carried out by senior judges. We have already mentioned that there should be a routine tribunal for everyone and that this should replace the current ad hoc arrangements. The role of the managers also seems to be out of date. Although good-hearted and useful in their role, they are an anomaly from the past. They should be combined with tribunals to provide a body of individuals who are able to regularly review the MHA at a local level and in a formal way.

The current supervised discharge order and its underling the supervision register seem to be useless as ways of enhancing good-quality mental health care. They were reactions to certain events in Parliament, they do not improve therapeutic activity and they are complicated to organise. For example, there are six separate forms to fill out for a supervised discharge order and just filling out one order takes nearly 45 minutes. Their sudden introduction highlights the need for considered MHA reform and how problems occur when legal changes take place in a hasty and slapdash fashion.

A new Mental Health Act?

In 2002 (June), the government published a draft version of its proposed new MHA, the outcome of a considerable period of review and consultation. As outlined in the previous section, there have been increasing calls for reform, this following the usual historical cycle of changes that are required every 20–30 years. There was no formal Inquiry Committee this time as there was in the 1950s prior to the 1959 MHA; however, a Scoping Committee chaired by a law professor was set up and a Green Paper and a White Paper (in December 2000) were published. These have all generated controversy, in particular the proposal to include the notion of dangerously severe personality disorder (DSPD; see Chapter 1) that was put into the latter document. With the publication of the draft bill in 2002 there was even more concern because of the very broad definition of 'mental illness' that it contained. It not only seemed as though the government was going to bring in powers to detain DSPD patients by stealth but also that it was going to be possible to detain drug- and alcohol-dependent and sexually disordered patients, patients who had been carefully (and wisely) excluded from the 1983 MHA.

The implications of these proposals were very much those of a public safety agenda, fears reinforced by various ministerial pronouncements and a rising tide of tabloid paranoia about paedophiles, psychotic murderers and pusillanimous psychiatrists. However, the opposition to the bill created an extraordinary alliance of professionals (doctors, lawyers, the police, social workers, nurses, psychologists, etc.), voluntary bodies and patient/user organisations. This Mental Health Alliance was so strong that the bill was dropped from the Queen's speech in both autumn 2002 and 2003 (i.e. it was taken out of the planned legislative programme for the coming year), although the then Secretary of State, Alan Milburn, insisted later that it would be found parliamentary time. The most important changes put forward in this draft, in terms of their effect on day-to-day practice, are outlined below:

1. No exclusion of patients because of alcohol/drug dependence, for example, using a broad definition of mental illness, of a nature or degree sufficient to require treatment.
2. Retention of the 72-hour (emergency) and 28-day (assessment and treatment) orders, as defined in the 1983 MHA Sections 4 and 2, but, after that, any further treatment to be decided by a tribunal.
3. All patients, therefore, to automatically have a tribunal hearing within 28 days, with appropriate reports to be provided for the tribunal's consideration. The tribunal still to consist of a legal chair, a psychiatrist and a layperson but with the possibility of a single lawyer sitting and taking advice only as he or she might require.
4. Powers to be given to the tribunal to enable it to order treatment for up to 6 months or even a year at a time via an agreed and essentially mandatory care plan. This could include regular medication, attendance at reviews and even day centre attendance, as well as (if deemed necessary) continued inpatient treatment. Such an order could be seen as a community treatment order.
5. Abolition of the role and powers of the hospital managers, now seen as a rather outdated aspect of an Act designed to be community oriented.
6. Extension of the ASW's specific role and powers to other appropriately qualified and trained professionals, such as nurses or occupational therapists, provided that they have had a suitable course of MHA training.
7. Broadly similar legislation in other areas of the MHA, including clarification of the dilemma around the 'Bournewood' ruling concerning patients unable to clearly state their wishes because of dementia or severe learning difficulties, for example.

Although these proposals have created concerns over a number of aspects of patient care and the likely heavy hand of the law in limiting the flexibility of many treatment regimes, a particular debate has centred around the notion of a community treatment order (CTO), which will, de facto, come into operation.

The publicly expressed fears have included somewhat unrealistic fantasies of people being forcibly injected on the kitchen table, as well as unacceptable intrusions into a patient's privacy. The arguments for and against CTOs are summarised in Box 9.1.

Box 9.1   Arguments for and against community treatment orders (CTOs)

For

- It is happening anyway under current law, i.e. Sections 41 and 3 (when on Section 17 leave), and supervised discharge
- In psychiatric care, a CTO is less restrictive than a hospital-based order, it avoids the unnecessary use of inpatient treatment and it is, therefore, in the interests of the freedom of the individual
- It acknowledges the focus on care in the community and is a logical extension of the whole community care philosophy
- It reflects the preferences and primacy of the patients and their families, especially those who consistently express their wish to stay out of hospital if at all possible

Against

- Fears are regularly expressed of the possibility of being forced to take treatment at home or of being over-medicated unnecessarily for longer periods of time
- The therapeutic relationship between a patient and a doctor or nurse could readily be undermined by the very fact of the order imposing a supervisory/risk-oriented approach
- The notion of social control predicts that such orders could be used increasingly widely to treat even those with relatively mild conditions – the thin end of the wedge, so to speak
- If current legislation already enables a CTO de facto, what is the point of bringing in new powers?
- Given the current shortages and staff limitations in psychiatric services, might a CTO not be used as a shortcut to mass treat patients without providing the personal support services that they really need?

Whatever the outcome of the legislation debate, it is clear that there are going to be substantial changes to routine practice over the next 2–3 years. This will mean that anyone working in the system will have to keep up to date, not only in terms of the 'rules of the game' but also more importantly in terms of the agreed procedures around ensuring patients' rights and keeping to the spirit of the law. It is also likely that community care workers will have to consider whether they wish to train as appropriately qualified health-care professionals, able to take on the role of an ASW as in the 1983 MHA. Some may see it as an advantage, adding new skills (and possibly item-for-service payments) to hard-won experience; others may see it as a burden, interfering with their day-to-day work and bringing a whiff of the legally assertive into what should be a voluntarily therapeutic relationship with those whom they are looking after. The important thing, as always, will be to do what best suits your skills and temperament, and what will best help the kind of patients that you are looking after.

Every community mental health worker needs to know about the MHA. It can be seen as part of one's terms of service and appropriate training programmes are a necessity. Routine seminars are particularly useful – we would suggest at least one a year – because once you start discussing the MHA, there's always another conundrum waiting around the corner. However, provided that everyone keeps in mind the following two basic principles, namely (i) first do no harm and (ii) the patient's best interests come first, good sense should prevail. Although, at times, the MHA may seem cumbersome in terms of its language and procedures, it does make you write reports, it makes you think twice, it makes you explain things to intelligent and legally trained minds and it makes you put on clean clothes (for tribunals especially). Never think of it as a burden but rather as a beloved treasure map, to take out and pore over every now and then as you come to yet another strange turning in the labyrinth of mental illness. It is the rules of the game, and those who know it generally get to look after their patients better.

Drugs and booze
(Or the addiction/dependence problem)

10

The tendency to put substances into our bodies to bring about a change in our mental state is deeply ingrained in human nature. Almost all of us do it; there is no society on earth that does not 'do drugs' in one form or another. History also tells us that, perversely, one of the best ways to encourage the use of any particular drug is to prohibit its use. The desire, or maybe the need, to get 'stoned' is one of the few things that separates man from most of the other creatures on the planet.

Legal or illegal, prescribed or over the counter, it is a safe bet that 99% of the patients on any caseload take drugs in one form or another. A core component of care worker skill, therefore, involves knowing what lies behind this all too human of behaviours. This chapter considers a patient's relationship with substances that are not taken in the prescribed or therapeutic sense (although, as we shall see, these too can carry street status) but in what is rather dubiously known as the 'recreational' sense. There is very little in the life of a crack addict that lives up to this sunny adjective, but it is a fact that the wine buff stirring to the plop of a cork from a bottle, the heroin addict thrilling at the pull of a tourniquet or the quiet pleasure that we get popping the foil on a fresh jar of instant coffee have more in common than most of us realise. Understanding what unites and separates a wine drinker, a crack head, a dope smoker, someone on 40 a day and a coffee freak is the first aim when working with anyone who has a 'drug issue'.

Every care worker, therefore, should have at least a basic understanding of the answers to these four questions:

1. Why do our patients take drugs?
2. What are the main types of drugs?
3. How can drugs affect the body and the life of the user?
4. How can we help people to understand and alter their drug-taking habits?

Why take drugs?

We take drugs to change our state of mind. This isn't quite as obvious as it sounds, because the way that any given drug exerts an effect upon the brain is only one part of the intoxication experience. The state of mind of the user before taking the drug, their expectations of the drug, their familiarity with its use and the setting in which they take it are just as important as the chemical effect in itself. This explains why some people will feel tipsy after drinking nothing but neat orange juice if they have been conned into believing that it has been spiked with vodka beforehand. It also explains why someone may have the time of their life on an LSD trip with a friend on a sunny day but can have a terrifying nightmare of a time on exactly the same drug while alone at a noisy party. Expectation and context play more of a role than most of us realise.

Most people take a drug to enhance their well-being, but perhaps a better way to understand this is to say that people take drugs to alter the way in which they experience and respond to the outside world. With the depressant substances, such as alcohol, benzodiazepines (tranx), the opiates and, to some extent, cannabis, this involves reducing psychological arousal – the mental and physical sensations of anxiety, tension and even sadness. This reduction in arousal is usually accompanied by a pleasurable sense of disconnection from things. Given that, for many of our patients, the world around them is a source of considerable grief, this seems understandable.

Stimulants, on the other hand, such as cocaine, amphetamines (speed) and caffeine, seem to give many users a subjectively greater sense of confidence in taking on the outside world, especially when it is boring. They result in comparatively little of the disconnection that is seen with the depressants but they do give a sense of being above and unbothered by problems. Hallucinogenic drugs are stranger still and seem to alter the very quality of the way that users perceives the outside world.

However, for more established users who are moving towards dependency, it is often the very absence of the drug itself that becomes the primary source of distress. Clearly, to understand what different drugs do to people, we need to have a basic idea of the ways in which they act upon the nervous system.

What different types of drug do to the brain

There are all sorts of way of classifying psychotropic drugs. Perhaps the most important classification has more to do with politics than brain chemistry: legal versus illegal. Societal proscription of a drug can do more damage than the chemical effect itself. Half a gram of cocaine found in a patient's pocket can have a bigger impact on the patient's life than if those same milligrams went up the patient's nostrils. This legal/illegal dichotomy also conveniently blinds us to the fact that two of the nastiest drugs in the world, nicotine and alcohol, are socially sanctioned. Therefore, do not be fooled into thinking that patients who are using illicit drugs have a worse problem than those using legal drugs. In what follows, we intentionally ignore this dichotomy; as far as the tissues of the central nervous system (CNS) are concerned, a drug is a drug is a drug.

Drugs that depress the central nervous system

In terms of sheer numbers, the depressant, or sedative, drugs are by far the most commonly used, because some 90% of the adult population consumes alcohol on a regular basis. And when it comes to alcohol, 'adults' start at around the age of 14. It is impossible to underestimate the significance of alcohol in our world. From 'wetting the baby's head' to the funeral wake, almost every event in our Westernised culture is associated with ingestion of this chemical, which also happens to be a good rocket propellant. Some 20% of the population will have trouble with this drug at some point in their lives and 5% will become dependent.

Alcohol, C_2H_5OH (also known as ethanol), is a tiny, colourless molecule that works its way into virtually every tissue in the body and, with chronic ingestion, causes damage throughout the body. Alcohol exerts its effects by stabilising all nerve membranes, making them less electrically responsive. Some parts of the brain, especially the inhibitory parts, are much more sensitive to this deadening effect. This accounts for the 'disinhibiting' effect of alcohol; in the early stages of intoxication, booze takes out the bits of our brain that say 'shouldn't' and 'shan't', the superego, strict parent bit, so to speak. The barbiturate tranquillisers, now virtually unobtainable, exert their effect in a very similar way. Alcohol is, of course, easy to make. Airborne fungi and yeasts will stop settling upon and fermenting fruit-borne sugars only when hell freezes over, and so alcohol seems set to remain the world's favourite drug for some time to come. Even chimpanzees drink it.

The other major group of depressant compounds are the benzodiazepines (benzos) and their cousins, the 'Z' drugs (e.g. zopiclone), which we encountered in Chapter 4. The dramatic growth in the use of these drugs over the last 30 years explains the disappearance of the barbiturates. Unlike alcohol, benzos work via a specific chemical messenger [gamma-aminobutyric acid (GABA)] in the brain, and so have a much more specific effect on arousal, attention and memory. They are, thus, much less toxic, but this cleanness of effect also makes them very moreish, especially to anxious people. As a rule, the shorter-acting compounds, such as lorazepam and flunitrazepam, are more moreish than their longer-acting cousins, diazepam and chlordiazepoxide. Benzo drugs that contain a halogen molecule, such as chlorine, fluorine or bromine, seem to be particularly potent disruptors of memory, although this may be more down to their reputation – flunitrazepam is the famous 'date rape' drug – than to any real chemical difference. Benzos do not occur naturally and can be made only via reasonably complex pharmaceutical processes. Thus, most benzodiazepines originate from medical prescriptions. Nevertheless, they are widely abused and carry a significant street value, especially among those who use them as an antidote to calm the effects of excessive indulgence in stimulants or to deal with withdrawal from other depressants.

Opiates, like the benzos, also exert their effects via a specific set of chemical messengers in the brain, the endorphin and encephalin systems. Unlike the more straightforward depressants, however, the effects are much more complex. This is probably a reflection of the intricate role of these chemical messengers throughout the spine and the brain. Whereas GABA seems to serve as a reasonably simple 'damping' system in higher parts of the brain, the endogenous opioids are right down there in the basic wiring of the CNS, overseeing processes such as pain, pleasure, reward and the initiation of learned behaviours. This probably accounts for their remarkable ability to induce dependency and the profound craving associated with withdrawal.

It takes the best part of a year to become totally dependent on alcohol (and even then you have to be going some), whereas it only takes a few weeks to become dependent on heroin or opium. Opiates have a particularly potent effect upon breathing; the parts of the lower brain that control breathing are rich in opiate receptors and so are particularly sensitive to the depressant effects of drugs such as heroin. This, and the fact that tolerance drops very swiftly after only short periods of abstinence, accounts for much of their dangerousness in overdose, as friends of Jimi Hendrix and countless others will testify. Opiates, like alcohol, are abundant in nature, coming largely from the sap of the opium poppy *Papaver somniferum*, a plant which grows nicely in Afghanistan and surrounding regions. Street heroin usually comes in the form of a soluble brownish or off-white powder, depending on what adulterating agents it contains.

Another tiny, nasty little molecule that gets deep down into the cogs of the CNS is nicotine, the principal active ingredient of tobacco. Like the opiates and the benzos, it works on a well-defined neurotransmitter system, the difference being that nicotinic receptors are found on nerve cells in virtually every part of the brain and the body. Again, this seems to account for the profoundly addictive qualities of the drug, which can both calm you and make you feel more alert. Because nicotine has such a wide range of effects on the CNS, it is hard to classify it as a straightforward depressant; however, it certainly increases activity in the parasympathetic or resting part of the autonomic nervous system. Nicotine addiction – smoking – is very common among people who have experienced a major mental illness; the smoking room is usually one of the most crowded places in any inpatient psychiatric unit.

Drugs that excite the central nervous system

These drugs also work, either directly or indirectly, on the transmitter systems in the brain that seem to play an activating role in arousal, attention, memory and what may be loosely termed 'mental energy'. The chief among these are the so-called brain monoamines: dopamine, noradrenaline (norepinephrine) and serotonin. The relative influence of each seems to account for interesting differences in the intoxication effect of the different drugs, as well as their propensity to induce dependence. Cocaine, for example, seems to have a powerful stimulating effect on the noradrenergic and dopaminergic systems, which are thought to play an important role in purposeful and learned behaviours. This may account for the very strong craving and psychological dependence that cocaine can swiftly induce.

Cocaine usually comes in the form of a white powder, cocaine hydrochloride (sometimes known as the base form of cocaine). This is reasonably soluble in water and, for many, the watery nasal mucus (i.e. the lining of your nose, close to lots of brain-bound blood vessels) does nicely as a place in which to dissolve the drug. Therefore, cocaine is commonly taken by nasal inhalation or 'snorting'. The absorption process is relatively slow, however, because the cocaine base is chemically quite tied up with the hydrochloric acid component. Many drug dealers get around this by mixing cocaine with an equal quantity of bicarbonate of soda, adding water and baking it to form a slab of 'rock-like' cocaine bicarbonate and sodium chloride. In this form, the cocaine holds on to its base far less avidly and, when heated, makes a cracking noise, freeing up the base cocaine. This makes it easier to smoke 'freebase', 'rock' or 'crack' cocaine. The effect is quicker, more intense and, as we will see when we consider lifestyles below, much more disruptive of the monoamine functions of the CNS, sanity included.

The amphetamines seem to work in pretty much the same way but appear to have a more powerful effect upon peripheral parts of the nervous system, leading to a higher pulse rate, tremor, restlessness and agitation. It is hard to be certain whether this is the result of a true difference between cocaine and the amphetamines or simply reflects the fact that recreational doses of amphetamines are relatively higher. Whichever is the case, it is surprising how many people report that the subjective effect of cocaine is 'smoother' and less 'raw' and that it is more pleasant to take than its amphetamine cousin. One genuine difference between these two types of drug is that amphetamines do not occur naturally whereas the coca leaf is harvested at great profit from the mountainous regions of South America. Cocaine-like compounds abound in nature. The humble betel nut, one of the ingredients of paan, a favourite drug of the Indian subcontinent, has a mild stimulant effect, whereas khat, a thick leafy plant that grows happily throughout the horn of Africa and the Arabian gulf, has an effect that is not entirely unlike the club drug ecstasy although rather more sedating. Khat is not illegal in the UK and its use is particularly popular among men originating from these regions, as anyone who has ever worked among a Somali population will testify.

There are many reasons why it is important for mental health workers to know about these stimulant drugs, especially in the inner cities where crack cocaine consumption is reaching epidemic proportions. Stimulants not only cause acute psychotic states but also seem to reduce the threshold for developing severe, longer-lasting psychotic symptoms in vulnerable individuals, even at lower doses. And, as if that isn't enough, the sheer pressure of the crack-addicted lifestyle is enough to cause sadness and madness in the hardiest of souls. We will return to this below.

The hallucinogens

The hallucinogens include LSD ('acid'), psilocybin (the active ingredient of magic mushrooms), cannabis (especially the stronger varieties, e.g. 'skunk') and mescaline. The effects of this group of drugs are just plain weird and remind us how little we know about the brain. For example, LSD is extremely potent – a few milligrams is enough to cause spectacular hallucinations – and, strangely, it appears to exert most of its effects long after the drug itself has left the body. Experimental subjects who swallowed LSD labelled with a small amount of radioactivity to track its whereabouts in the brain carried on tripping for hours after the Geiger counter had stopped crackling. Hallucinogenic drugs act in very complex ways upon higher functions of the brain compared with the relatively crude effects of the stimulants and depressants. Thus, hallucinogenic drugs alter perception, memory, emotion, the sense of time passing and even the entire subjective sensation of consciousness itself. Small wonder, then, that people refer to the effects of the hallucinogens as a 'drug experience'.

They also appear to have a lower propensity to cause dependence, in the physical sense of this much misunderstood word (see below). That is, abrupt discontinuation does not lead to marked physiological changes such as those seen with alcohol, nicotine and the opiates (see below). Again, this probably underscores the complexity of the effects that they have on the CNS. However, from the care worker's point of view, these drugs are important as they have a propensity to induce short-lived psychotic states that can closely resemble an acute episode of schizophrenia. Knowing how to distinguish one from the other is an important psychiatric skill.

Cannabis

This drug belongs in a class of its own for two reasons: first, because it is far and away the most widely used of all street drugs and second, because its range of effects is so varied that it defies simple classification. Cannabis (or dope, grass, weed, bush, green, ganga, kif, hash and countless other names) is derived from the leaves and flowering tips of *Cannabis sativa*, a sturdy plant that grows to a remarkable size in hot climates where it is cultivated on an industrial basis. The Caribbean countries, for example, probably produce more dope than sugar cane. It also grows quite well in milder, European climates, a fact not lost upon what one expert has referred to as 'the optimistic sowers of cage-bird seed'.

263

Cannabis is not so much a drug as a group of drugs having different effects. This variety is compounded by the fact that cannabis reaches the user in many different strengths and preparations, for example the dried leaves and flowers of the plant (grass) or the resin drawn from crushed tips (hashish). Thus, cannabis has a varied and sometimes curious effect on the user. It is, in part, a stimulant, consumers noting mental arousal with disorganised thinking and distractibility. It also has a euphoriant effect and a relaxant effect. Many patients swear blind that they cannot doze off at night without the help of a joint. It is also a mild hallucinogen of virtually every perceptual modality, with users noting particular enhancements of visual, auditory and somatic sensations. And, as if that isn't enough, it also has an odd propensity to stimulate appetite. Individuals affected by 'the munchies' have been known to empty a fridge at one sitting; experiments are under way to exploit this as a treatment for the nauseating side effects of cancer chemotherapy.

Another chemical curiosity of cannabis concerns its solubility. Unlike most other drugs, which are water soluble, the main active ingredients of cannabis are oily substances that dissolve well in fatty tissues, of which the brain has plenty. Thus, cannabis builds up in body tissues with prolonged use and this seems to cause an interesting change in the way that cannabis intoxication varies over time. The first few joints always have the most acute effect on mood, thought and perceptual distortion. After a few days of regular use, the more sedating effects seem to take over, as many regular cannabis smokers will attest.

From the care worker's point of view, cannabis is important not only because of its sheer ubiquity (it is probably no exaggeration to say that some 50% of an inner-city caseload will have cannabis in their bloodstream) but also because it appears to increase the risk of developing psychotic illness with prolonged usage. In smaller amounts, on the other hand, it may even do some good, i.e. as a relaxant.

Other drugs

Because mankind has been getting stoned on one sort of drug or another since coming out of the caves, it is a safe bet that we will continue to do so for the foreseeable future. Drug fashions will always come and go, and the novelty of each new arrival on the drug scene will, to some extent, determine its popularity. More sophisticated manufacturing techniques will also play a part in the development of new 'designer drugs'. An example of where this has already happened is in the refinement of the standard amphetamine molecule to incorporate a side chain of methylene dioxide, so creating methylenedioxymethamphetamine or MDMA, better known as ecstasy. Few pundits on the drug scene in the early 1980s could have predicted the way that this stimulant, with its powerful mood-altering properties, would explode in popularity, particularly amongst young visitors to nightclubs, parties and raves.

Countless other drugs abound, for example ketamine, GHB (gamma-hydroxybutyrate) and nitrates, each attracting its own nickname and connoisseurs. Whatever their differences, they all work on the same target organ, the brain, and it seems reasonably certain that, barring some unanticipated breakthrough, they will continue to work via one or more of the mechanisms described above. As we will consider in Chapter 11, this never-ending availability of drugs will pose a major challenge to the care worker of the future. It is already a core skill of the care worker of the present to know what drugs their patients are taking and why (Fig. 10.1).

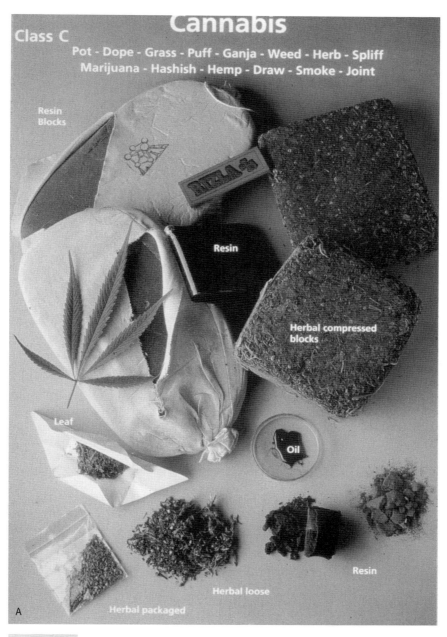

Figure 10.1 ● Well-known street drugs: (A) cannabis (Class C); (B) hallucinogens (Class A); (C) opiates (Class A); (D) cocaine (Class A).

(Continued)

Figure 10.1 ● (Continued)

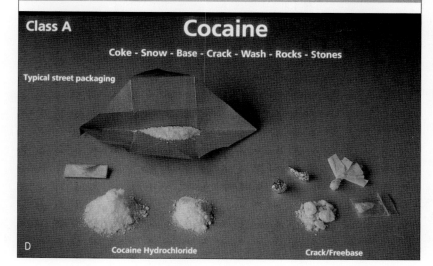

Dependence and withdrawal

People often refer to an individual as being 'addicted to drugs' without being clear what they mean. Drug dependence is a much misunderstood concept that has not particularly gained in clarity from the attempt to break it down into the twin notions of physical and psychological dependence. A lot of hot air has been generated by this half-correct distinction, which has its roots in our old enemy, the mind/body split. As we have observed throughout this book, the mental is the physical, and addiction demonstrates this neatly. Few of us have a problem understanding that nicotine and heroin produce profound changes in the minds and bodies of almost everyone who uses them when their supply of the drug is interrupted. We refer to this state as 'withdrawal' and psychiatrists state that they are observing a 'withdrawal syndrome'. The key features of withdrawal associated with common drugs are shown in Box 10.1.

Box 10.1 Characteristic withdrawal features of commonly misused drugs

Alcohol The most serious of all withdrawal syndromes, can be fatal. Early-stage features include vivid dreaming, insomnia and restless irritability. Mid-stage features include anxiety, tremulousness, sweating, palpitations, nausea, dilated pupils, epileptic convulsions. Late-stage features include panic, extreme agitation and a terrified psychotic state with visual and tactile hallucinations (so called 'delirium tremens').

Opiates Appears worse than it is. Rarely fatal. Resembles mild 'flu; runny nose, sneezing, yawning, shivering, gooseflesh (so-called 'cold turkey'), myoclonic jerks (so-called 'kicking the habit'), nausea, vomiting, diarrhoea, pronounced dysphoria, anxiety, craving for opiates.

Benzodiazepines Similar to alcohol withdrawal, especially with diazepam and chlordiazepoxide, but usually less severe and less commonly progresses to delirium. Chronic anxiety and insomnia common. May be prolonged over months.

Stimulants (cocaine, amphetamines, MDMA) Need for excessive sleep, mental slowing, irritability, poor concentration. Dysphoria may be more intense and prolonged with MDMA, appearing to peak 1–2 days after use. Often there is a craving for the drug, especially with cocaine and crack cocaine.

Cannabis The existence of a clear cannabis withdrawal syndrome remains disputed, but many regular heavy users individuals report nausea/loss of appetite, irritability, insomnia and vivid dreaming.

Hallucinogens No clear withdrawal syndrome has been consistently reported for these drugs, but some users report a sense of detatchment from surroundings. LSD is occasionally associated with poorly understood 'flashback' phenomena, which involve sudden, short-lived perceptual distortions weeks or months after the last use of the drug.

But what about those drugs whereby discontinuation does not lead to any instantly recognisable psychophysiological display of symptoms? Many people can stop using cocaine, MDMA or cannabis, even after many years of regular use, with relatively little in the way of a recognisable withdrawal syndrome. Does this mean that they are not 'dependency forming'? And what about a frail elderly woman recovering from a hip replacement, who feels afraid and unsteady when she leaves her walking stick behind for the first time since the operation? Are curved pieces of wood addictive? It is probably simpler to say that anything that can cause pleasure or reduce discomfort is addictive, and that some substances, especially those that have relatively straightforward effects on the CNS, are more likely to cause a specific, recognisable withdrawal syndrome.

We have come a long way in our understanding of dependency syndromes over the past 50 years. Indeed, it is probably no exaggeration to state that dependency is one of the few areas of brain science where we have a good understanding of just what is going on mentally, physically and socially, all at the same time. The fact that this wisdom hasn't allowed us to come up with any effective new treatments tells us something very important about addiction in particular and human nature in general: science only comes up with big answers when it is married to philosophical issues of morals and agency. Or, to put it another way, to overcome an addiction, you have to really want to stop.

This biopsychosocial integration of knowledge is useful to the care worker, both in learning to recognise and gauge the severity of a drug problem and in helping a patient to do something about it. It tells us what signs to look for in the bodies of our patients, in their thoughts and actions and in the sorts of lives that they lead. More specifically, it tells us to look out for a constellation of features that together form a 'dependency syndrome'. The defining features of such a syndrome are shown in Box 10.2 and are worth considering in some detail.

Box 10.2 Core features of addiction (substance dependence syndrome)

1. *Tolerance*: a need for larger quantities of the drug to obtain the same effect
2. *Withdrawal*: symptoms that clearly follow discontinuation of the drug
3. *Salience of drug-seeking behaviour*: users spend increasing time and effort obtaining, taking and recovering from drug
4. *Narrowing of the repertoire of drug-taking behaviour:* as dependence worsens, the drug consumption tends to become more stereotyped
5. *Decline in social function*: drug use gets in the way of living
6. *Internal struggle*: subjective awareness that drug is doing harm and nagging awareness of need to do reduce intake
7. *Reinstatement*: swift return to problematic patterns of use after a period of abstinence

Dependency on a drug – or on anything else come to that, even climbing mountains or watching news broadcasts – only happens once someone has been doing it for a while. This truism hides a deeper truth: you don't have to be addicted to have a serious drug problem. Countless imperilled drug dabblers hide behind the rationalisation that 'I'm not an addict'. One-fifth of the adult population has an alcohol problem, but only a small fraction of these people are alcohol dependent. Dependency takes time to form and occurs more quickly with some drugs than with others. Over this time, the body, like all living systems, adapts to the effects of the substance and so becomes 'tolerant'. We considered this acquisition of tolerance in Chapter 4 when we looked at the dependency-forming effect of benzodiazepines. Tolerance and its corollary, withdrawal upon discontinuation, comprise the core physiological elements of the dependence syndrome.

Another more puzzling physical hallmark of dependence is the reinstatement effect. It takes a good few years of heavy boozing to become dependent on alcohol, but, within a few weeks of stopping, most people are well over withdrawal and back into a state of stable, symptom-free abstinence or (more rarely) controlled drinking. However, if they start to drink heavily again, their tolerance shoots up almost overnight. A chemical adaptation that previously took years now takes only a couple of days. It is as though the CNS has some sort of chemical memory for the effects of alcohol, or whatever drug is being taken. Reinstatement is seen with almost all drugs and suggests that the old adage of Alcoholics Anonymous – 'once an alcoholic, always an alcoholic' – may be biologically true.

Although these processes happen at the tissue level, more complex behavioural changes also start to occur. Activities that centre upon the drug – getting it, taking it and recovering from it – gradually take precedence over other behaviours. In technical jargon, this is called 'primacy' of drug-taking behaviour. In a similar way to tolerance first time around, this takes time and usually leads to a clear decline in the person's ability to function effectively as a parent, friend, employee, etc. Early on, a heroin-addicted mum will still give priority to her crying baby; 5 years later, she's too zonked to make it to the school gate.

We can pose this as a useful question in our work with our patients, i.e. to what extent is drug taking in general dominating their lives. If the answer is 'quite a bit', you have an addict on your caseload. Another telltale change over time is the drug-taking behaviour itself, which tends to become less varied and more stereotyped as the problem becomes established. We can also pose this as a useful question: how much can our patient vary their drug-taking behaviour? Usually, the narrower the range of drug-taking behaviour, the greater the problem. Thus, instead of drinking wine, beer, sherry or malt whisky, depending on the time and the occasion, the true alcoholic just drinks whatever keeps his or her alcohol level up.

Very few people get into trouble with drugs without a nagging suspicion that they are doing so somewhere along the way. This awareness of losing control over one's behaviour and, therefore, damaging oneself always causes discomfort, which some people may go to extraordinary lengths to avoid. Some deal with it by simply taking more of the drug and spiral rapidly out of control. Others simply deny that there is any problem, even when confronted with overwhelming evidence, for example an angry spouse's discovery of empty vodka bottles behind the wardrobe. The human capacity for self-deception is truly staggering, and addicts have it in spades.

Few people are able to live with the effort of such denial all of the time and this is reflected in another cardinal feature of the addicted mind: the internal struggle against the urge to go on using. Many individuals can spend years in this 'precontemplative' state. Mark Twain, who knew a thing or two about human nature, hit the nail of nicotine addiction on the head when he said: 'Giving up smoking is the easiest thing in the world. I know, because I've done it thousands of times.' This internal wrestling with the self breeds discomfort, which in turn generates guilt, irritability and half-hearted promises to do something. These psychological principles underpin one of the most useful acronyms in the caring business: CAGE. Box 10.3 shows what we mean.

> ## Box 10.3 CAGE questionnaire
>
> Alcohol dependence is likely if the patient gives two or more positive answers:
>
> - Have you ever felt you should **c**ut down your drinking?
> - Have people **a**nnoyed you by criticising your drinking?
> - Have you ever felt bad or **g**uilty about your drinking?
> - Have you ever had a drink first think in the morning to steady your nerves or get rid of a hangover (**e**ye-opener)?
>
> The CAGE questionnaire was developed by Dr John Ewing, founding director of the Bowles Center for Alcohol Studies, University of North Carolina at Chapel Hill. CAGE is an internationally used assessment instrument for identifying problems with alcohol. 'CAGE' is an acronym formed from the italicised letters in the questionnaire. From Ewing JA (1984) Detecting alcoholism: the CAGE questionnaire. *J Am Med Assoc* 252, 1905–1907.

The lifestyles of people with drug problems

As we have seen, the lifestyle of a person using drugs changes as the drug, or rather the drug-taking behaviour, takes a firmer hold on them. A useful way to look at this is to consider the relative physical and social elements of the problem at various points in its course. We can conceive of this as two overlapping horizontal wedges, one physical and one social (see Barry's story in Fig. 10.2). The width of the wedge at any given point indicates its relevance to the patient's life. At the outset, social factors play by far the most important role in a person's drug taking, as well as their life in general, which is usually varied in all the normal, human sorts of ways. At this point, the physical processes of tolerance, dependence and tissue damage contribute relatively little to the person's difficulties. By the end of the process, however, it is the other way around. Physical issues are everything, as much of the person's time is spent robbing, lying, scoring, getting stoned and doing whatever is necessary to stave off yet another wave of withdrawal. By this stage, the person's social repertoire is as narrow – no partner, no job, no mates – as their pattern of drug taking. The same basic pattern is repeated day after day after day until they do something about it. Or they die.

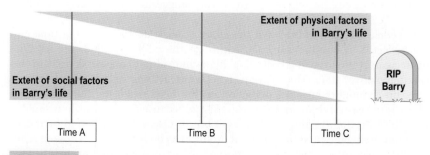

Figure 10.2 ●Barry's story.

Spotting this gradual decline into dependence, and knowing how to identify it as early as possible, are key skills of a competent care worker. To be able to do this properly, the care worker needs to know about more than just the effects of the drugs. We must also develop some understanding of what might be called 'drug culture' – matters that are relevant to drug use in the broadest sense. Knowing how much any given substance roughly costs, what it is called, how and where it is obtained, how it is taken, in whose company, how often and where is invaluable when it comes to convincing your patient that you know what you are talking about. This is worth considering briefly here.

The routes by which drugs make their way into the body may seem reasonably obvious to most people. You don't have to be a reader of the *Daily Mail* to know that most drugs are inhaled, swallowed, snorted or injected. As far as the authors are aware, suppositories have not hit the UK drugs black market in a big way just yet. The point of entry into the body can leave all sorts of telltale marks that are well worth looking out for. A smoker's cough and nicotine stains on the dominant hand (left-handers rarely smoke with their right hand) are pretty obvious, but the not-so-obvious marks are just as important. Glue and solvent sniffers often have a slight area of roughened redness around their lips or nose from the application of the vessel holding the drug, a common skin irritant. Someone who has just taken a line of cocaine often sniffs and then edgily touches their nose in a sort of casual wipey gesture. The forearms of regular heroin injectors often bear signs of 'tracking' that run along the arm veins. The redder the most recent needle point, the more recent the use. Heavier scarring of the arms often indicates infected injection sites, or even a history of self-harm, a behaviour that is not uncommon in the chaotic life of many drug users. When arm veins appear fully used up, drug users will often move on to their groin or feet or even the major jugular veins of the neck. Once dependency has a hold, it is amazing to what lengths some folk will go to get their favourite molecule into their body.

Every drug requires the use of some sort of device to get it into the body and it pays to know a little about drug paraphernalia; there is a fair chance that spotting something on a home visit, hastily half-hidden, may be an early sign that something is up. Heroin, cannabis and crack can easily be smoked, rolled as a 'joint' mixed with tobacco. The famous 'Rizla' packet of cigarette rolling papers is often torn and rolled into a little homemade cardboard filter, or 'roach', which is stuffed into the end of the joint. Torn-off Rizla packets are often forgotten and left lying around, a reasonably sure sign that someone around is using something. Smoking drugs in joints or 'spliffs', however, is a pretty ineffective way of getting them into the lungs, especially when the drug is expensive and does not burn easily mixed in with tobacco, as is the case with heroin and cocaine, crack or straight. Much of it goes up in smoke between 'lugs' or inhalations.

The amount of drug that reaches the brain is increased if it is heated unmixed and the smoke hoovered up with some sort of tube. This is the case when 'chasing' the pungent bluish smoke that curls up from burning heroin or the thinner greyish smoke from burning crack, or when burning it over a piece of perforated tinfoil and sucking it down through some sort of makeshift tube, such as the cardboard core of a toilet roll, a drinks can or a plastic bottle. You will be surprised how often you will find such items lying around when you visit the homes of some of your more disorganised customers if you look out for them. Occasionally, a patient will leave them lying around as a way of trying to tell you something.

With injected drugs, most commonly heroin, the drug has to be converted from a semi-soluble brownish powder (which can contain anything from crushed paracetamol to baking powder) into a liquid suitable for injection. This is usually done by heating it in a spoon with a small amount of water. The heat also sterilises the solution making it (slightly) safer to inject. Usually, it is drawn up into a small plastic syringe via a makeshift filter, often a blob of cotton wool or a cigarette filter, to exclude the more gravelly, undissolved bits from the syringe. The resulting filtrate is then injected into a vein that has been swollen (to make it easier to receive the needle) by means of a tourniquet made from almost anything.

Established addicts will tell you that this preparatory ritual is extremely pleasant and forms almost as important a part of the drug taking as the 'hit' of the drug itself. This underscores the powerful way that the human mind makes associations between specific stimuli (the pop of the cork, the pull of the tourniquet, the 'plik' of the coffee jar) and the arrival of a chemical reward a few moments later. In the world of substance misuse, we all act like Pavlov's dogs.

The social environment, that is the role played by other people, is also an important part of someone's drug-using behaviour, whether they are dependent or not. We do not have to dive into the drug underworld to understand that 99% of all drug-taking behaviour is a supremely social enterprise; a trip to a pub or a tea dance at a retirement home will do. Surprisingly few people take drugs in complete isolation except, perhaps, in the later stages of an addiction career, as we saw with Barry at the thin end of the wedge (Fig. 10.2). Therefore, it is always worth finding out who is around when a patient takes their drugs. Many of those with more severe enduring mental illness live sparse social lives and, for them, a trip to 'score' some grass or crack, for example, may be the highlight of their week, usually the day on or after the giro comes. Sudden changes in pecuniary status, emptying of the fridge or the 'disappearing television' may be subtle indicators that a dealer has decided to call in a debt.

The world of the drug user (and, sadly, many of our patients) is particularly feral, thanks to the illegal environment in which drugs are taken. One nasty manifestation of this, becoming sadly more common in the crack-infested nooks of our inner cities, is the way that users and dealers parasitically prey upon vulnerable people, using their homes as dens for dealing, using and whatever other colourful activity they choose to partake in. Often, the host is a vulnerable person with a chronic illness and few friends who at first is only too grateful for the company, the excitement and maybe even the odd free smoke; however, as the cuckoo grows in the nest, this soon changes. To see what we think should be done about it, see the film *Dead Man's Shoes* and read Chapter 11.

Talking to people about their drug use and helping them to change it

The ambitious title of this section is really beyond the scope of this chapter but a few points are worth mentioning here. From what we have said above, it is part of the care worker's job to know a fair bit about the world of drug use and misuse, which, after all, reflects the world that we all inhabit. For many, including the less experienced care worker, it is easy to be seduced by the cool fashion of the entire scene. We are all raised on a diet of gangsta films, rap videos and countless more subtle affirmations of the idea that bad is good (ask anyone under the age of 25 what 'wicked' means) and it is rather easy for a care worker, picking delicately along the edges of the real-world scene, to feel as if they are involved in something that is not entirely undramatic. This can lead to all sorts of slips, some more serious than others.

Be careful, for example, when using local vernacular to talk to your patients about drugs. Whatever your familiarity with your patient's 'homies' and 'bloods', you will not be broadcasting on a professional frequency if you resort to such colourful argot and may send an implicit message that you accept, or even approve of, an activity that is both illegal and, more importantly, the opposite of what you are trying to achieve. Familiarity with a person's problem does not mean that you have to share their values about that problem. A larger version of this mistake is to share drugs with your patients. Never, *ever* try to get onside with patients by taking drugs with them or being around when they are dealing. However much you may think that one of the few pleasures a patient has in life is smoking a spliff, partaking is going way beyond the rules of clinical engagement. The converse is equally true: don't preach. We all have opinions about the quintessentially human activity of self-intoxication and it can become easy for our moral judgements to hamper our caring efforts.

Before you can begin to help someone with a drug problem you have to first satisfy yourself that they have a problem (not that difficult) and then get them to accept that they have a problem (much more difficult). Psychology comes in handy here. Consider the stages by which most of us face up to any problem. First, we spend time realising that something is different. This often starts as a vague, nagging feeling that only slowly evolves into an idea that something is wrong. In our heads, we start to come up with all sorts of explanations of what this might be and why it might be so. Some of these reasons are more honest, and often more uncomfortable, than others.

Imagine, for example, that you sought an explanation for your inexplicable urge to binge on alcohol, crack and valium until you collapse. Which of the following would you rather tell yourself: 'I like to go a bit over the edge every now and then' or 'Whenever I am reminded of the way my father used to abuse me I get totally wasted'? For most people, a central part of a drug problem, whether dependent or not, is about putting off the moment that they have to think about even thinking about what it is that is really upsetting them. Most of us deal with the more pressing problems in our lives by erecting all sorts of interesting barriers against the core truth that says 'do something'. People with drug problems have found a way of doing this that appears to come out of a bottle or a small paper bag. A really skillful care worker can cut to the core of these thoughts and deeds using an interviewing technique known as 'motivational interviewing'. We recommend that you check this out.

There are all sorts of interesting shortcuts to this core. In Chapter 8, we looked at ways of talking to suicidal people that cut to the central question of whether or not they really wanted to die. There are a number of tricks that, in their own way, are just as helpful when assessing whether or not someone has got what it takes to do something about a drug problem. The CAGE questionnaire is one. Another is to exploit the moment. Very few people suddenly decide to disclose a concern about their substance use out of the blue, without having struggled with the issue privately beforehand. The point at which they begin to talk about it, often after weeks of what feels like pulling teeth, is usually the culmination of months of worry, doubt and self-reproach. This can often be discerned from their behaviour over the time prior to presentation. Just as a tree trunk can reveal all sorts of things about the climate over the years, so a carefully elicited history can tell you how a patient feels about making inroads into their drug-taking behaviour.

Start by asking patients how much of their drug they have consumed in the last 24 hours. Generally, the worse the problem, the more they will underestimate this. Then, ask about their intake over the previous week. This is not as difficult as it sounds if you take it day by day and give little cues to aid recall: 'Were you in the pub?' or 'Did you have a smoke with your dealer?' Then, try over a month. This method cuts down on underestimation, or can at least give you a feel for the extent of their self-deception, and gives you a reasonable idea of just how much of the stuff they are taking. From this, the severity of the dependence is relatively easy to guess. Also look out for a recent decline in intake – a sure sign of internal struggle – and try to get a feel for the extent of their drug tolerance. For dangerous drugs such as heroin, where the tolerance changes quickly, this can be lifesaving. Keep your eyes, ears and nose open for the physical and social consequences of dependence. With drug injectors, always ask about sharing 'works' or needles and make sure that they know the score with hepatitis B, hepatitis C and HIV.

That is the easy bit. Now, the real work begins. What you are trying to do, in essence, is to persuade someone to persuade themself that they need to give up a tried and cherished method of self-destruction that they have spent a large part of their time justifying to themself. Working with a drug problem is a bit like a mediaeval siege. You can storm the ramparts (watch for boiling oil), you can surround the place and sit it out or you can try hurling the occasional dead sheep into the courtyard. Do what Hippocrates told you to do 2000 years ago: get the patient's friends and family onside and harness the heat that is generated by the countless tragedies, large and small, that drug misuse entails. Near misses of personal tragedy make very good dead sheep.

Another variant of the dead sheep strategy is to get the patient to see their problem in a different way, for example to think of the problem not in terms of the drug but in terms of the cash. Asking a smoker to think of his habit as £50 per week instead of 40 a day can sometimes prompt change, especially if you can get them to keep this thinking up. Diaries are often very useful in addiction work. In the case of alcohol or any other drug that comes in different forms, for example the benzodiazepines or cannabis, try substituting a favourite form for a less salubrious equivalent, matching unit for unit. An inebriate young mother of two might insist that two bottles of Chardonnay a night is 'just a drink with friends', but the observation that she is getting through the equivalent of three bottles of vodka a week or five cans of Tennant's Super each night can set a few balls rolling. Know your units of alcohol and have a rough idea of the strengths of the most common drugs, legal and illegal. Drug work, with its clearly measurable outcomes, high stakes and siege psychology, is often great fun and, barring some disastrous rewriting of the Mental Health Act, you hardly ever have to grapple with the dilemmas of compulsory treatment. If someone does decide to stop, well done, but graded detoxification (in or out of hospital) is usually best, especially for alcohol and smack (heroin).

However, working with people who have drug problems is also exasperating. Don't fall into the amateur's trap and expect results. No matter how good your relationships and how persuasive your oratory about the hell fires of crack addiction, you are talking to those who have devoted a large part of their lives to this particular behaviour. People hardly ever give up overnight except in films and, if they did, they probably wouldn't be talking to you in the first place. It is a sobering thought that about 95% of people who sort out a drug problem of one sort or another do so without any professional help at all. Explaining this to an addictions worker is a fun way to spend a wet Friday afternoon. The general mental health care worker doesn't have to be an addictions specialist, but he or

Box 10.4   Useful sources of support and information for people with addiction problems

- Release: www.release.org.uk; tel: 0207 729 9904
- Alcoholics Anonymous: tel: 01904 644026
- Narcotics Anonymous: tel: 0207 730 0009
- HIT: www.hit.org.uk; tel: 0870 990 9702
- NHS Smoking Helpline: tel: 0800 169 0169
- Lifeline: tel: 0161 839 2075

she should know someone who is. This is not usually difficult. Drug and alcohol problems are so overwhelmingly common that every town in the country has its own drug helplines, detox units, counselling services and Alcoholics Anonymous and Narcotics Anonymous groups, all beavering away alongside the statutory and nationwide services. Some useful contact details are given in Box 10.4; their local equivalents should be either in your head or your office. Cultivate a good relationship with these people. They are siege masters.

The challenges of the future

11

As we have shown, caring for mentally ill folk in the community – largely away from institutions – is a complex and rewarding task. It requires personal skills and emotional maturity; a knowledge of medicine, psychiatry, nursing and social work; an awareness of both history and the most modern of ideas; and, above all, an abounding interest in people and what they do. How can those of us working in mental health really make things better? How can we escape the unhelpful stereotypes attached to this kind of work? The first person to coin a term to define the 'community mental health worker' of the 21st century will be a real hero because, by coming up with a defining term or phrase, it will be possible to help the public grasp what mental health really means. However, there is no point in producing some politically correct euphemism, because obscure language simply reduces the public's trust.

The standard community mental health team (CMHT) – or variant thereof, for example assertive outreach team (AOT), home treatment team (HTT), etc. – presently consists of people from different disciplines. The nurse, the social worker, the psychologist, the occupational therapist and the psychiatrist are all put together and given some team-building exercises and it is assumed that things will click. Yet, the training programmes for this disparate group of individuals vary enormously and there is little or no cross-fertilisation of teaching. Recently, the idea of patients themselves being integrally involved in education has gained ground, something that is much to be welcomed. Having someone describe what it really means to be depressed or diabetic or arthritic (or all three) can only help to give us a broader understanding of the problems that our patients face. Just as important, this approach highlights the areas of knowledge that should be common to all community mental health workers. Although professional training, such as nursing registration or a social work qualifying certificate, provides the obvious entry into the role of community mental health worker, developing a series of 'core competencies' (to use the modern phrase), perhaps via a diploma programme, seems vital for the future.

What are these 'core' skills? We would suggest that the previous 10 chapters have summarised them to a large degree; they are not difficult to acquire if someone wants to learn, wants to reflect on their practice and wants to know about mental health. These skills include knowing about the causes and nature of psychiatric illnesses, the various treatments (psychological, social and pharmacological), how services work (or why they don't work) and mental health law, and being up to date on the complexities of housing, benefits, educational systems and who does what within them. Being able to relate to individuals who vary widely in terms of their professional, cultural and attitudinal backgrounds is also part of the game. In particular, there is room for touches of creativity and even theatricality, as well as a limitless curiosity about how the world works. The following broad topics seem to us to be at the heart of the future agenda.

Fighting stigma

As we have emphasised throughout this book, the greatest problem for a Cinderella service such as mental health is dealing with people's attitudes. Stigma is everywhere; in our language, our television shows, advertising, insurance payouts and job applications. The stigmatisation of mental disorder is so subtly pervasive that it is easy to miss; if we lived at the bottom of the sea, would we have a word for wet?

In spite of our cultural pretensions to be modern, ancient fears of mental illness still cause us to mock the mentally ill, attack them or marginalise them. This can lead to avoidance of effective help and ready exploitation by quack therapists. It can bring family shame and suicide. It can also lead to chronic underfunding of services. When it comes to the crunch, no matter how many times the Chancellor says he wants to improve mental health care (usually after some eye-grabbing incident), the money usually doesn't get there. The NHS has an extraordinary capacity to undedicate those officially dedicated mental health funds and rework them as they pass through the system. Then, hey presto, it's a fertility clinic or a weight-loss clinic rather than a community team for those less appealing patients with chronic schizophrenia or a day centre for the frail elderly with early dementia (who aren't quite enough of a hassle to alarm the Health Minister).

How do we really address stigma? There have been several campaigns (e.g. the Respect campaign by the mental health charity MIND and the Changing Minds campaign of the Royal College of Psychiatrists) and there is some evidence that people are becoming more open and liberal – at least in some places – towards mental illness. Even that notorious tabloid *The Sun* changed its front page when covering the boxer Frank Bruno's admission to hospital (with an acute mental illness), thanks to vociferous and articulate complaints. But campaigns have to be persistent, consistent and from the bottom up. They need to start in school, with children regularly taught about health, including mental health, in the wider sense. Every school child loves talking about bodily functions. Why shouldn't the amazing functions of the brain be on the curriculum? This need not be difficult or expensive. Imaginative cartoons, from *Tom and Jerry* to *The Simpsons*, literally show how characters think and feel and act.

A real challenge here is to cure that 17th century hangover, 'Cartesian dualism'. This phrase derives from the work of the Renaissance philosopher René Descartes (1596–1650), who suggested that the body was a machine, with the soul or mind sitting in it as a kind of ghostly operator that separates after death. However, research shows again and again that what and how you think affects what you do and how your body works, and vice versa. The mind is the body; taking exercise can, literally, improve your mood. Active unwinding through practiced meditation can eliminate tension headaches. Yoga can slow the heart rate. So, why differentiate between physical illness and psychiatric disorder? Why sign a plaster cast on a broken leg yet ignore someone who has survived an overdose? The drive to create a caring attitude for the mentally ill, equivalent to the kind of care elicited by, for example, a bald child with leukaemia or a blind man with a white stick, needs to be carried on into adult life. Many excellent films have sympathetically portrayed mental illnesses: *A Beautiful Mind* is a film about schizophrenia with a happy ending; *Girl, Interrupted* showed that caring can help in borderline personality problems. In the early 1990s, the TV soap *Eastenders* ran the Jo Wicks storyline that sold to over eight million people the idea that combined drug and social treatments for schizophrenia really work. We should expect, and demand, these attitudes everywhere.

Some people feel that even the word stigma is itself stigmatising and that we should view the matter instead as one of simple discrimination. Society has certainly changed its attitudes to discrimination in many other areas of life. Consider how, over the last 30 years, we have changed our reactions to all but two of the words in Box 11.1.

Box 11.1 Changing patterns of stigma

Paki

Coon

Spastic

Wog

Nigger

Queer

Poofter

Madman

Schizo

Antidiscrimination law has led to many successful lawsuits but it is still likely that you will not be shortlisted if you tick yes to a history of mental illness when applying for a job. Look at the small print of travel insurance and you will see mental illnesses and their associations carefully excluded. Of course, if you can prove that your mental illness has a clear physical cause, for example you developed hallucinations secondary to the anti-malaria tablets that you took on holiday (which can happen), then that's okay. It's as if there is a lingering suspicion that mental symptoms in isolation are either made up or suggest that, if you weren't so spineless, you would have sorted it out yourself.

We have also described the effects of the inquiry culture, whereby anyone involved in looking after someone who kills themselves (or even someone else) is automatically seen as blameworthy. In the UK, 10 people a day die on the roads, one-third of them because of alcohol abuse, but that is somehow seen as being acceptable in a society that enjoys driving fast and drinking hard. Deaths from cancer, heart attacks and strokes are accepted (by and large) as being untreatable, as 'terminal events' for example. The notion that someone simply has a malignant mental illness, which could lead them to take their own – or even other people's – life, regardless of the quality of their care, does not chime in the same way with public opinion. Of course, poor care should be shown up for what it is but singling out mental illness for special treatment is, by definition, stigmatising.

Can we ever really banish the stigma of mental illness? It's been around for so long that many of us might despair. However, the community mental health worker of the future is going to have to crack this one because, without it, we're going to go on foundering. Depression may be at the top of the list of illnesses that have the most impact on human lives (according to the World Health Organization), but its recognition, and the resources to treat it, remain seriously limited. Should we introduce, perhaps, some sort of national community service so that anyone leaving school spends time working with the chronically ill (the elderly, the physically handicapped, those with schizophrenia)? This way, people would learn at first hand the meaning and the sheer humanity of psychological suffering, and mental health could seamlessly take its place in the wider agenda of sickness and health.

The biopsychosocial approach (doing stuff and the meaning of life)

This juggernaut of a word has informed approaches to mental illness for 30 years or more but it still doesn't stop people from hiding in their own preferred corner of the biological, psychological and social triangle. In many ways, this reflects the way that people deal with most problems of bewildering complexity – by retreating into the false comfort of something that feels simpler. This retreat is all the easier if your refuge is justified by a professional framework – medicine, nursing, psychology, social work – to make it feel as if that is where you belong professionally. As we have tried to argue throughout this book, effective mental health work can really only begin once we crawl out of our various disciplinary hidey-holes. The whole point is that you have to look at all three views together to really understand and help someone with a mental illness. If you don't understand how their body works, you can't detect the often subtle abnormalities in their capacity to think, feel, remember, choose and act. If you don't have a good grasp of the world that they live in, you will never win their trust, and if you don't have some basic psychological understanding of the way that their mind works, then even talking to them, let alone helping them, is nigh on impossible.

This kind of understanding doesn't just relate to how people become ill. It also relates to how we get them better because, in the end, that's all that really matters. You can theorise all you want about how someone arrived at their particular level of handicap or isolation, and that may help you find a road back for them; however, true community mental health workers should be able to think on their feet and go to work on any patient's demoralisation there and then. They should be a kind of one-stop shop, able independently to do some CBT (cognitive behavioural therapy), fill out the DLA (disability living allowance) form, haggle with housing and prescribe an SSRI (selective serotonin reuptake inhibitor) antidepressant.

And out of all this, the good worker needs to find a way of making patients feel better about themselves and their lives. Having something meaningful and useful to do on a regular basis is about as close as we can get to an answer to the meaning of life. It doesn't really matter what it is – making music, going to a day centre, typing letters, visiting your mum, building a customised car, bungee jumping – 'doing stuff' is crucial to staying alive. The nastiest of the mental illnesses, the chronic negative states of psychotic illness or the severe dementias, boil down to just this: an inability to do stuff. In our society, with its emphasis on individual ability, skill, achievement and productivity – i.e. doing stuff – we hold people who have problems with doing stuff in very low regard. It is our old enemy, stigma, popping up again in a different guise. And there is no real reason why it has to be this way, either. In many so-called 'developing countries' (heaven knows what we expect them to develop into!), patients with severe mental illness maintain much more of a foothold in society. Surprisingly, even though stigma abounds just as viciously in these cultures as it does in our own, such people are still conferred a degree of value and worth that the 'mad folk' of our world are not. And, surprise, surprise, look at their better longer-term prognoses for illnesses such as schizophrenia.

Trying to create a sense of acceptance and belonging for each of the patients on our caseload is, in effect, one of the central goals of all care work. We saw how this applies to all treatments everywhere in Chapter 4. There are good reasons to be optimistic here, too. Our culture is slowly becoming more tolerant of difference, and we are beginning to realise that people with diverse mental disorders can be well suited to some role or other if they are given half a chance. This doesn't have to be patronising. For example, psychopathic personalities, with their ability to discount their emotional state, have been found to make excellent bond traders. There is a strong correlation between emotional sensitivity and depression, and an even stronger bond between creativity and bipolar disorder, as well as some personality types. Anxious people can learn to channel their fearful energies to remarkable ends. Aloof, avoidant or schizoid individuals – including many with psychotic illnesses – can thrive in environments where social stimulus is minimal, allowing them to perform individual task-based work, for example accountancy, filing or typing. Finding the right nook or cranny for each and every patient is the core target for the care worker of the 21st century.

Getting just one individual out of hospital, living independently and doing something that he or she likes is a major achievement. Staying supportive of people, even though they may have dropped out of many programmes, can still be rewarding. In truth, every patient who doesn't get better is a challenge to us to get better at the job. This can often feel like an uphill struggle but it doesn't need to be if we remember the point of Chapter 4: treatment – what we are doing with our patients – is a never-ending experiment that we are constantly reviewing, tweaking and relaunching in a new direction. With care work, you can never have tried everything. How best to convince that lousy locum doctor about the sexual side effects that discourage a patient from taking medication? What extra knowledge do I need to help another find a place in a 24-hour supported home? And what if I do an anxiety management course and take a fresh look at someone suffering from panic attacks? Harmonising our approach is the key to making mental health care a modern and attractive profession.

What are you/we going to do about illicit drugs?

At present, in the UK, there are many substances that are illicit or, to put it more crudely, can get you nicked. The severity of punishment will depend on whether a substance is seen as being Class A, B, C or various legal definitions in between and these, of course, keep changing. The opiates, the stimulants and the hallucinogens are taken in staggering quantities throughout the world – some half a million ecstasy tabs every weekend in the UK alone. Like alcohol and cigarettes, their consumption is controlled by availability, price and fashion but, unlike booze and fags, they subject their users to all the mess and mischief of the criminal playground known as the drug scene.

In an odd way, the use of most psychotropic drugs reflects the main reasons why people go to see their GP anyway: because they have some sort of pain, are feeling tired or are bored. All of these may be variously expressed as physical symptoms, such as a headache, or the complaint of being depressed or stressed, but they are the core signs of a major problem that confronts our society: there are millions of people out there who feel an unpleasant gap between the way that their life is and the way that they want it to be. Whether what they want is a good thing, or even available, is beside the point. People use drugs to numb this nasty sense of not feeling right.

Because there is such a large overlap between mental health problems and drug use, any community mental health worker must have an understanding of how drugs affect people, what can realistically be done to help them and how to differentiate between illness and acute drug effects. Some people literally go psychotic just for a day or two because, for example, they've smoked too much strong hashish (so-called 'drug-induced psychosis'). Others seem to be very depressed, which may be because they have run out of crack cocaine (and the money to get any more for several weeks). As we have seen, many patients with long-term schizophrenia are easy prey for crack dealers, and a patient's home may be taken over as a kind of 'crack house'. The combination of dependence, the worsening of symptoms, impoverishment and harassment, and sometimes overt bullying and assaults, can be very frightening to deal with.

What is to be done? Should we try to set strict rules and refuse to provide support or even help with benefit forms if patients go on abusing drugs? Should we be sympathetic and try to turn a blind eye? If you are too strict, patients will simply keep away and so you won't be able to help at all but, if you sympathise, your manager or even the police may start coming down on you for going along with illegal activities. Many people consider that criminalisation of drugs is a complete waste of time, anti-therapeutic and brings the law into disrepute. Working to get legislation changed would certainly help our patients, by getting them away from the demeaning embrace of the criminals and the gangsters. But laws, and the attitudes of the people who ultimately change them, shift only slowly and, right now, there are literally thousands of people, not just on run-down council estates but all over the place, who are living through their own version of hell because of some drug or other.

At the moment, let's face it, the outlook for a really useful answer to the problem posed by illegal drugs is not very good. Most people are quite pessimistic about the effectiveness of treatments, and the rising tide of drug and alcohol use seems to point to the lack of impact of the so-called 'war on drugs'. There are reports of a possible vaccination being developed, which would make one immune, for example, to the effects of cocaine (so presumably people wouldn't take it). The substances buprenorphine and antabuse block the effects of opiates and alcohol, respectively, and produce bad effects (e.g. nausea) if taken at the same time as the drug. The increasing use of specialist rehabilitation programmes in prisons (and at least two-thirds of prisoners have a significant drug problem) and drug and testing treatment orders (DTTOs) may be a way forward. Our view is that it will take a combination of these approaches, used consistently over the next 20 years or more (i.e. for a whole generation of adults), to get the drug problem under control. There is no simple one-fix solution but a peek into the world of the future, say 20 years on, could look like this.

2028: One possible vision

1.   All drugs are legalised, marketed in agreed and safe amounts, taxed and sold with health warnings and health promotional material.
2.   Advertising of drugs that can be a health risk or cause dependence is allowed but only if the same amount of money is spent on health promotion/warnings before and after the drug advertisement.

3. A range of vaccines and blocker drugs are readily available and used as part of legal/court mechanisms for those who carry out antisocial behaviour (e.g. multiple burglaries) to feed their habits.
4. Cleaner, 'smarter' medications are available to deal with conditions such as depression and schizophrenia, without the side effects or limitations present so often today.
5. There is a general acceptance that occasional drug use, like occasional alcohol use, is not necessarily bad for you, can help unwind distress and isn't necessarily linked to street-fighting culture.

This world would look a little different from the one that most of us inhabit today. This relaxation of current proscriptions, and honest acceptance that it is an epidemic that affects us all, would at first lead to an increase in the visibility of drug problems. It would also, almost certainly, lead to an increase in the total number of drug problems overall, especially at first, but this would probably subsequently decline. Such a change would be met with much huffing and puffing from the indignant and complacent who would prefer to continue with the delusion that our current approach is effective. It would also provide a field day for the newspapers and could be powerful enough to topple a government brave enough to try it. Drug-induced psychotic admissions to hospitals might also rise but since when did the indignant, complacent classes ever worry about that? They would, by then, have turned their thoughts to the far more dramatic drop in the numbers of burglaries and muggings.

How are we going to deal with risk?

The culture of risk management, and its offspring 'risk assessment' and 'risk-assessment tools', has been described in some detail, especially in Chapters 1 and 8. If this seems to be something of an obsession of the authors, you have been paying attention. In our view, it is the single most pernicious change in the delivery of mental health care in the last 20 years. Its rise has been poorly documented and is in need of much greater understanding. Its protagonists are lawyers and hindsight junkies who are, in essence, creaming a living from the random misfortunes that happen to mentally ill people in a complex, individualistic and unrealistic society. When we start using risk as the basic criterion for whether we see or help someone as a mental health worker, we essentially become psychological dustcart drivers. People who need help but aren't at 'risk' will be overlooked, even though they comprise the vast majority of those with mental health problems. Billions of pounds will instead be spent on a small group of possibly 'risky' individuals.

Our view is that proper assessments of patients, in terms of their social situation, their mental state, what they do and what they say, must always include some understanding of at-risk behaviour as a potential outcome. Risk should be confined to the warp and woof of day-to-day practice but it shouldn't have a heading of its own. Once you have developed a risk-assessment tool and 'trained' someone to tick the boxes, then what? If all the boxes carry double ticks, the only logical solution is to bang the person up and throw away the key. However, if there are only partial, scant hints from the past, ticking boxes doesn't help. In fact, it might appear as if something has been done – the form has been filled in – but nothing has actually been done therapeutically. Your patients will feel as if you are just accentuating the negative and blighting their fortunes into the bargain.

283

Questionnaires and risk-assessment tools have sprouted up like mushrooms (perhaps the guy found running down the road yelling 'mushrooms, mushrooms, mushrooms', referred to in Chapter 3, is a sane care worker!). No doubt more will be devised, meant to be of greater specificity and sensitivity. Whether these are something that a mental health care worker should be using routinely is a moot point. There are accepted rules of good practice in terms of recognising danger signs, being aware of symptoms, knowing when to disengage, not visiting alone, etc; however, in our view, these should be built into the regular care plan and not made something different or extra.

In particular, we consider that the 'risk agenda' is likely to have troubling consequences for the future. Two obvious issues that it will have an impact on are new mental health legislation (see below) and the notion of reinstitutionalisation (see below also). The rising tide of risk aversion and the increasing numbers of fences, cameras, security guards, special constables, police, etc. are the natural consequences of marked differences in wealth between different groups in society. Obviously, the lone mental health care coordinator can do little to turn back this social tide but being realistic about the whole 'risk business' is most important for your peace of mind. There are sensible things to do, there are difficult patients, there are malignant illnesses, and no one can – or should – supervise anyone on a 24-hour 'man to man marking', one-to-one basis.

Remember, if enough people within the practical, front-line mental health services don't do something, it doesn't get done. The classic example of this was the introduction of the supervision register in the mid-1990s, as already outlined. This was meant to be a wonderful way for us, the mental health workers, to draw up a register of all those patients who might be seriously ill, pose a potential public risk and, therefore, be in need of 'supervision'. This list of 'suspects' was somehow meant to enhance our understanding of these patients by making it easier to keep an eye on them and was accompanied by the Patients in the Community legislation designed to do this.

In fact, very few patients were put on the supervision register and even fewer were placed under Section 25 orders as outlined in the Act. This was largely thanks to the heroic inactivity of the great majority of doctors, nurses, social workers and other therapists who could simply see no point in going through all this rigmarole. The whole thing has been quietly dropped, to everyone's benefit. It is, therefore, worthwhile being critical about the risk agenda, in whatever way you can. By all means fill in the forms, talk the talk and embed it in your day-to-day practice when thinking about how to cope with individual patients. But the history of psychiatry shows very strongly that when those working in it are seen as helpers and therapists rather than jailers or social controllers, their lot is much better. Their views are taken on board, the conditions they manage are considered more sympathetically and they are even portrayed in positive roles on television and in films. The long-term battle to make sure that care of the mentally ill stays in the Department of Health rather than the Home Office has to be carried out at all levels of the care system.

A new Mental Health Act?

We have already discussed in Chapter 9 the kind of things that might be introduced in a new Mental Health Act, something that has been bubbling up through the parliamentary process (Scoping Committee, Green Paper, White Paper) since the beginning of the 21st century. Perhaps the most unique outcome to date has been the forging of a Mental Health Alliance between the many disparate, interested bodies, both statutory and voluntary, to oppose the government's attempted legislation. Remarkably, professional bodies such as the Royal College of Psychiatrists and the British Association of Psychologists, as well as many patient and carer organisations such as MIND and Rethink, now stand united in opposition. This is a highly ironic coalition of people who have usually never agreed on anything, a lack of coherence that has been a problem for mental health reformers down the ages.

Why has such an alliance been formed? The answer lies in at least two major features of the published drafts of the Act. These are the notions of the category of dangerously severe personality disorder (DSPD) and the very broad categories (with no exclusions) of people who could potentially be designated as 'mentally ill'. Both involve widening the net so that mental health professionals could be empowered – bullied even – to rein in the undesirables of society. Previous legislation, for example in 1983, had carefully excluded people with sexual deviations and alcohol and drug dependence from being sectionable, whereas those with the largely socially determined traits of 'personality disorder' could only be treated against their will if they were genuinely 'treatable'. This was known as the 'treatability clause' and its inclusion in the 1983 Act was to make sure that treatment against one's will was only given for conditions that could be seen as proper, treatable 'illnesses' rather than variations in socially accepted behaviour.

At the time of writing it is unclear how things will pan out. It seems most unlikely that the present generation of psychiatrists will be persuaded to detain people on the basis of the spurious notion of a dangerously severe personality disorder, not least because this category has no place as a specific diagnosis in psychiatric textbooks or psychiatric understanding of personality disorder. The same is true for drugs and alcohol. Previous attempts at detaining people, for example in the 19th century, for 'chronic inebriation' – a nice phrase for being drunk all the time – proved a waste of time and resources. In countries such as New Zealand where compulsory treatment of addiction is supported by law, these laws are hardly ever used and reflect the simple truth of addiction treatment: you can lead an alcoholic to water, but you can't make him drink. Having such exclusions and safeguards in mental health legislation makes sense in terms of targeting treatment and the resources required to those who can really benefit. Even more important, the notion of detaining someone against their will and depriving them of their freedom, not because they have broken the law but because they have the potential for breaking the law, really is something out of *1984* or *Minority Report.*

However, in our view, some of the new legislation could be of real benefit. For example, a community treatment order is something that has been used in other parts of the world (e.g. New Zealand, parts of the USA); it means that, even though they have no insight, people can be treated without having to bring them into hospital. The whole point of modern treatment is that it doesn't necessarily require being 'in hospital', as recognised by the massive expansion in community-based care. Likewise, giving everyone a routine tribunal within 28 days of admission means that proper care plans have to be drawn up and everyone gets a second opinion. Separating out treatment and social control should also benefit mental health workers, who can be seen as therapists and helpers rather than versions of the thought police. The continental European custom of using courts and tribunals for any kind of detention has meant that mental health workers there have not had the demoralising impact of an inquiry and blame culture heaped upon them.

Even more germane to our case is the acceptance that any suitably quali-fied mental health care worker (that clumsy phrase again) can be part of the Mental Health Act. At present, doctors (specially approved under Section 12, i.e. reasonably experienced psychiatrists) are required to write up the recom-mendations for detention and approved social workers actually carry out the application for detention. Even the most experienced community psychiatric nurse, occupational therapist or psychologist has no role at all to play. Yet, there is no rea-son why such expertise, which will be required for the new tribunals, should not be part of the Act in itself. Of course, some workers may prefer to stay uninvolved because of fears of breaking the therapeutic relationship by signing a section order. However, the evidence, both research-based and personal, is that patients very rarely take it out on a care worker personally if they have been part of a Mental Health Act detention. They may vociferously disagree, stop their treatment as soon as they are discharged and go on disagreeing that they have any kind of illness, but that doesn't mean that they won't come and see you. This curious dis-sociation reflects the complex nature of the illnesses we treat. Either way, the new legislation is likely to usher in a notion of a generic mental health worker, suitably trained and experienced, who can take on the role of applying for detention, just like today's approved social worker.

As far as legislation goes, the future, therefore, will again be rather up to us. The Mental Health Alliance has perplexed the government, which is used to the old 'divide and rule' approach towards many specialist and professional organi-sations. In the end they need *us* to carry out the tasks of assessment, treatment and, if necessary, detention, and by sticking together, some sensible rules may come through. In this broader sense as well, the breaking down of the boundar-ies between different specialities within mental health can only be of benefit, not unlike workers uniting against the bosses.

Reinstitutionalisation?

As the notion of risk and the spread of forensic establishments darken our hori-zons, there is increasing evidence, Europe-wide at least, that reinstitutionalisation is back. For those not sure what this means (and the history is all in Chapter 1), it essentially has a physical and a psychological component. The physical one is quite straightforward: it means 'bricks and mortar'. When the asylums were being furi-ously built in the later part of the 19th century, a despairing medical editor talked about this as the 'bricks and mortar solution'. Building large (institutional) build-ings has a peculiar fascination for some. It's good for the building trade, good for the catering trade who have to supply the institutions and good for the civil servants who have to organise it. It sustains the comfortable illusion that there is a real dif-ference between the mad and the not mad. The presence of a physical separation also invites the notion of 'normals' possibly being liable to being infected by having mad folk among them!

At present, of course, the official line is that acute beds are closing and are not needed. The line is that, thanks to all the new community care teams, there is no need to admit people. But, in the background are what one might call 'the new long-stay', those who go in and out of hospital via the revolving door, sometimes via prison and the streets, because of the severity of their illnesses. Care homes, rehabilitation units, forensic low dependence units (many of them in the private sector) and, of course, the medium secure units (MSUs) themselves (ever rising in number) are part of this genesis. It is as if the old asylum, having been broken up and scattered, is slowly coming together again like the bad guy in *Terminator 2*. The number of beds is difficult to count because they are under so many different categories and the reasons given for them are so various: public safety, risk management, structured care, long-term psychosocial interventions, etc.

More fundamentally, the bed-closure programme has gone too far. As bed numbers declined around 1980, detentions under the Mental Health Act (which had been declining in parallel) suddenly started to rise again (see Fig. 1.5). Around the same time, changing economic circumstances led to increased homelessness and, since the 1990s, prison numbers have soared. These factors cannot be entirely separated. The fact of the matter is that some forms of mental illness, even today, have only a limited response to treatment and sufferers need to be looked after. In a similar way to supermarkets, economies of scale mean that group homes rather than individual residences will, in the end, always win out; off we go on the same old journey that the Victorians travelled as their asylums got bigger and bigger.

The problem with reinstitutionalisation is that large institutions, whether hospitals, prisons or schools (or even monasteries and nunneries), tend to take on certain characteristics, particularly when money is short. These include the degradation of the environment to the barely acceptable (in terms of paint, curtains, food, space), the setting up of rules to structure the day for everyone and the petty tyrannies that can flourish behind walls. The phrase 'out of sight out of mind' emphasises the disposal aspects of this and, in part, the drive to reinstitutionalisation panders to the public wish not to be reminded of troubled folk. Consider, for example, the apparent success of the New York police in reducing mugging and crime in that city over the last 10 years. By removing, at the slightest pretext, people not behaving correctly in public, for example beggars, squeegee merchants and rowdies, they saw themselves as removing the social 'undergrowth' behind which serious crime was hiding. To some extent they were right but, of course, the USA now has the largest proportion of its population in jail, nearly 2 million in total, out of all the countries in the world.

There is also a sense in which reinstitutionalisation can be seen as a state of mind. We have established AOTs to engage with the more difficult cases and hopefully keep them out of hospital but the team members have to be 'assertive' for it to work. They try to insist on a patient having a structured day, taking their medication, living in a certain place, etc. and so, in a sense, they impose themselves on a patient's day-to-day activities. This is generally a good thing because many of those with chronic illnesses often lack motivation, social contact and initiative and are easily exploited (by drug dealers for example, as outlined above). Such patients can live much richer lives when supported thus. Although this can't really be seen as true institutionalisation, in a similar way to being stuck in a building with set rules and regulations, there are elements of this approach that demand conformity to social norms. The move back to institutions, therefore, can be seen as reflecting the pressures to conform within modern society (led largely by the advertising industry and style labels), as well as reflecting the risk agenda and intolerance. Furthermore, the likelihood is that, given the swings and roundabouts of history, this process will go on for another generation or so before someone once more rediscovers the negatives. Then the pendulum will swing back to community care and 'normalisation', no doubt propelled by a fresh host of institutional scandals.

Is it all over for the community mental health team?

Although it developed as the natural corollary to the closing of the asylums, the CMHT emerged more by luck than judgement. It was originally devised in the USA to provide ongoing care to all those leaving the asylums. In fact, it failed to achieve this because the workers preferred to talk to younger, more interesting people with troubled souls than chronic, whiffy, ageing schizophrenics. In the UK, things were more practical but it still took time for the various components of a modern CMHT to come together. Psychiatrists didn't really want to leave their offices (whether in the asylums or the hospitals); social workers were employed by the local boroughs; CPNs (community psychiatrist nurses) were mainly there to give injections and a brief word of sympathy; and the psychologists were in short supply and, quite reasonably, more interested in delivering the therapies of the time rather than token economy systems for socially disabled psychotics. The mainstay of modern clinical psychology, CBT, hadn't caught on back then.

As a set of tasks emerged, and as community care increasingly realised that it was struggling, (and was told that it was 'failing' by all and sundry, including a senior health minister), the notion of a multidisciplinary team gathered momentum. Different workers started talking to each other, at least a little. Across the land, with great variations in custom, practice and timing, the notion of the CMHT slowly emerged through the 1980s. However, its role then began to be questioned. Should it be attached to primary care (i.e. each GP has a pet CPN and social worker)? Should it confine itself to crisis assessments and home treatment? Should it apply itself to aftercare for discharged patients? Because the CMHTs were perceived to be failing, the National Service Framework and the NHS Plan decided that specialist teams were required. These included AOTs, crisis intervention teams, HTTs and early intervention services (EIS). Essentially, the functions of the CMHT were chopped up into what were seen as the key components, with good and bad results.

The good has been that the government has provided more staff in community mental health services by enhancing the resources in these teams. Likewise, services can now provide a better quality of care that is targeted more at individual needs, such as those people who have proven hard to engage (they get assertive outreach) or those needing brief support without hospitalisation (HTTs). Aiming to care for people at the beginning of a severe mental illness – as the Roman poet Ovid said – makes sense in trying to ameliorate its long-term consequences. However, there are still many patients in between these well-defined groups who seem to be missing out. They include those who are still going in and out of hospital because of the brittle nature of their illness; those who remain highly dependent and vulnerable; the acutely ill homeless who are, by definition, not suitable for home treatment; those who see their GP most of the time but who need specialist help from time to time; and those who are so challenging, disorganised and intoxicated (and sometimes all three) that even an AOT can't keep track of them.

How long these shiny new teams will survive is uncertain. By being so specialist, staff can become rather de-skilled; if all you are doing is, say, looking after first-onset psychotic illness, how will you know what to do for people 20 years down the track? Only doing crisis intervention can easily lead to burnout, whereas just looking after long-term chronic illness can again lead to loss of skills in acute management. All of these specialisations miss having a general overview of things. Some suggest that better staffing of CMHTs and covering smaller patches would be better, with one or two specialists working across teams (e.g. dual diagnosis) to provide support. Others suggest taking all these disparate teams and putting them in one building all together.

Another problem with having multiple teams is that they have borders and 'interfaces', and boundary disputes are the bind of many organisations. Whose responsibility is this person? But he lives over there, doesn't he? Is this really a crisis? Why do *we* seem to be dealing with all the difficult cases? The classic difficulty often occurs between a CMHT and a forensic outreach team. Analysis of the clientele of each shows that they are exactly the same; although the forensic people have done nastier things in the past, their behaviours and illnesses are not much different today. Managing them might now actually be easier because the powers given by, for example, a restriction order (Section 41 of the current Mental Health Act) make it absolutely mandatory that they live where they are told, have their injections, etc. Social institutionalisation generates control.

Our own view is that the CMHT, if properly constituted and led, can provide a good service. Its difficulties have arisen because it was there in the front line and open to all. So many diverse demands have been made upon it that, just like the acute ward, it has been swamped. Having no boundaries that were discernible, CMHTs have found themselves taking on drug addicts, criminals, head injury cases, the homeless, rowing couples, asylum seekers and countless combinations thereof. In this regard they provided an excellent assessment service because their combination of skills made it possible to define just what a patient's needs might be; however, no one else was willing to take up the move-on requirement. It was as if a casualty department had been set up in a tent in the high street and then been blamed for being full of people all the time because there were no hospital beds to put them in.

If we assume, therefore, that CMHTs should: (i) see everyone of a particular age group (e.g. from 18 to 65) referred for mental health problems; (ii) be able to reach a diagnosis and look at social needs and treatment needs; and (iii) either arrange the treatment themselves or move patients on to the appropriate agency, this seems reasonable. Treatment can take place at a day centre, in the patient's home or in a ward. The best CMHTs operate with their own ward integrated in terms of staff (i.e. the same doctors, nurses, occupational therapists and so on) and have a good working relationship that sees the ward as a part of the team rather than an interface to be managed. Out of all this comes what we consider to be the tasks of the new generic mental health worker. And, if we look at what these tasks are, we can describe the appropriate training needed to carry them out.

The all-singing all-dancing generic mental health worker?

So what does the generic mental health worker (GMW) have to learn and what does she or he have to do? We have seen how people from a wide range of backgrounds can take on the role of a GMW but we have also seen how the good GMW goes well beyond the narrow remit of, say, nursing or social work and puts it all together when helping the patient on their journey. Apart from knowing your local Care Programme Approach (CPA) guidelines or the Mental Health Act, what do you really need to know about? The list of topics is literally endless but the following describes what we feel are the main ones.

Social psychology

We stress the word 'social' in this respect because 'no man is an island, entire of itself' (as John Donne put it). Half of the problem facing the mentally ill lies in their inability to find a role in society. They are isolated by their symptoms, find it hard to make friends and don't know how to behave correctly, even down to the simple business of buying a pack of cigarettes. Knowing something about how individuals react and how they react to people reacting to them, whether in twos and threes or in larger groups, is central to understanding how patients can be integrated more. For example, many people with schizophrenia suffer from what we might call 'neophobia' (i.e. a fear of the new or different), so taking someone along to the day centre doesn't just mean introducing them once, it means taking them on a regular basis until they get so used to it that it becomes custom and habit.

Neurophysiology

This is difficult stuff. Brains are complicated pieces of hard and soft wiring, have a consistency of mushy toothpaste and no one really knows how they work. Electricity, hormones, chemicals and gravity all have an effect, and the whole point about people with serious mental illnesses is that they do have some abnormal brain function. In our view, trying to understand unusual behaviours or experiences (e.g. hearing voices) in this way, rather than judging people morally, is more helpful in getting them better.

Sociology

This has a ring of the 1970s about it but the combination of understanding sociology and ethology (how animals or humans inter-react in groups) has been most helpful in many aspects of psychiatry. We use group therapy extensively but understanding family structure and networks, for example in terms of high expressed emotion (EE), and the way that this affects vulnerable patients is also important. Likewise, it helps us understand the way in which networks develop across geographies and genders and ages and the ways in which people develop because of their sociocultural background.

Psychopharmacology

This has been the biggest 'breakthrough' in mental health care since the 1950s. Some may not like the apparent medicalisation of troubled souls but the fact of the matter is that people have left asylums after decades of confining psychotic symptoms. Mood swings can be reduced, or even abolished in some cases, by lithium, valproate and other stabilisers. Benzodiazepines can break a crippling cycle of anxiety long enough for psychological treatments to take hold. Antidepressant drugs can work wonders for some people with major depression. This is not to say that we shouldn't be very cautious about 'big pharma', given that trying to fit diagnoses to the drugs available, rather than the other way round, has been one of their rather obvious games of late. Nevertheless, the amount of money put into research by big pharmaceutical companies and the extraordinary breakthroughs made in managing untreatable illnesses cannot be ignored. If you do not know about medication, how it works, its side effects and the possibilities for new medications, you are not really involved in a key part of community care.

Therapeutics

In particular, one of the most important things for any community care worker to understand must be the effects of therapy. Most people tend to believe that if you are ill and are given something (a yellow pill, vitamin C, an antibiotic, a course of psychotherapy) and you then get better, it must have been the treatment that made you better. But the more robust philosophical position to hold is that just because B comes after A doesn't mean that A caused B. So, just because you gave Mr Smith an injection of antipsychotic and 3 days later he is no longer psychotic, it doesn't *necessarily* mean that it was the antipsychotic that did it. This is where double-blind studies, randomised controlled trials and all the paraphernalia of proper modern science are needed. Being sceptical about new claims, understanding the basis for research methodology and asking for help if you don't understand the statistics are all just as important.

Stigmatology

The good care worker will be an influential stigmatologist in both their professional and their personal life. Patients are not aliens from another planet, nor are they dangerous beings to be herded like prisoners or children to be treated with benign despair and occasional chocolate bar handouts. It is far better to think of patients, particularly those with the more severe mental illnesses such as schizophrenia, as heroes of evolution, the quality of whose existence is a measure of the quality of our civilisation. This isn't easy; being robust in countering negative comments about 'nutters' or 'psychos' in an argument when you are outnumbered takes quite a lot of courage.

Politics

Even if you are a dedicated clinician who prefers seeing people to writing notes or going to meetings, don't ignore the roles of management and administration. Managers and administrators may always think that they are doing something new when, in fact, it was usually done 5 years ago (everything goes round in 5-year cycles, roughly speaking, in the NHS), but their enthusiasm is important to grasp. They have only a 1- or 2-year 'window' to get something done in terms of 'change' so they tend to change things regardless. When doing this, they can sometimes attract funds from various labelled projects, which means more money and staff for your services, even if you have to call them by a new name. Take these on board, don't get too worked up about the details, let the managers move on and gradually reintegrate the service you once had, hopefully now with extra resources. There has always been politics in health care and it is useful to have a

291

hunch about what the next important policy initiative is going to be so that, when you put your bid in for a new worker or service, you get the right phrases smartly embedded in the proposal. Terms such as 'social exclusion', 'service user agenda' or 'robust communication initiatives' always go down well. Follow the news and watch for the eye-catching stories, often the major drivers of change.

Traveller

In putting together all these roles, it is important to remember that, just as every patient takes a strange, personal journey from illness towards some form of health (hopefully), so everyone who works in mental health takes a parallel journey. We usually start off with one or two prejudices about how best to do things, perhaps believing that psychotherapy and counselling will solve all and that medication is just a big pharma myth, or vice versa, but most of us reach different conclusions every few years. In time, we realise that these conclusions themselves are nothing more than staging posts en route to yet another conclusion, and so it goes on. After a while, this can become exhilarating. The secret is to *keep learning* because if psychotherapy really can change brain activity and if exercise really does make you happy, how can we harness the essence of these kinds of changes? The adage that the wiser you get, the less you really know may be a cliché but it also happens to be true. The more time that you spend in different places talking to different people, be it patient, carer, colleague or public, the more you will find yourself taking different positions. Write about it. Reflect on it. Be prepared to change. Be sceptical about fancy new treatments. Watch out for gurus. Just because most people think something, doesn't mean it's necessarily true. Every patient is different, no matter what they appear to share, and every patient is someone to be learned from. Always try to see beyond what the patient looks like – you never know, he or she might just be a tabloid journalist on the lookout for a good story. But most of all, treat patients like your own mother or brother and think how you'd like to be helped if you couldn't think straight. Our business is unique and wonderful and the journey never ends.

Index

$101.95